ATLAS OF MICROVASCULAR SURGERY

ATLAS OF MICROVASCULAR SURGERY

Anatomy and Operative Approaches

Berish Strauch, M.D.
*Professor and Chairman
Department of Plastic and
 Reconstructive Surgery
Albert Einstein College of Medicine
 and Montefiore Medical Center
Bronx, New York*

Han-Liang Yu, M.D.
俞漢良
*Assistant Professor
Department of Plastic and
 Reconstructive Surgery
Albert Einstein College of Medicine
Bronx, New York
Attending Orthopedic Surgeon
Zhong Shan Hospital
Shanghai Medical University
Shanghai, People's Republic of China*

with

Zhong-Wei Chen, M.D.
陳中偉
*Professor and Chairman
Department of Orthopedics
Zhong Shan Hospital
Shanghai Medical University
Shanghai, People's Republic of China*

Ralph Liebling, M.D.
*Director, Plastic and Reconstructive
 Surgery Service
Bronx Municipal Hospital Center
Assistant Professor
Department of Plastic and
 Reconstructive Surgery
Albert Einstein College of Medicine
 and Montefiore Medical Center
Bronx, New York*

Illustrated by

Li-Guo Liang
梁利國
*Coordinator of Medical Illustration
Department of Plastic and Reconstructive Surgery
Albert Einstein College of Medicine
and Montefiore Medical Center
Bronx, New York*

1993
THIEME MEDICAL PUBLISHERS, Inc. New York
GEORG THIEME VERLAG Stuttgart • New York

Thieme New York
333 Seventh Avenue
New York, New York 10001

Atlas of Microvascular Surgery
Berish Strauch, M.D.
Han-Liang Yu, M.D.

Library of Congress Cataloging-in-Publication Data

Atlas of microvascular surgery : the anatomy of operative techniques /
Berish Strauch . . . [et al.] ; illustrated by Li-Guo Liang.
    p.   cm.
    Includes bibliographical references and index.
    ISBN 0-86577-436-6. — ISBN 3-13-783001-X
    1. Blood-vessels—Surgery—Atlases.   2. Blood-vessels—Anatomy—
Atlases.   3. Microsurgery—Atlases.   4. Flaps (Surgery)—Atlases.
I. Strauch, Berish, 1933- .
    [DNLM: 1. Blood Vessels—Anatomy & histology—atlases.
2. Microsurgery—methods—atlases.   3. Vascular Surgery—methods—
atlases.   WG 17 A88435]
RD598.5.A78   1992
617.4′13059—dc20
DNLM/DLC
for Library of Congress   92-401
                                                                              CIP

Copyright © 1993 by Thieme Medical Publishers, Inc. This book, including all parts thereof, is legally protected by copyright. Any use, exploitation or commercialization outside the narrow limits set by copyright legislation, without the publisher's consent, is illegal and liable to prosecution. This applies in particular to photostat reproduction, copying, mimeographing or duplication of any kind, translating, preparation of microfilms, and electronic data processing and storage.

Important note: Medicine is an ever-changing science. Research and clinical experience are continually broadening our knowledge, in particular our knowledge of proper treatment and drug therapy. Insofar as this book mentions any dosage or application, readers may rest assured that the authors, editors, and publishers have made every effort to ensure that such references are strictly in accordance with the state of knowledge at the time of production of the book. Nevertheless, every user is requested to carefully examine the manufacturers' leaflets accompanying each drug to check on his own responsibility whether the dosage schedules recommended therein or the contraindications stated by the manufacturers differ from the statements made in the present book. Such examination is particularly important with drugs that are either rarely used or have been newly released on the market.

Some of the product names, patents, and registered designs referred to in this book are in fact registered trademarks or proprietary names even though specific reference to this fact is not always made in the text. Therefore, the appearance of a name without designation as proprietary is not to be construed as a representation by the publisher that it is in the public domain.

Printed in the United States of America.

5 4 3

TMP ISBN 0-86577-436-6
GTV ISBN 3-13-783001-X

To Mom Strauch and Mom Feuerstein, for all of the long years of guidance and encouragement.

Berish Strauch, M.D.

To my wife, Hui-Zhu, my son, Yue, and all my teachers.

Han-Liang Yu, M.D.

CONTENTS

Preface ix

Introduction 1
    Definitions..1
    Training in Basic Microsurgical Techniques 1
    Exposure of Recipient Vessels 2
    Microsurgical Anatomy and its Variations 3
    Donor Sites..3
    Flap Design 4
    Harvesting Techniques 4
    Comment and Insights..4

Part 1   Upper Extremity

1   Shoulder, Arm, and Axilla 8
    Deltoid Flap 8
    Medial Arm Flap 12
    Lateral Arm Flap 17
    Posterior Arm Flap..22
    Recipient Site Exposures......................................26
    Bibliography 43

2   Forearm Region..44
    Forearm Flaps...44
    Radial Forearm Flap..49
    Radial Forearm Flap for Penile Reconstruction 57
    Reversed Radial Forearm Island Flap.....................61
    Radial Forearm Osteocutaneous Flap 63
    Radial Forearm Tendinocutaneous Flap 67
    Ulnar Forearm Flap...69
    Recipient Site Exposures 74
    Bibliography..82

3   Hand and Wrist..84
    Anatomy of the Radial Artery—Deep Palmar
       Arch System 84
    Anatomy of the Ulnar Artery—Superficial Palmar
       Arch System 85
    Recipient Site Exposures......................................88

Part 2   Lower Extremity

4   Gluteal Region..102
    Gluteus Maximus Flap..102
    Superior Gluteus Myocutaneous Flap 104
    Gluteal Thigh Flap (Based on the Inferior
       Gluteal Vessels)...107

    Vascularized Iliac Bone Graft (Based on the
       Superior Gluteal Vessels)...............................111
    Recipient Site Exposure 116
    Bibliography 118

5   Groin Region 120
    Groin Flaps...120
    Iliac Flap and Inferior Epigastric Flap..................120
    Iliofemoral Flap 123
    Iliac Flap...129
    Osteocutaneous Groin Flap (Based on the SCIA) ...130
    Composite Groin Flap with "Tendon" Transfer......132
    Lower Abdominal Flap......................................136
    Iliac Flap (Based on the Fourth Lumbar Artery).....139
    Vascularized Iliac Bone Graft 142
    Vascularized Iliac Bone Graft (Based on DCIA) 145
    Iliac Osteocutaneous Flap (Based on DCIA).........154
    Internal Oblique Flap 159
    Bibliography 164

6   Thigh Region 166
    Gracilis Flap 166
    Gracilis Muscle Flap..168
    Gracilis Myocutaneous Flap 171
    Tensor Fascia Lata Flap 174
    Tensor Fascia Lata Myocutaneous Flap................176
    Tensor Fascia Lata Osteomyocutaneous Flap 179
    Rectus Femoris Flap..180
    Rectus Femoris Muscle Flap...............................182
    Rectus Femoris Myocutaneous Flap....................185
    Thigh Skin Flaps 187
    Medial Thigh Flap 187
    Lateral Thigh Flap 190
    Anterolateral Thigh Flap 194
    Anteromedial Thigh Flap 197
    Recipient Site Exposures....................................201
    Bibliography 216

7   Lower Leg and Knee..................................218
    Fibula and Adjacent Tissue Transfer 218
    Vascularized Fibula Bone Graft.........................221
    Peroneal Flap (Lateral Leg Skin Flap) 228
    Fibular Osteocutaneous Flap 233
    Fibular Osteomuscular Transfer......................238
    Gastrocnemius Flap 244
    Medial Gastrocnemius Muscle Flap 245
    Lateral Gastrocnemius Muscle Flap 250
    Saphenous Flap 252
    Leg Skin Flaps 257
    Anterior Tibial Flap 257

Reverse Anterior Tibial Island Flap 262
Medial Leg Flap...264
Posterior Leg Flap..270
Recipient Site Exposures................................275
Bibliography 312

8 Ankle and Foot 314
Dorsalis Pedis Flap...314
Dorsalis Pedis Skin Flap 320
Dorsalis Pedis Osteocutaneous Flap with
  Second Metatarsal......................................326
Dorsalis Pedis Tendinocutaneous Flap with
  Extensor Tendons 332
Extensor Digitorum Brevis Flap 336
Extensor Digitorum Brevis Muscle Flap............337
Medial Plantar Flap 341
Free Toe and Toe Tissue Transfers 347
Free Big Toe Transfer 350
Free Second Toe Transfer...............................356
First Web Space Skin Flap..............................361
Wrap-Around Flap 364
Modified Wrap-Around Flap 367
Free Pulp Flap 372
Vascularized Joint Transfer.............................373
Second and Third Toe Transfer En Bloc............378
Recipient Site Exposures................................379
Bibliography 385

Part 3 Trunk

9 Thorax 390
Pectoralis Major Flap 390
Pectoralis Major Muscle Flap..........................393
Pectoralis Major Myocutaneous Flap 398
Pectoralis Major Osteomyocutaneous Flap 400
Clavicular Segment of the Pectoralis Major
  Muscle Flap 402
Pectoralis Minor Muscle Flap 408
Serratus Anterior Flap 414
Serratus Anterior Muscle Flap 415
Serratus Anterior Myocutaneous Flap 420
Composite Serratus-Latissimus Muscle Flap 422
Serratus Anterior Costo-Osteomuscular Flap........424
Revascularized Costal Bone Graft and
  Intercostal Flap..426
Vascularized Rib Graft (Based on the Posterior
  Intercostal Artery) 427
Lateral Intercostal Skin Flap 430
Posterior Costal Osteocutaneous Flap 433
Vascularized Rib Graft (Based on the
  Anterior Intercostal Artery) 435
Anterior Costal Osteocutaneous Flap 438
Lateral Thoracic Flap (Axillary Flap) 440
Bibliography 446

10 Abdominal Wall and Cavity.....................448
Rectus Abdominis Flap..................................448
Rectus Abdominis Muscle Flap (Based on
  the Inferior Epigastric Vessels)....................451
Rectus Abdominis Myocutaneous Flap
  (Based on the Inferior Epigastric Vessels).......454
Lower Transverse Rectus Abdominis
  Myocutaneous Flap 455
Modified Lower TRAM Flap 458
Thoracoumbilical Flap....................................459
Greater Omentum Transfer 462
Free Omentum Transfer 464
Extending Greater Omentum 467
Composite Flap of Stomach and Omentum.........468
Free Jejunum Transfer 472
Recipient Site Exposure 477
Bibliography 480

11 Back 482
Latissimus Dorsi Flap.....................................482
Latissimus Dorsi Muscle Flap 487
Latissimus Dorsi Myocutaneous Flap 493
Bilobed Split Latissimus Dorsi Flap 496
Lateral Split Latissimus Dorsi Flap 498
Rib-Latissimus Dorsi Osteomyocutaneous Flap ...501
Scapular and Parascapular Flaps 504
Scapular Flap..506
Parascapular Flap..512
Scapular Osteocutaneous Flap.......................514
Scapular and Parascapular Combined Flap 517
Scapular and Latissimus Dorsi Combined Flap 519
Bibliography 522

Part 4 Head and Neck

12 Head and Neck..526
Temporoparietal Flap 526
Temporoparietal Fascia Flap 528
Bilobed Temporal Fascia Flap 532
Temporocalvarial Osteofascial Flap.................534
Free Scalp Skin Flap 536
Superficial Cervical Flap 538
Submental Flap...544
Recipient Site Exposures................................550
Bibliography 553

General References 555

Index 557

PREFACE

Donor sites are as important for microvascular surgeons as fabric materials are for tailors.

It has been almost three decades since microvascular surgical techniques have been clinically applied. In the initial period of the 1960s, successful replantations of the upper extremities were reported in the United States and China. The development of replantation spurred the improvement of optical equipment, suture materials, and instruments, as well as the refinement of anastomotic techniques for microvascular surgery. These developments also set the stage for attempts at free tissue transfer in the early 1970s. Limited series of free toe transfers and free skin flaps were subsequently carried out.

In the 1970s, in addition to free toe transfers and free skin flaps, revascularized muscle, bone, and nerve grafts, as well as composite tissue transfers, were developed, and many of the useful donor sites were discovered in this decade, based on anatomic investigations and clinical trials. Microvascular surgery grew as an ancillary development of general surgical, plastic surgical, and orthopaedic techniques and obtained a firm foothold in medical science.

In the 1980s, the techniques matured with further anatomic investigations and clinical applications. Many surgeons mastered these microsurgical techniques, which were then popularized and became more effective in patient management.

Seeking to make the techniques of free tissue transfer convenient for surgeons to approach rather than hiding them in relatively obscure references, this *Atlas of Microvascular Surgery: Anatomy and Operative Approaches* has the following goals.

1. This is a comprehensive work and includes 43 donor sites with detailed anatomy, and 98 basic and varied techniques of flap design, harvesting or fabrication, as well as 39 procedures for exposure of the recipient vessels. Almost all of the necessary anatomic information and surgical techniques for reconstructive microsurgery are described and illustrated.

2. This book is concise and precise. An enormous amount of literature has been collected and reviewed relating to reconstructive microsurgery. The essentials have been selected and combined with our anatomic investigations and clinical experiences, and the results have been condensed into short, clear, and succinct descriptions.

3. The *Atlas* is relatively easy to peruse and to understand. There are approximately 570 illustrations that present clear anatomy and variations thereof, for step-by-step operative procedures. We have avoided the use of photographs, as we have not generally found them as instructive as detailed drawings. Each flap is preceded by a description of the relevant anatomy. The first of each set of drawings for every flap described lists all of the anatomic structures that will be discussed or indicated for that particular flap. All figures following list only the structures specific for that drawing.

In addition to describing the anatomy and detailed harvesting of all the flaps, we have also attempted to describe the anatomic approaches to the major vascular recipient sites. These sections are found at the end of each anatomic area.

4. We hope that the work will prove to be a valuable reference for those who are actively involved in microsurgery. In addition to general anatomy and operative techniques, variations in arterial anatomy are emphasized, and clinical comments are added for each donor site. Even for the experienced surgeon, briefly reviewing related chapters before attempting a specific microvascular transfer should prove very helpful: details of the related anatomy and specific procedure will thereby be recalled, and reminders of clinical advantages and disadvantages should allow a review of the clinical applications.

Even a quarter of an hour spent on the relevant information will provide additional confidence to the microsurgeon.

We consider this work as an international collaboration and extension of knowledge between the United States and China, as well as a collaborative effort between plastic and orthopaedic surgeons, in whose specialties a great deal of microvascular surgery is performed.

Our special thanks for making this book possible go to Dr. R.D. Landres, Director of Academic Affairs, Department of Plastic and Reconstructive Surgery, Albert Einstein College of Medicine and Montefiore Medical Center. She has provided invaluable editorial assistance in the preparation of the text. We also gratefully acknowledge the extensive drawings of Li-Guo Liang, the artist and coordinator of the medical illustrations.

This book is dedicated to all the pioneers in microvascular surgery, whose tireless and brilliant efforts have resulted in the disclosure of donor sites for wide clinical application.

Berish Strauch, M.D.
Han-Liang Yu, M.D.

ATLAS OF
MICROVASCULAR
SURGERY

INTRODUCTION

DEFINITIONS

In certain operative procedures, the naked eye is not sufficient for the most precise and accurate results. Surgeons need improved visualization under microscopic magnification, along with the utilization of accompanying microsurgical instruments.

Microsurgery is a surgical territory in which incisions, sutures, dissections, ligations, osteotomies, etc., are performed under the microscope. Within this territory are included, for example, techniques for suturing the cornea in ophthalmologic procedures and fenestration for otosclerosis in ear procedures.

Microvascular surgery is a particular area of microsurgery, in which small vessels, with diameters of less than 2.5 mm, can be repaired for limb or tissue revascularization. This area of techniques includes both replantation and reconstructive microsurgery.

Reconstructive Microsurgery

Reconstructive microsurgery comprises a surgical category utilizing revascularized tissue transfer to repair acquired or congenital defects or malformations. The objective of these reparative procedures is the restoration of function or the improvement of appearance, or both. Acquired defects or malformations are usually the result of traumatic injury, burn destruction, or malfunction incident to disease or the surgical resection of tumor or other affected tissue.

Reconstructive microsurgical procedures generally consist of the following steps:

1. Preparation of the recipient site, including resection of tumor or other diseased tissues, and exposure of the recipient artery and veins, as well as nerves, tendons, or bony structures, as required.
2. Elevation of donor tissues on a vascular pedicle, keeping the circulation intact.
3. Transfer of the elevated tissues from the donor to the recipient site for replantation by vessel anastomoses. Sometimes, bony fixation and repair of nerves or tendons may be needed as, for example, in a toe-to-hand transfer.

In reference to the measures just mentioned, harvesting of donor tissues and the exposure of recipient vessels are key techniques for any individual case involving reconstructive microsurgery. For this reason, this book will focus particularly on these two issues, especially on the harvesting of donor tissues.

In textual descriptions and figure legends, the anatomic terminology follows *Gray's Anatomy;* numbers in the text following anatomic terms represent and parallel the structures illustrated, so that the reader can easily match the text with the figures.

TRAINING IN BASIC MICROSURGICAL TECHNIQUES

We emphasize that the surgeon must be well trained in microvascular techniques on animal models in the laboratory before attempting clinical trials. A goal of crucial importance to the success of revascularized tissue transfer is the patency of vessel anastomoses. To this end, we suggest training in the following areas.

Mastering Microsurgical Instruments. The surgeon should be comfortable in handling all microsurgical instruments under the operating microscope, with hands and eyes cooperating adroitly.

Adjusting the Operating Microscope. Eye pieces for both eyes should be adjusted to obtain a stereopsis that facilitates operative maneuvers. The surgeon should also be skilled in controlling the foot pedals to keep the focus sharp, and should be able to change magnification at will, whenever required during the procedure.

Different operative maneuvers require varying magnifications. We suggest that low magnification (5× to 9×) is best used for vessel preparation (dissection, clamp application, trimming of adventitia, irrigation) and knot tying in a wide-view field. Moderate magnification (10× to 17×) is suggested for suture placement; and high magnification (18× or more) should be used for inspection.

Suture Selection. Depending on the diameter of the vessel used for anastomosis, a proper-sized suture should be selected. Commonly, 10-0 monofilament nylon is used for vessels with diameters of 0.8 to 1.5 mm; 9-0 is used for vessels with diameters of 1.6 to 2.5 mm; and 11-0 is used for vessels with diameters of less than 0.7 mm.

Course of Training. Training should proceed in an orderly and step-by-step fashion. When beginning practice in suturing and knot tying on a silicone sheet, end-to-end anastomoses are performed on the carotid artery of rats, with gradual advancement to the rat femoral artery and vein. Bypasses can then be undertaken in the femoral artery with grafts of the saphenous artery to practice end-to-side anastomoses. Finally, successful executions of ear replantation in the rabbit and free epigastric flap transfer to the neck in a rat model, should produce expertise and confidence.

To reach a desired level of training, the surgeon needs at least 3 months of practice, as well as patience and focused effort.

Producing Secure Anastomoses. To attain a high patency rate subsequent to performing anastomoses, the surgeon should attend consistently to the following requirements:

1. An atraumatic technique is employed, with gentle handling of vessels with adventitia; avoiding damage to the intima is crucial.
2. Proper trimming of the adventitia is important, so that there is no interference with the anastomosis.
3. An appropriate tension is beneficial for anastomotic patency. If the tension is excessive, an interpositional vein graft should be considered.
4. Depending on vessel diameter, appropriate and equal intervals between stitches are required, and, according to vessel-wall thickness, appropriate marginal distances between the point of suture insertion and the transected vessel edge must be determined.
5. During the anastomosis, all possible effort should be directed toward the successful eversion of the intima of both transected vessel edges, and inversion should be avoided.

Since details of the basic microsurgical techniques have been provided in published descriptions and illustrations of both experimental and clinical microsurgery, we recommend some of these works for the novice microsurgeon, rather than repeating available materials:

- Acland RD: *Microsurgery Practice Manual.* Louisville, KY: University of Louisville Microsurgery Laboratory, Price Institute of Surgical Research, Department of Surgery, Health Sciences Center, 1977.
- Ballantyne DL, Razabone RM, Harper AD: *Microvascular Surgery: A Laboratory Manual.* New York: Institute of Reconstructive Plastic Surgery, New York University Medical Center, 1980.
- Berger A, Tizian C: *Atlas of Microsurgical Technique.* Norfolk, VA: Hampton Press Publishing, 1987.
- Chen ZW, Yang TY, Chang TS: *Microsurgery.* Berlin, Heidelberg, New York: Shanghai Scientific and Technical Publishers and Springer-Verlag, 1982.

EXPOSURE OF RECIPIENT VESSELS

As was mentioned before, the exposure of recipient vessels is of significant importance in reconstructive microsurgery, as well as in replantation microsurgery, for determining the main vessels. However, as far as can be determined, there is a dearth of published information concerning recipient-vessel exposure. For this reason, our book will describe the relevant techniques for the surgeon's reference.

For general use, incisions and procedures will be described and illustrated in normal vessels: in reality, there are commonly defects and deformities at the recipient site. We urge surgeons to adjust or modify the described techniques for each individual case. Preoperative Doppler examination or angiography may be useful for confirming the existence and condition of recipient vessels.

MICROSURGICAL ANATOMY AND ITS VARIATIONS

A knowledge of the anatomy of donor-tissue blood supply is absolutely indispensable for harvesting procedures. In addition, anatomic investigations have always been prerequisites for clinical applications of every revascularized tissue transfer. In our literature searches, we found that arterial anatomy and its variations have been the most complicated and difficult subjects in donor-site descriptions. Such descriptions have been complex and confusing, with insufficient information, and often even with disagreement among authors.

According to our investigations and experience, we have tried to make such descriptions well-organized and accurate, as well as concise and practical. We also have attempted more detailed anatomic descriptions of commonly applicable donor sites than have appeared previously. Vessel diameter and pedicle length measurements, as provided in the text or tables, refer to the average in adults; variations in children are also provided. In addition to normal cases, variations in the arterial anatomy are emphasized, so that the surgeon will have some idea of proper management in abnormal anatomic variations that may arise intraoperatively.

The morphology of relevant muscles, bones, and nerves, as well as of venous drainage, is clearly described, as related to each specific donor site.

Revascularized tissue transfer consists mainly of the free skin flap, free muscle flap, revascularized bone graft, and free toe transfer, as well as revascularized nerve graft, etc.

The free skin flap comprises three patterns, according to the nature of the blood supply:

1. The axial skin flap is supplied by its direct cutaneous vessels, e.g., the groin flap.
2. The musculocutaneous flap is supplied by its musculocutaneous perforators, e.g., the latissimus dorsi musculocutaneous flap.
3. The fasciocutaneous flap is supplied by its septofasciocutaneous perforators, e.g., the radial forearm flap.

The revascularized bone graft usually needs nourishment from the nutrient artery included in its vascular pedicle; it can also be nourished by the vascular network on the periosteum only.

DONOR SITES

It is widely known that there are numerous donor sites in the body that can provide materials for restoration of function or appearance at other sites, with little or no morbidity. The descriptions of donor sites in this atlas concentrate on tissue transfer involving revascularization by microvascular anastomosis. Pedicle tissue transfers (even those with vascular pedicles) are not included. However, most of the donor sites described in this book can be used with vascular pedicles for local transfers in indicated cases.

Tissues for microvascular reconstruction include the free skin flap, free muscle flap, revascularized bone graft, revascularized joint graft, and free toe transfer, as well as free omentum and free jejunum transfer, among others. Tendons, fascia, nerves, or nail and hair can be included in composite flaps, used as vascularized grafts, with certain indications.

There may be several techniques for harvesting the various tissues supplied by a donor site. Following anatomic description, the first tissue-harvesting procedure, which is usually the basic technique at this donor site, is described in detail.

The terms "free" and "revascularized" have also been omitted in most chapters to avoid redundancy; we believe that readers will understand this omission and supply the necessary adjectives.

Donor sites are as important for microvascular surgeons as fabric materials are for tailors. Surgeons should be familiar with the properties of all donor sites, so that both donor materials and their related techniques can be correctly chosen to meet recipient site requirements.

FLAP DESIGN

After a donor site and its related properties are clearly understood, the design of the flap should be carefully considered. On occasion, angiography or Doppler flowmetry may be required.

Usually, an axis should be first drawn for the skin flap. An axial skin flap uses the course of the direct cutaneous artery as the axis, while that of a fasciocutaneous flap is along the septum of compartments where septofasciocutaneous perforators emerge. In contrast, the area of a musculocutaneous flap involves the underlying muscle.

The design of flap shape and size must be in accordance with the defect at the recipient site; we suggest that a template be routinely used. Generally, the size of the flap should not be more than 1 cm larger than the defect. Flap size depends on the blood supply capacity of the vascular pedicle, which may be estimated according to the diameter of the pedicle vessel, age, general patient condition, etc. The "maximum size" mentioned in the text for each flap derives from case reports in the literature. Such measurements are given only for reference; the surgeon should be circumspect in considering these maximum measurements.

HARVESTING TECHNIQUES

Especially for surgeons with less experience, a detailed review of the anatomy and its variations, careful consideration of indications, and accurate flap design are suggested before flap elevation.

If the donor site is on an extremity, a tourniquet is applied while the extremity is elevated; full exsanguination is not necessary, so that the vascular structures can be clearly identified during dissection. An incision extending from a side of the designed flap is usually used for full exposure of the neurovascular pedicle.

Harvesting procedures are described step by step and can be easily followed as the flap is raised. On occasion, dissection of the neurovascular pedicle and flap elevation can be alternated, according to the surgeon's experience or the situation during the procedure at the time. The pedicle should be carefully protected during either dissection or elevation, and any excess tension on it should be avoided. At the donor site, any potentially valuable main nerves and vessels should be preserved, and care should be taken to minimize morbidity as much as possible.

After flap elevation, the tourniquet is released, and flap circulation evaluated before the vascular pedicle is divided. In general, mechanical dilation of the pedicle vessels is not advocated.

Two surgical teams for donor site harvesting and recipient site preservation are required in the interest of saving time. There is the additional benefit in the two-team approach in that the procedure at the donor site may be adjusted, as required, while the recipient-site defect is being prepared. The pedicle should not be divided until complete preparation at the recipient site is completed, in order to minimize flap ischemia.

Direct closure at the donor defect should be attempted, if at all possible. Undermining and applying retention sutures may contribute to the approximation of wound edges. However, if the defect is too extensive, direct closure might cause excessive tension and result in a crisis in limb circulation or in subsequent wound dehiscence. In this case, a split-thickness skin graft or local rotation skin flap should be applied.

A few specific donor-defect closures are included directly after descriptions of flap-harvesting techniques.

COMMENT AND INSIGHTS

As we mentioned before, there is a parallel between donor sites for the microsurgeon and various materials for the tailor: each donor site, as each tailoring material, has its own specific properties, allowing the flap to meet whatever special requirements are necessary. For example, the bulkiness of the gluteal muscle flap is acceptable in breast reconstruction; the thick keratotic skin of the medial plantar flap is usable in reconstruction of the weight-bearing heel area or palmar area.

Instead of the use of simplified "advantages and disadvantages," the *Comment and Insights,* which appear throughout this book, are objectively based on the authors' knowledge and experience with each donor site, according to its popularity in clinical use. This is based on pragmatic clinical concepts for each donor site and summarizes vascular anatomy, tissue property, donor morbidity, and general clinical application. There are four considerations in the evaluation of popularity:

1. The flap has been developed over time and is still commonly and widely applied, e.g., the latissimus dorsi flap, radial forearm flap, revascularized fibula bone graft, among others.
2. The flap has been developed over time and was previously more widely used; although still in use, its applicability has lessened, e.g., the groin flap.
3. The flap is newly developed and its application is growing, e.g., the lateral arm flap.
4. The flap is newly developed, but its reliability and applicability need further anatomic investigation and clinical trials, e.g., thigh flaps and leg flaps.

For reliable clinical use, items 1 and 3 are recommended. If there appear to be strong indications, item 2 may be prudently considered. As to item 4, we suggest that the surgeon would do well to carry out cadaveric anatomic investigations and maneuvers before the first clinical application.

In general, flap reliability depends on adequate vascular anatomy. Knowledge of the arterial variations should give a surgeon more confidence, and evaluation of pedicle length should make anastomosis and dissection easier. Measurement of vessel diameters will usually represent the capacity of the blood supply to the flap; however, septofasciocutaneous or musculocutaneous perforators arising from the pedicle vessels should also be evaluated for fasciocutaneous or musculocutaneous flaps.

Part One
UPPER EXTREMITY

1 SHOULDER, ARM, AND AXILLA

Deltoid Flap

Anatomy (**Fig. 1-1**)

The *posterior circumflex humeral artery* [6] branches from the axillary artery distal to the origin of the subscapular artery at the lower border of the subscapularis. It runs backward around the surgical neck of the humerus through the quadrangle space [4] that is bounded by the teres minor [2] above, the teres major [3] below, the long head of the triceps [5] medially, and the surgical neck of the humerus laterally.

The *cutaneous branch* [7] of the artery arises near the quadrangle space and passes into the areolar tissue, emerging in the deltoid-triceps groove to supply the skin over the deltoid muscle.

There are two venae comitantes accompanying the arterial system.

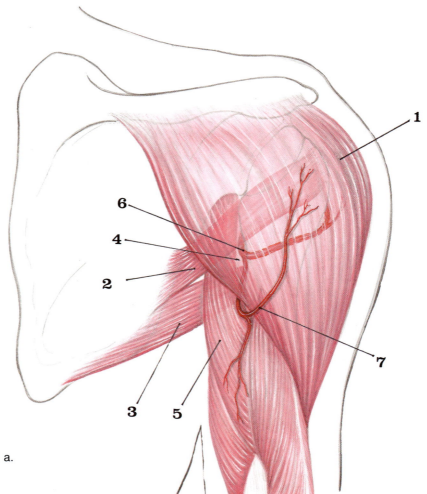

1. Deltoid m.
2. Teres minor m.
3. Teres major m.
4. Quadrangle space
5. Long head of triceps m.
6. Posterior circumflex humeral a.
7. Cutaneous branch

Innervation

The upper lateral cutaneous nerve of the arm issues from the inferior division of the axillary nerve and accompanies the cutaneous vessels. The nerve provides sensibility to the skin over the posteroinferior two thirds of the deltoid and the upper portion of the triceps.

Measurements of the Neurovascular Anatomy

		Diameter (mm)
Posterior circumflex humeral	Artery	2.0–3.0
	Vein	3.0–4.0
Cutaneous branch at emergence	Artery	0.8–1.0
	Vein	1.0–1.3

Variations (Fig. 1-2)

At the emergence of the neurovascular cutaneous branches in the deltoid-triceps groove, there may be some variation. At times, two pedicles enter the flap, with a common origin from the posterior circumflex humeral vessels (early bifurcation), or, rarely, the major pedicle penetrates the lower portion of the deltoid muscle to enter the overlying skin.

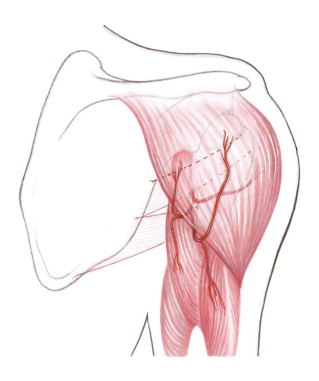
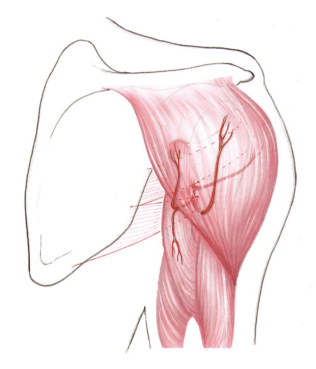

COMMENT AND INSIGHTS

The neurovascular anatomy is quite constant, although there may be some variations in the cutaneous branches that affect vessel caliber. The basic elevation of the flap is fairly simple. Pedicle length and vessel diameter are quite satisfactory for microvascular transfer. The donor site provides a relatively thin, pliable, fasciocutaneous flap with sensibility.

Skin area for flap transfer is relatively large (up to 35 × 15 cm), whereas the area of sensibility innervated by the upper lateral cutaneous nerve of the arm varies from 13 × 6 to 19 × 15 cm, with an average of 15 × 10 cm.

This flap is applicable in reconstructions of soft tissue defects of the head, neck, and extremities. The color match is especially acceptable for the head and neck.

The donor defect is usually covered with a split-thickness skin graft. When the width of the defect is less than 6 cm, primary closure is possible. The skin-grafted donor site has a noticeable scar and depression that may be unacceptable to some patients.

A potential risk of axillary nerve damage can be minimized by careful dissection.

Harvesting Technique

(**Fig. 1-3**) A line is drawn from the acromion to the medial epicondyle of the elbow as the axis of the flap, so that the emergence of the neurovascular cutaneous branches is approximately near the point at which the line intersects the posterior edge of the deltoid muscle. The largest reported size of this flap is 33 × 13 cm.

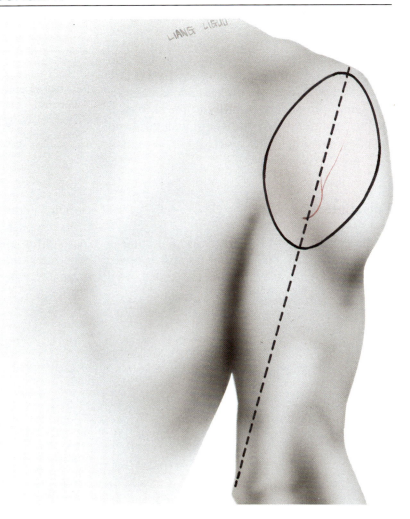

1. Deltoid m.
2. Triceps m.
3. Cutaneous branch of posterior circumflex humeral a. and upper lateral cutaneous n. of arm
4. Posterior circumflex humeral a. and axillary n.
5. Teres minor m.
6. Teres major m.
7. Surgical neck of humerus
8. Deltoid-triceps groove

(**Fig. 1-4**) The superior portion of the flap is elevated in a plane deep to the deltoid muscle fascia. Dissection is carried out toward the pedicle [3] that is usually visible on the undersurface of the flap. Attention should be paid to preserve all of the branches near the anticipated emergence in the deltoid-triceps groove [8], since variations may appear there.

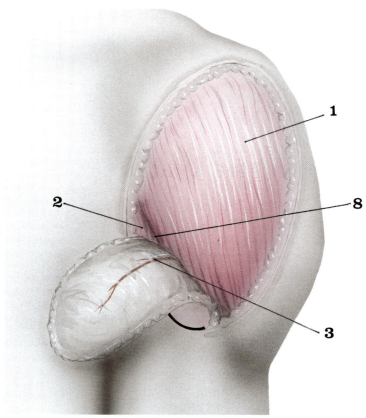

1. Deltoid m.
2. Triceps m.
3. Cutaneous branch of posterior circumflex humeral a. and upper lateral cutaneous n. of arm
8. Deltoid-triceps groove

(**Fig. 1-5**) After the emergence of the neurovascular cutaneous branches [3] is identified and isolated, the skin flap is circumferentially completed.

2. Triceps m.
3. Cutaneous branch of posterior circumflex humeral a. and upper lateral cutaneous n. of arm
8. Deltoid-triceps groove

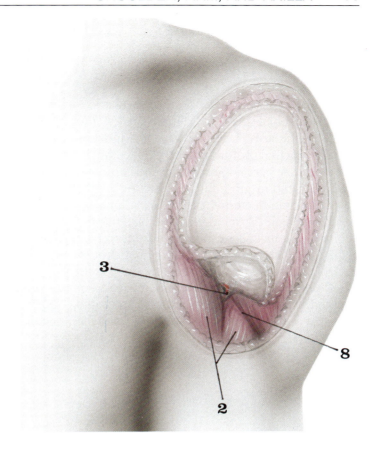

(**Fig. 1-6**) After retracting the deltoid muscle [1] superoanteriorly and the triceps [2] posteriorly, the neurovascular pedicle is dissected in the quadrangle space to expose the posterior circumflex humeral vessels and the axillary nerve [4]. The posterior circumflex humeral vessels are divided distal to the takeoff of the cutaneous branches, and the upper lateral cutaneous nerve of the arm [3] is separated from the axillary nerve. Extreme care should be taken not to injure the axillary nerve [4] during this procedure.

A long neurovascular pedicle, reaching 6 to 8 cm, can be developed by further dissection and transection of the posterior humeral circumflex artery.

1. Deltoid m.
2. Triceps m.
3. Cutaneous branch of posterior circumflex humeral a. and upper lateral cutaneous n. of arm
4. Posterior circumflex humeral a. and axillary n.
5. Teres minor m.
6. Teres major m.
7. Surgical neck of humerus

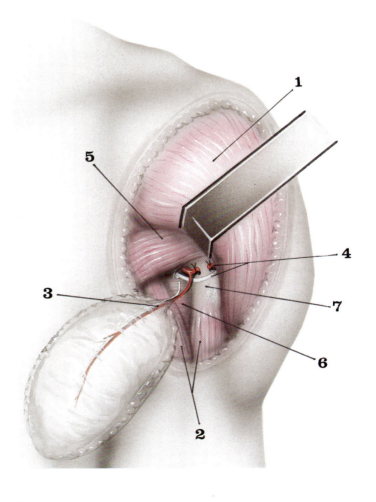

Medial Arm Flap

Anatomy (Fig. 1-7)

The *superior ulnar collateral artery* [11] arises from the brachial artery [9], slightly below the middle of the arm. Occasionally, it originates from the brachial profundus artery. It accompanies the ulnar nerve, pierces the medial intermuscular septum at about the junction of the lower and middle thirds of the arm, and descends between the medial epicondyle and the olecranon. In its course, it gives off one to four cutaneous branches [12] to the medial skin of the arm. However, in 13% of cases, there is no cutaneous branch from the artery; instead, an enlarged musculocutaneous branch from the biceps or a direct cutaneous branch from the brachial artery appear.

The superior ulnar collateral artery has a diameter ranging from 1.0 to 2.5 mm, with an average of 1.7 mm at its origin, and the size of the cutaneous branches varies from 0.5 to 1.4 mm.

Venous drainage is provided by two venae comitantes and the basilic vein.

Innervation

The medial cutaneous nerve of the arm (2 mm in diameter) descends along the medial side of the brachial artery and basilic vein to the middle of the upper arm. At this point, it pierces the deep fascia and is distributed to the skin of the medial side of the lower half of the arm.

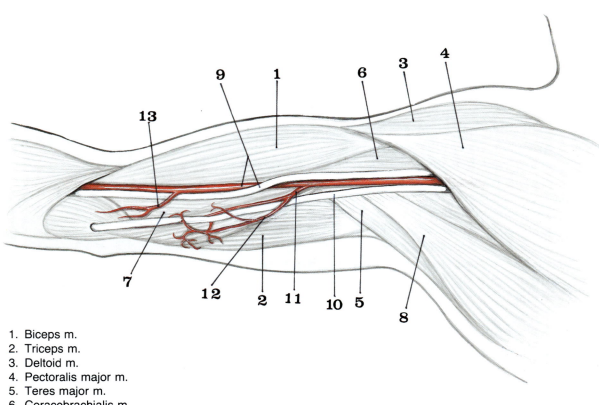

1. Biceps m.
2. Triceps m.
3. Deltoid m.
4. Pectoralis major m.
5. Teres major m.
6. Coracobrachialis m.
7. Brachialis m.
8. Latissimus dorsi m.
9. Brachial a. and median n.
10. Ulnar n.
11. Superior ulnar collateral a.
12. Cutaneous branch
13. Inferior ulnar collateral a.

COMMENT AND INSIGHTS

There have been several cases of free medial arm flaps reported. This flap is a septofasciocutaneous flap based on the superior ulnar collateral artery in the medial septum of the arm. Since there is a certain variation in the superior ulnar collateral artery, the medial cutaneous nerve of the forearm is usually sacrificed, causing anesthesia of the medial side of the forearm after flap harvesting. The skin territory of the flap is generally limited and the flap is not widely used clinically.

However, the skin texture of the territory of this flap is usually thin, elastic, and quite hairless, and it is provided with sensibility through its constant cutaneous nerve. Therefore, it still can be considered for use in facial reconstruction and in hand resurfacing.

If the width of the flap is less than 7 cm, the donor deficit can be closed primarily. Cosmetically, the donor site of the flap is well hidden and morbidity after harvesting is generally minimal, except for a loss of sensibility in the forearm.

Harvesting Technique

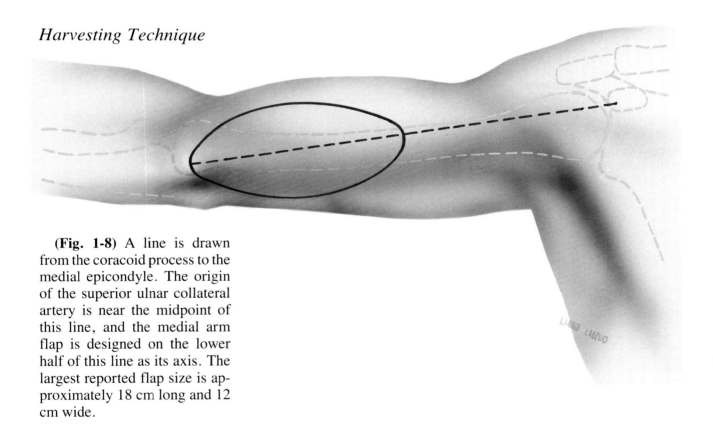

(Fig. 1-8) A line is drawn from the coracoid process to the medial epicondyle. The origin of the superior ulnar collateral artery is near the midpoint of this line, and the medial arm flap is designed on the lower half of this line as its axis. The largest reported flap size is approximately 18 cm long and 12 cm wide.

1. Biceps m.
2. Brachial a. and median n.
3. Superior ulnar collateral a.
4. Basilic v.
5. Ulnar n.
6. Medial cutaneous n. of arm.
7. Triceps m.
8. Brachialis m.
9. Medial cutaneous n. of forearm

(Fig. 1-9) The anterior part of the flap with deep fascia is raised from the biceps [1] toward the medial intermuscular septum. Before reaching the septum, dissection proceeds carefully to identify a major cutaneous branch from the septum to the flap. Occasionally, it may emerge from the posteromedial aspect of the biceps muscle. The major cutaneous branch is traced to the superior ulnar collateral artery [3] or directly to the brachial artery [2]. All other small fasciocutaneous branches should be kept intact with the septum and the skin flap.

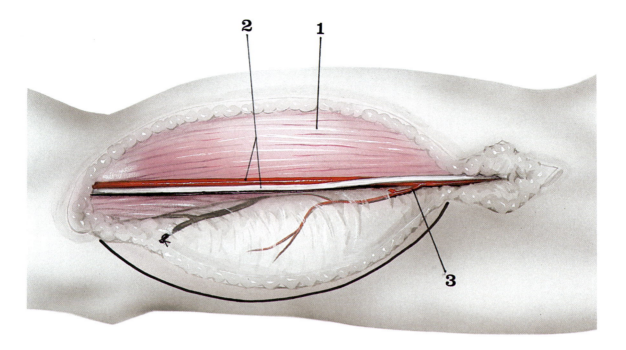

1. Biceps m.
2. Brachial a. and median n.
3. Superior ulnar collateral a.

(**Fig. 1-10**) The posterior part of the flap is incised. The medial cutaneous nerves of the arm [6] and forearm [9], and the basilic vein [4], are identified and included in the flap. (The medial cutaneous nerve of the forearm is usually sacrificed.) The ulnar nerve [5] is isolated from the septum and the superior ulnar collateral vessels, leaving it in the arm.

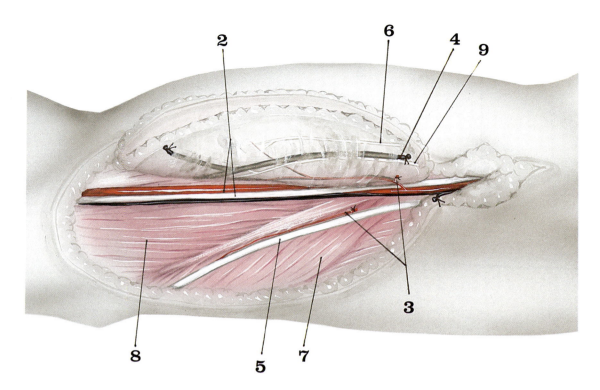

2. Brachial a. and median n.
3. Superior ulnar collateral a.
4. Basilic v.
5. Ulnar n.
6. Medial cutaneous n. of arm
7. Triceps m.
8. Brachialis m.
9. Medial cutaneous n. of forearm

16 ATLAS OF MICROVASCULAR SURGERY

(**Fig. 1-11**) Keeping the septum intact with the flap, the medial intermuscular septum is separated from the brachial vessels and the median nerve [2], distal to proximal. The major cutaneous branch and the superior ulnar collateral vessels [3] are further dissected to the origin from the brachial vessels. Simultaneously, the medial arm flap is isolated on the superior ulnar collateral vessels [3], the basilic vein [4], and the medial cutaneous nerve of the arm [6].

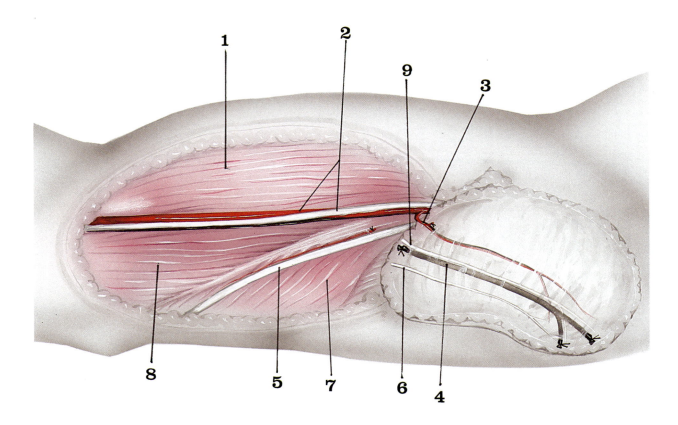

1. Biceps m.
2. Brachial a. and median n.
3. Superior ulnar collateral a.
4. Basilic v.
5. Ulnar n.
6. Medial cutaneous n. of arm
7. Triceps m.
8. Brachialis m.
9. Medial cutaneous n. of forearm

Lateral Arm Flap

Anatomy (Fig. 1-12)

The *deep brachial artery* [6] divides into two terminal branches while it is coursing in the groove of the radial nerve. The middle collateral artery descends in the substance of the medial head of the triceps, whereas the radial collateral artery [8] continues to accompany the radial nerve. Once the *radial collateral artery* appears on the anterolateral aspect of the triceps, it divides into anterior and posterior branches. The *anterior branch* [10] continues to accompany the radial nerve deeply between the brachialis [4] and brachioradialis [5], while the *posterior branch* [9] enters the lateral intermuscular septum between the brachioradialis [5] and the triceps [3]; the posterior branch continues to run toward the lateral epicondyle.

In its course, the posterior branch of the radial collateral artery gives off two or three fasciocutaneous branches, to supply the lower lateral skin of the arm. The most proximal of these branches is closely related to the posterior cutaneous nerve of the forearm.

Venous drainage is supplied by one (25% of cases) or two (75% of cases) venae comitantes and the cephalic vein.

Innervation

The lower lateral cutaneous nerve of the arm, a branch of the radial nerve, perforates the lateral head of the triceps, just behind the insertion of the deltoid. It then passes to the front of the elbow, lying close to the cephalic vein, and supplies the skin of the lateral part of the lower half of the arm.

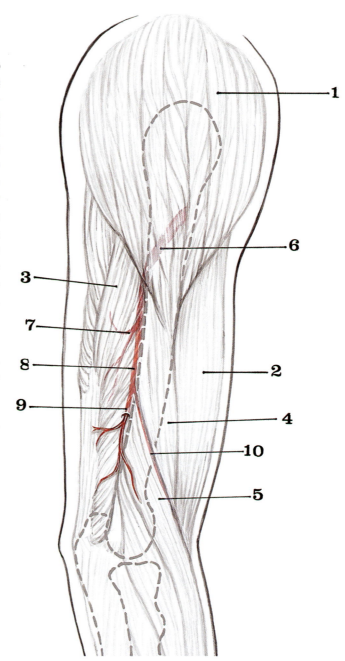

Measurements

		Diameter (mm)
Deep brachial	Artery	1.7
	Vein	2.0
Radial collateral	Artery	1.3
	Vein	1.9
Cephalic vein		3.2

1. Deltoid m.
2. Biceps m.
3. Triceps m.
4. Brachialis m.
5. Brachioradialis m.
6. Deep brachial a.
7. Middle collateral a.
8. Radial collateral a.
9. Posterior branch
10. Anterior branch

COMMENT AND INSIGHTS

Since the very first case of the lateral arm flap was reported, it has become one of the more popular flaps clinically in the last decade, because of its constant arterial anatomy, reliable harvesting technique, and its adequate size and length of the vascular pedicle.

This flap is a septofasciocutaneous flap based on the radial collateral artery in the lateral intermuscular septum of the arm. The skin texture of the flap is usually thin and elastic, but there is a tendency to hairiness in males. The flap can be provided with sensibility through its constant cutaneous nerve.

Clinically, the lateral arm flap is used in reconstructions of the head and neck and in resurfacing of the hand. In addition to a neurosensory fasciocutaneous flap, this donor site can be transferred as fascia alone or in a tendofasciocutaneous pattern with a central strip of 1.5 cm width of triceps tendon.

The skin territory is adequately large (up to 14 × 20 cm). However, if the width of the flap is less than 6 cm, the donor deficit can be closed primarily. Cosmetically, the donor site of the lateral arm flap is conspicuous, especially when a split-thickness skin graft has been used for closure of the defect.

Generally, donor site morbidity for the flap is minimal, but harvesting may sacrifice some sensibility to the lateral side of the forearm.

Harvesting Technique

(Fig. 1-13) A line is drawn from the insertion of the deltoid to the lateral epicondyle as the axis of the flap; the flap is centered on this line. Flap territory can include the distal half of the lateral aspect of the arm and the proximal fifth of the forearm. The maximum flap size is 20 × 14 cm, but for primary closure, the width of the flap should be less than 6 cm.

1. Triceps m.
2. Radial n. and radial collateral a.
3. Anterior branch
4. Posterior branch of radial collateral a. and posterior cutaneous n. of forearm
5. Lateral cutaneous n. of arm
6. Lateral epicondyle
7. Biceps m.
8. Brachialis m.
9. Brachioradialis m.
10. Cephalic v.

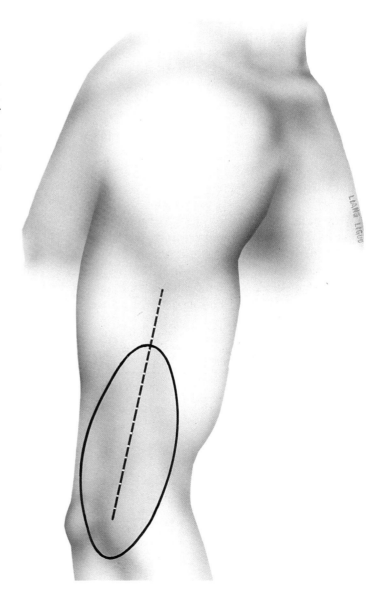

(**Fig. 1-14**) First, the posterior part of the flap is raised with its underlying deep fascia from the triceps muscle [1]. Once the lateral intermuscular septum is encountered and the branches from the septum to the triceps are ligated, the posterior branch [4] of the radial collateral artery [2] and the posterior cutaneous nerve of the forearm [4] are exposed in the septum by retracting the triceps muscle posteriorly. At the posterior proximal edge of the flap, the lower lateral cutaneous nerve of the arm [5] is identified and preserved with the flap.

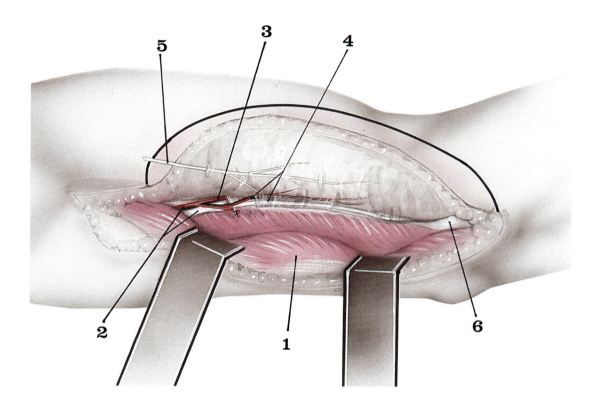

1. Triceps m.
2. Radial n. and radial collateral a.
3. Anterior branch
4. Posterior branch of radial collateral a. and posterior cutaneous n. of forearm
5. Lateral cutaneous n. of arm
6. Lateral epicondyle

(Fig. 1-15) The anterior part of the flap is elevated subfascially toward the lateral intermuscular septum. Once the posterior branch of the radial collateral artery [4] can be seen from both sides, the septum is detached from the humerus, starting distally. The posterior cutaneous nerve of the forearm [4] is usually sacrificed. The anterior branch of the radial collateral artery [3] is divided.

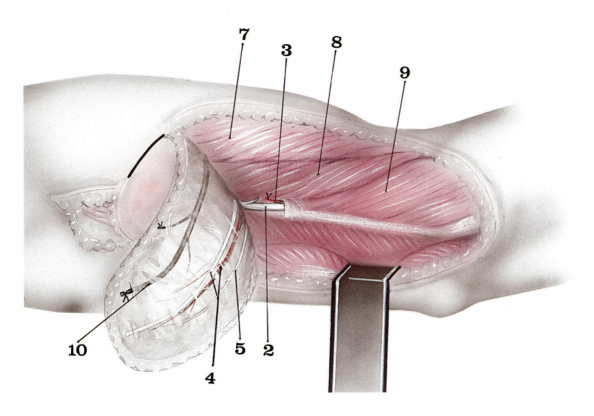

2. Radial n. and radial collateral a.
3. Anterior branch
4. Posterior branch of radial collateral a. and posterior cutaneous n. of forearm
5. Lateral cutaneous n. of arm
7. Biceps m.
8. Brachialis m.
9. Brachioradialis m.
10. Cephalic v.

SHOULDER, ARM, AND AXILLA

(Fig. 1-16) Dissection proceeds proximally toward isolating the vascular pedicle. After ligating the anterior branch, the radial collateral vessels [2] are dissected for greater pedicle length and larger vessel caliber. Pedicle lengths vary according to flap design, ranging from 4 to 8 cm.

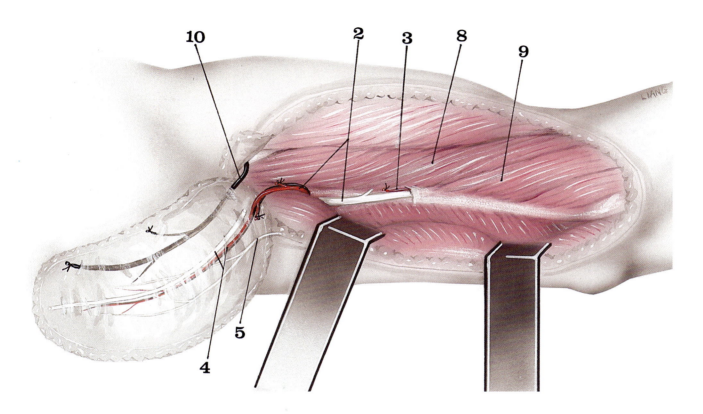

2. Radial n. and radial collateral a.
3. Anterior branch
4. Posterior branch of radial collateral a. and posterior cutaneous n. of forearm
5. Lateral cutaneous n. of arm
8. Brachialis m.
9. Brachioradialis m.
10. Cephalic v.

Posterior Arm Flap

Anatomy (Fig. 1-17)

An unnamed artery [7] arises from the medial side of the brachial artery [6] near the deep brachial artery. At times, it can arise from the deep brachial artery itself. After giving off a branch to the medial head of the triceps, the unnamed artery runs through the brachial aponeurosis under a fibrous band that is located at the angle formed by the medial head of the triceps and the tendon of the latissimus dorsi. Subsequently, as a cutaneous branch, it courses along the axis of the triceps muscle [1].

Before the artery pierces the aponeurosis, it is joined by one or two veins that enter the basilic vein.

Innervation

The posterior cutaneous nerve of the arm, a branch of the radial nerve, follows the unnamed artery to supply the posterior skin area of the arm.

Measurements

		Diameter (mm)
Unnamed artery	Artery	0.8–1.2
	Vein	1.0–1.5

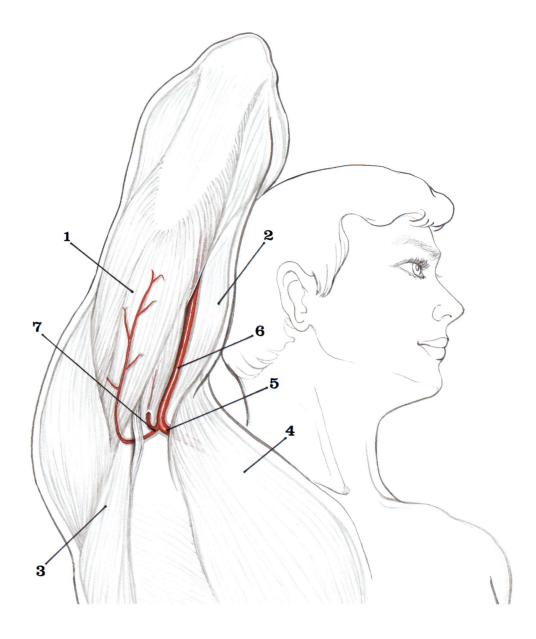

1. Triceps m.
2. Biceps m.
3. Latissimus dorsi m.
4. Pectoralis major m.
5. Axillary a.
6. Brachial a.
7. Unnamed a.

COMMENT AND INSIGHTS

There have been relatively few cases of the posterior arm flap reported; its reliability needs to be further clarified by anatomic investigation and clinical application. This flap is not recommended for routine use.

The flap is an axial cutaneous one.

The skin texture of the flap is usually thin, elastic, and quite hairless, and it is provided with sensibility through its cutaneous nerve. Its use in reconstruction of the hand and foot has been reported. However, the skin territory provided by the flap is generally limited, the largest reported size being 13 × 9 cm.

If flap width is less than 7 cm, the donor defect can be closed primarily. Cosmetically, the donor site is somewhat hidden, and donor site morbidity is minimal.

Harvesting Technique

(Fig. 1-18) The patient lies on the back, keeping the shoulder upward at a right angle. The flap is designed along the triceps muscle, with the proximal flap edge placed near the angle of the medial head of the triceps and latissimus dorsi. The skin territory can be 13 cm in length and 7 cm in width.

1. Long head of triceps m.
2. Medial head of triceps m.
3. Latissimus dorsi m.
4. Brachial a.
5. Unnamed a.
6. Posterior cutaneous n. of arm.
7. Radial n.
8. Deep brachial a.

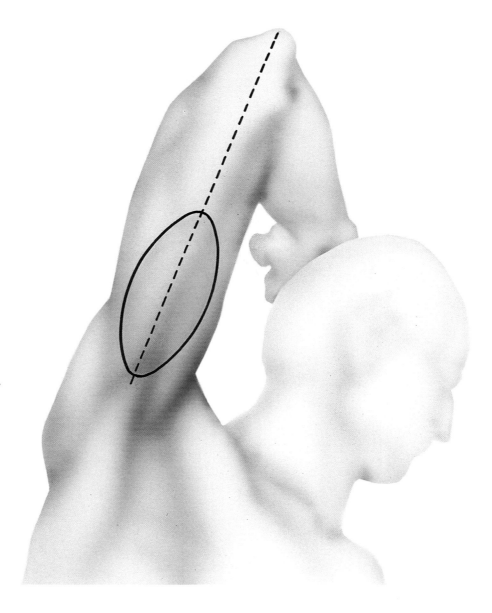

24 ATLAS OF MICROVASCULAR SURGERY

(Fig. 1-19) The flap, including the triceps muscle aponeurosis, is raised starting distally, while flap elevation proceeds proximally. The neurovascular bundle [5,6] becomes visible under the deep fascia.

1. Long head of triceps m.
2. Medial head of triceps m.
5. Unnamed a.
6. Posterior cutaneous n. of arm

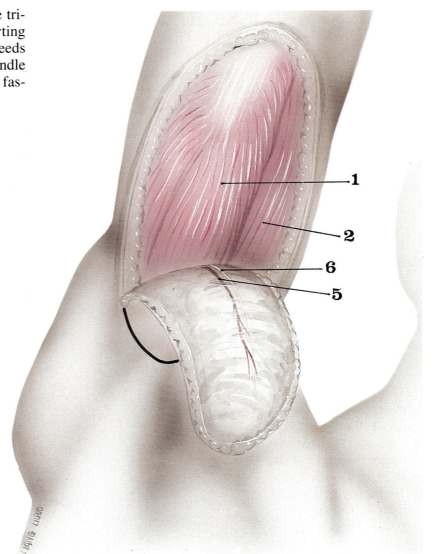

SHOULDER, ARM, AND AXILLA

(**Fig. 1-20**) The proximal edge of the skin flap is carefully incised. Tracing and protecting the neurovascular bundle, the fibrous band at the angle of the triceps [1] and latissimus dorsi [3] is identified and divided, to reach the brachial artery [4]. The neurovascular pedicle is dissected further, ligating the branch to the medial head of the triceps. Pedicle length can reach approximately 6 cm, with a range from 4 to 8 cm.

1. Long head of triceps m.
2. Medial head of triceps m.
3. Latissimus dorsi m.
4. Brachial a.
5. Unnamed a.
6. Posterior cutaneous n. of arm
7. Radial n.
8. Deep brachial a.

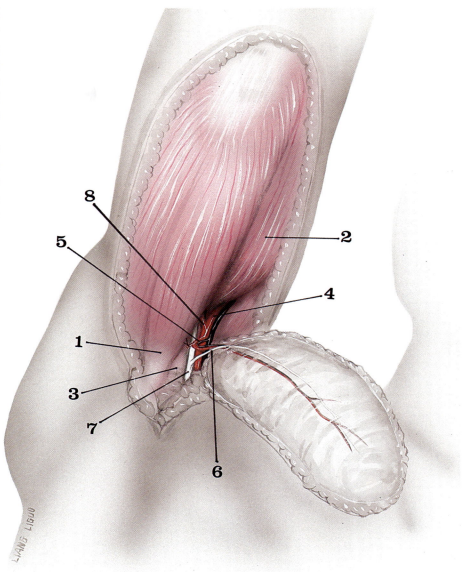

RECIPIENT SITE EXPOSURES

Axillary Artery (Fig. 1-21)

The axillary artery begins at the outer border of the first rib and ends at the lower border of the teres major. The pectoralis minor crosses the vessel and divides it into three parts: proximal, posterior, and distal, to the muscle.

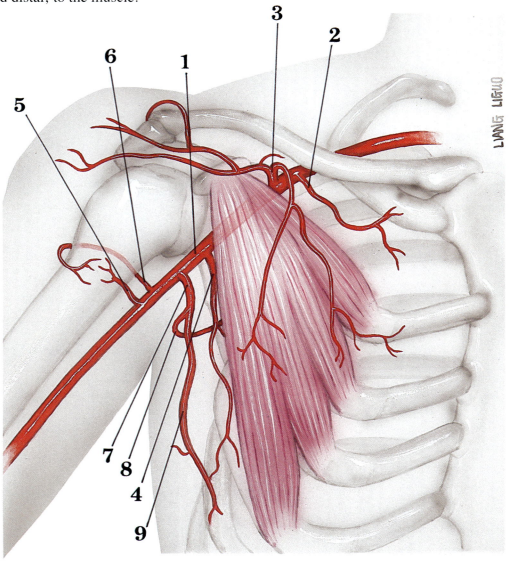

1. Axillary a.
2. Superior thoracic a.
3. Thoracoacromial a.
4. Lateral thoracic a.
5. Anterior circumflex humeral a.
6. Posterior circumflex humeral a.
7. Subscapular a.
8. Circumflex scapular a.
9. Thoracodorsal a.
10. Common circumflex humeral a.

SHOULDER, ARM, AND AXILLA

Variations in Branches from the Axillary Artery **(Fig. 1-22)**

A. Typical branching pattern
B. Common origin of lateral thoracic [4] and thoracoacromial arteries [3]
C. Common origin of the lateral thoracic [4] and subscapular [7] arteries
D. Origin of the posterior circumflex humeral artery [6] from the subscapular artery [7]
E. Common origin of anterior and posterior circumflex humeral arteries [10,5,6]

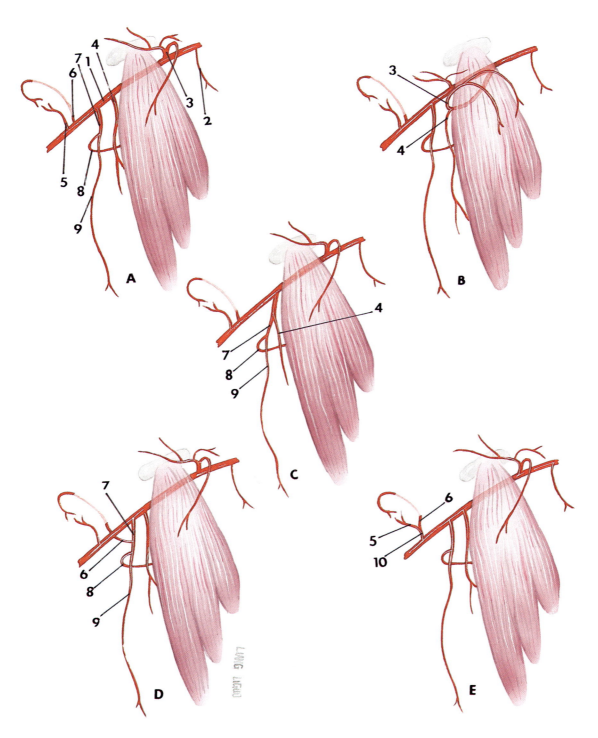

1. Axillary a.
2. Superior thoracic a.
3. Thoracoacromial a.
4. Lateral thoracic a.
5. Anterior circumflex humeral a.
6. Posterior circumflex humeral a.
7. Subscapular a.
8. Circumflex scapular a.
9. Thoracodorsal a.
10. Common circumflex humeral a.

Exposure of the First and Second Parts of the Axillary Artery

(Fig. 1-23) With the arm abducted to a right angle, an incision is made 1.5 cm below and parallel to the clavicle, from the coracoid process to about 3 cm lateral to the sternoclavicular joint.

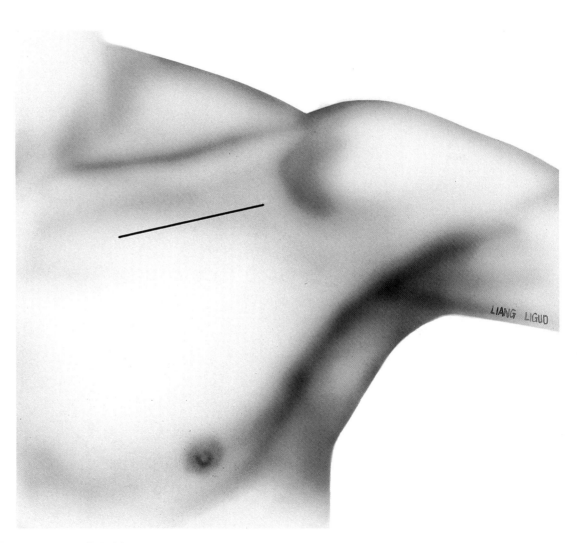

1. Thoracoacromial a.
2. Pectoral a.
3. Deltoid a.
4. Clavicular a.
5. Lateral pectoral n.
6. Cephalic v.
7. Deltoid m.
8. Pectoralis major m.
9. Pectoralis minor m.
10. Clavipectoral fascia
11. Axillary a. and v.
12. Brachial plexus

SHOULDER, ARM, AND AXILLA

(**Fig. 1-24**) After incising the pectoral fascia transversely, the muscle fibers of the clavicular head of the pectoralis major [8] are split to expose the clavipectoral fascia. The pulsation of the axillary artery can be palpated with a finger, medial to the coracoid process and the pectoralis minor, below the middle part of the clavicle.

The lateral pectoral nerve [5] lies in the fascia anteriorly, crossing the axillary artery and vein. It should be dissected and protected. The thoracoacromial artery [1] emerges through the clavipectoral fascia [10] at the medial edge of the pectoralis minor [9]. The cephalic vein [6], accompanied by the deltoid branch [3] of the thoracoacromial artery, crosses the pectoralis minor to enter the infraclavicular fossa.

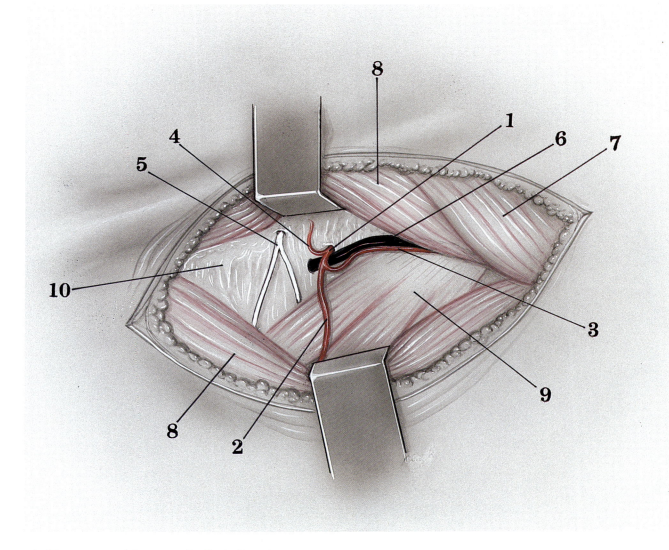

1. Thoracoacromial a.
2. Pectoral a.
3. Deltoid a.
4. Clavicular a.
5. Lateral pectoral n.
6. Cephalic v.
7. Deltoid m.
8. Pectoralis major m.
9. Pectoralis minor m.
10. Clavipectoral fascia

(Fig. 1-25) The thoracoacromial artery [1] is isolated near the edge of the pectoralis minor. Its acromial, clavicular, and deltoid branches are ligated, if a better exposure is required.

The vascular sheath is carefully divided along the pulsation line, to expose the axillary artery [11]. The axillary vein [11] lies below and medial to the artery, and the cephalic vein [6] joins it at the middle of the wound. The brachial plexus [12] is located above the axillary artery. The tendinous attachment of the pectoralis minor [9] can be divided for a further exposure of the second part of the axillary artery.

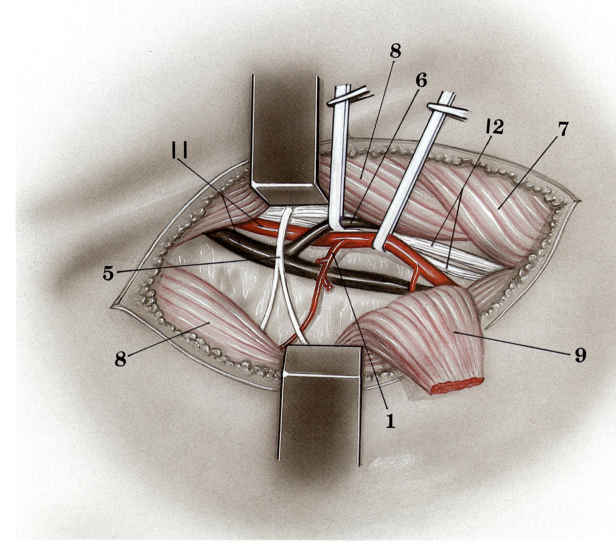

1. Thoracoacromial a.
5. Lateral pectoral n.
6. Cephalic v.
7. Deltoid m.
8. Pectoralis major m.
9. Pectoralis minor m.
11. Axillary a. and v.
12. Brachial plexus

Note. The thoracoacromial artery with a diameter of 2.3 to 4.1 mm usually can be used for end-to-end anastomosis. The cephalic vein is available for venous drainage of a vascularized graft. The axillary artery should be used only for an end-to-side anastomosis.

Exposure of the Second and Third Parts of the Axillary Artery

(Fig. 1-26) The arm is placed in an abducted position, with the palm upward. An incision is made along the medial side of the deltoid muscle and the deltopectoral groove, ending at the midpoint of the clavicle.

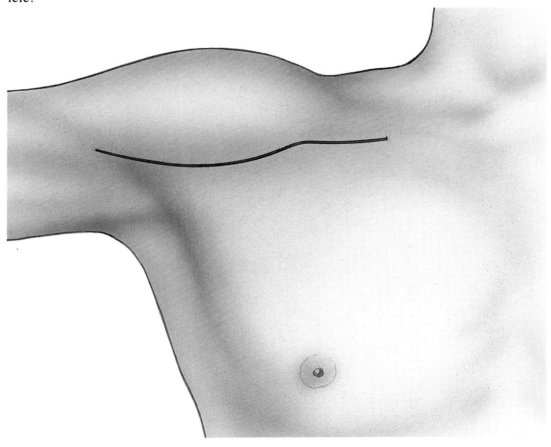

1. Deltoid m.
2. Short head of biceps m.
3. Coracobrachialis m.
4. Pectoralis major m.
5. Pectoralis minor m.
6. Cephalic v.
7. Axillary a.
8. Axillary v.
9. Brachial plexus
10. Subscapular a.
11. Lateral thoracic a.
12. Thoracoacromial a.
13. Anterior and posterior humoral circumflex a.
14. Median n.
15. Musculocutaneous n.
16. Latissimus dorsi m.
17. Subscapularis m.

(Fig. 1-27) The cephalic vein [6] is identified in the deltopectoral groove and retracted superiorly. The pectoralis major [4] is divided near its insertion and reflected inferiorly, to expose the contents of the axilla, the coracoid process, and the insertion of the pectoralis minor [5].

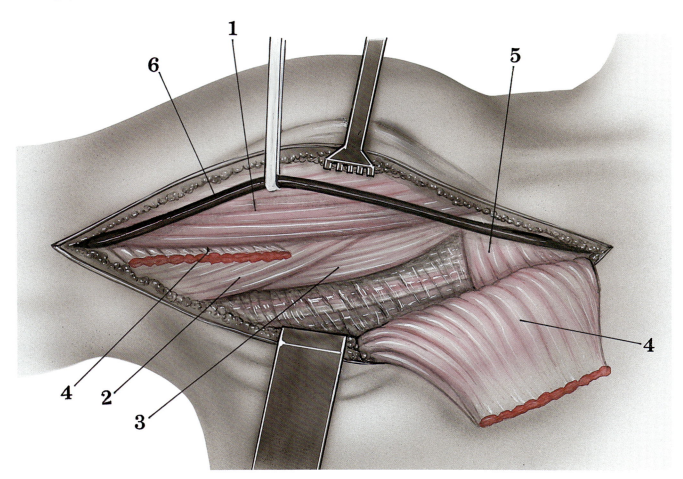

1. Deltoid m.
2. Short head of biceps m.
3. Coracobrachialis m.
4. Pectoralis major m.
5. Pectoralis minor m.
6. Cephalic v.

SHOULDER, ARM, AND AXILLA

(**Fig. 1-28**) Dissection proceeds to identify and protect the brachial plexus [9]. The axillary artery [7] is isolated by incising the vascular sheath along its line of pulsation. The axillary vein [8] is below the artery.

There are several branches arising from this part of the artery. The lateral thoracic artery [11] follows the lateral border of the pectoralis minor; the subscapular artery [10] arises at the lower border of the scapularis [17], running downward; the posterior humeral circumflex artery [13] arises near the takeoff of the subscapular artery, running backward; and the anterior humeral circumflex artery [13] originates from the distal part of the artery, running horizontally.

The tendinous insertion of the pectoralis minor [5] can be divided to get a fuller exposure of the second or even the first part of the artery, if necessary.

The lateral thoracic artery is 1.5 mm in diameter; the subscapular artery is 3 to 4 mm.

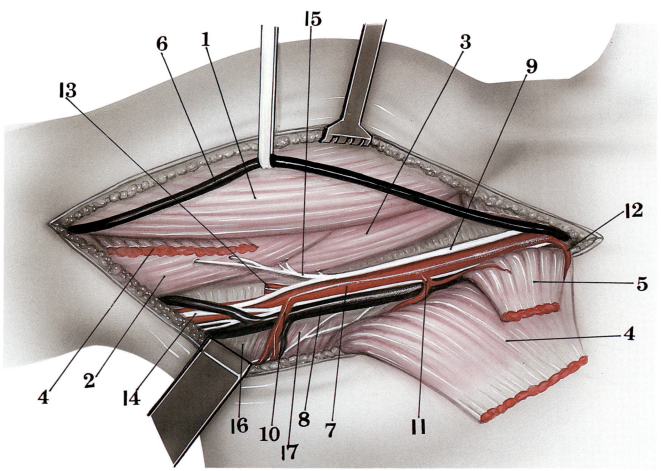

1. Deltoid m.
2. Short head of biceps m.
3. Coracobrachialis m.
4. Pectoralis major m.
5. Pectoralis minor m.
6. Cephalic v.
7. Axillary a.
8. Axillary v.
9. Brachial plexus
10. Subscapular a.
11. Lateral thoracic a.
12. Thoracoacromial a.
13. Anterior and posterior humeral circumflex a.
14. Median n.
15. Musculocutaneous n.
16. Latissimus dorsi m.
17. Subscapularis m.

Brachial Artery

The artery begins at the level of the lower border of the teres major and ends in the cubital fossa at the level of the neck of the radius, by dividing into the radial and ulnar arteries.

Medial Approach to the Proximal Part of the Brachial Artery and Deep Brachial Artery

(Fig. 1-29) The arm is abducted at a right angle in maximal supination. The skin incision begins in the axillary fossa and runs along the lower border of the pectoralis major and the groove between the coracobrachialis and the long head of the triceps.

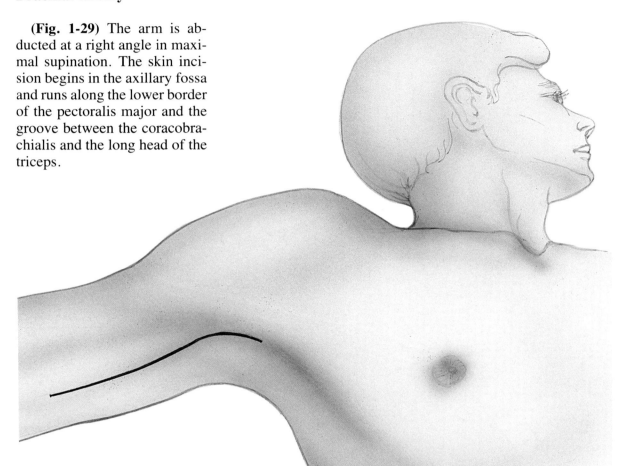

1. Coracobrachialis m.
2. Short head of biceps
3. Pectoralis major m.
4. Triceps m.
5. Teres major m.
6. Latissimus dorsi m.
7. Sheath of brachial a.
8. Brachial a.
9. Brachial v.
10. Deep brachial a.
11. Median n.
12. Ulnar n.
13. Radial n.
14. Musculocutaneous n.

(**Fig. 1-30**) Deepening the incision through the subcutaneous and fascial layers, the coracobrachialis muscle [1] is exposed between the biceps [2] and triceps [4], and the neurovascular bundle can be identified by its pulsation at the lower border of the coracobrachialis.

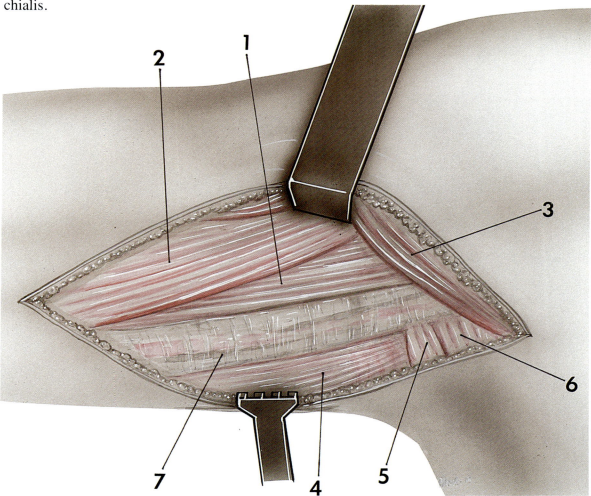

1. Coracobrachialis m.
2. Short head of biceps
3. Pectoralis major m.
4. Triceps m.
5. Teres major m.
6. Latissimus dorsi m.
7. Sheath of brachial a.

(Fig. 1-31) Retracting the coracobrachialis [1], the musculocutaneous nerve, the median nerve [11], and the ulnar nerve [12] are carefully dissected out, in a direction anterior, medial, and posterior to the artery, respectively. The brachial vein [9] courses more superficially in the lower portion of the wound.

Retracting the median nerve anteriorly, the proximal part of the brachial artery [8] is isolated. Just below the lower border of the teres major [5], the deep brachial artery [10] arises from the posterior aspect of the brachial artery, accompanies the radial nerve [13], and runs backward. The deep brachial artery, with a diameter of 2.5 mm, is available for end-to-end anastomosis.

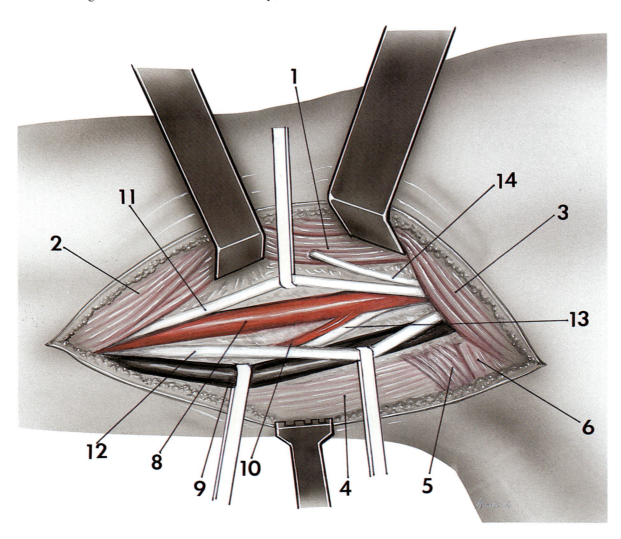

1. Coracobrachialis m.
2. Short head of biceps m.
3. Pectoralis major m.
4. Triceps m.
5. Teres major m.
6. Latissimus dorsi m.
8. Brachial a.
9. Brachial v.
10. Deep brachial a.
11. Median n.
12. Ulnar n.
13. Radial n.
14. Musculocutaneous n.

Exposure of the Middle Part of the Brachial Artery

(Fig. 1-32) An incision is made over the groove between the biceps and the long head of the triceps in the midportion of the arm.

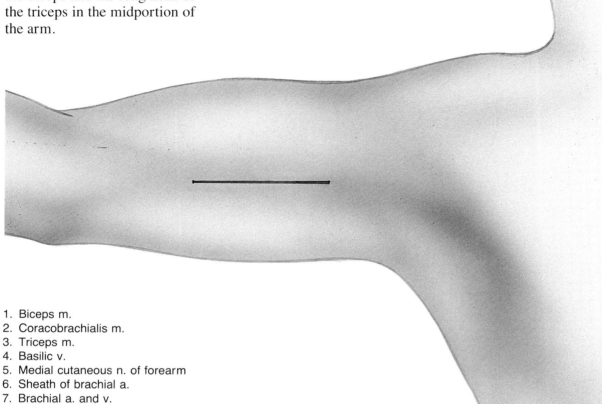

1. Biceps m.
2. Coracobrachialis m.
3. Triceps m.
4. Basilic v.
5. Medial cutaneous n. of forearm
6. Sheath of brachial a.
7. Brachial a. and v.
8. Median n.

(Fig. 1-33) The deep fascia is carefully incised over the groove. The basilic vein [4] usually perforates the deep fascia and joins the brachial vein in this region. The medial cutaneous nerve of the forearm [5] accompanies the basilic vein and lies medial to the brachial artery in the upper half of the arm.

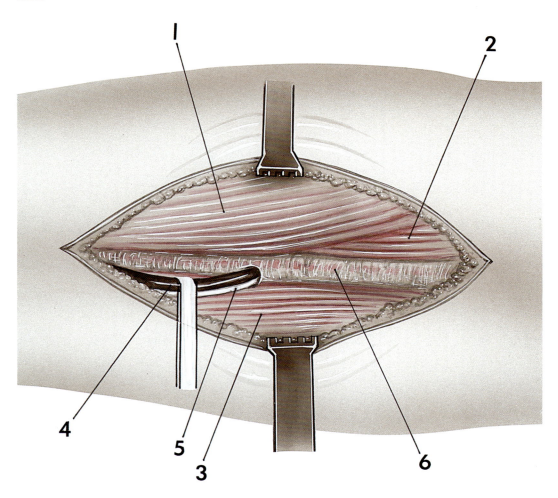

1. Biceps m.
2. Coracobrachialis m.
3. Triceps m.
4. Basilic v.
5. Medial cutaneous n. of forearm
6. Sheath of brachial a.

(Fig. 1-34) The neurovascular sheath is divided. The median nerve [8] crosses the artery from anterior to posterior, and it is retracted anteriorly. Dissection proceeds to isolate the brachial artery [7].

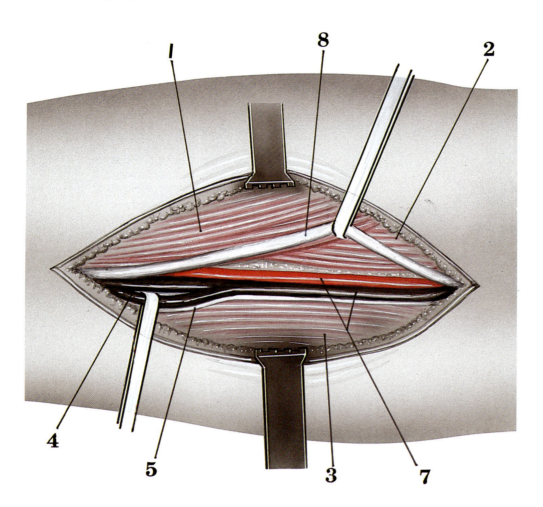

1. Biceps m.
2. Coracobrachialis m.
3. Triceps m.
4. Basilic v.
5. Medial cutaneous n. of forearm
7. Brachial a. and v.
8. Median n.

Posterior Approach to the Deep Brachial Artery and the Proximal Portion of the Brachial Artery

(**Fig. 1-35**) An incision is made on the lateral edge of the long head of the triceps, beginning 5 cm below the acromial angle and running distally to the olecranon for 8 to 10 cm.

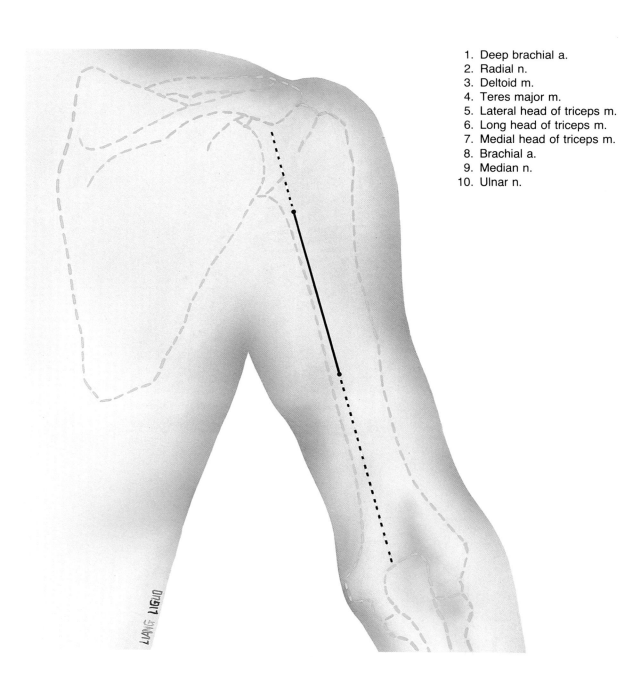

1. Deep brachial a.
2. Radial n.
3. Deltoid m.
4. Teres major m.
5. Lateral head of triceps m.
6. Long head of triceps m.
7. Medial head of triceps m.
8. Brachial a.
9. Median n.
10. Ulnar n.

(**Fig. 1-36**) Dividing the deep fascia below the posterior edge of the deltoid [3], the septum between the long and lateral heads of the triceps [5,6] is identified and entered with blunt dissection, and then developed distally with sharp dissection. At this stage, the deep brachial artery [1] and the radial nerve [2] appear below the teres major [4], running obliquely on the medial head of the triceps [7] from medial to lateral and disappearing between the lateral and medial heads of the triceps [5,7].

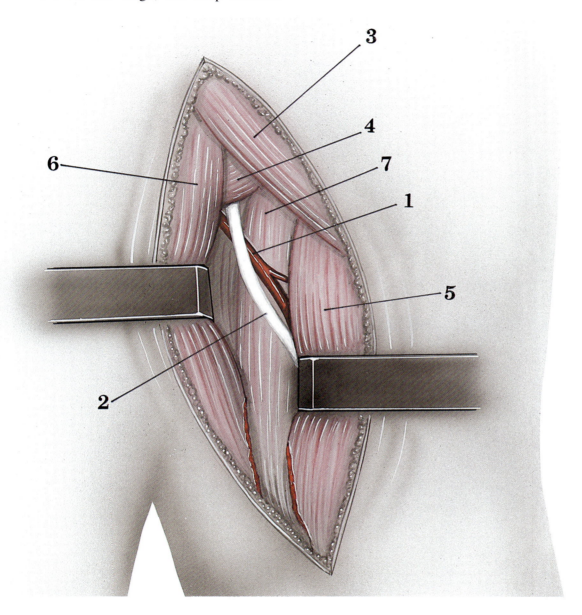

1. Deep brachial a.
2. Radial n.
3. Deltoid m.
4. Teres major m.
5. Lateral head of triceps m.
6. Long head of triceps m.
7. Medial head of triceps m.

(Fig. 1-37) The deep brachial artery [1] and radial nerve [2] are displaced laterally and protected. Retracting the long head of the triceps [6] medially, the medial edge of the medial head of the triceps [7] is identified, and then separated from the long head of the triceps. The brachial artery [8] can be found behind the ulnar nerve [10]. During the procedure, attention should be paid to protect the branch of the radial nerve to the long head, which runs more transversely than its parent trunk.

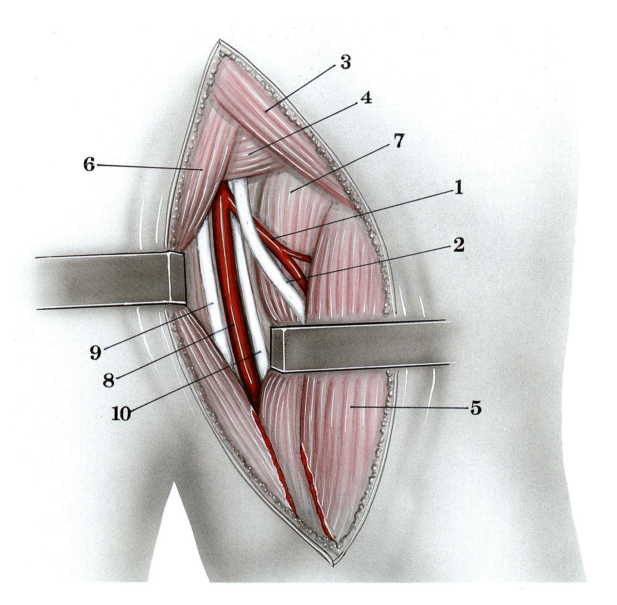

1. Deep brachial a.
2. Radial n.
3. Deltoid m.
4. Teres major m.
5. Lateral head of triceps m.
6. Long head of triceps m.
7. Medial head of triceps m.
8. Brachial a.
9. Median n.
10. Ulnar n.

BIBLIOGRAPHY

Budo J, Finucan T, Clarke J: The inner arm fasciocutaneous flap. Plast Reconstr Surg 73:629, 1984.

Cormack GC, Lamberty BGH: Fasciocutaneous vessels in the upper arm. Application to the design of new fasciocutaneous flaps. Plast Reconstr Surg 74:244, 1984.

Daniel RK, Terzis J, Schwartz G: Neurovascular free flaps. Plast Reconstr Surg 56:13, 1975.

Dolmans S, Guimberteau JC, Baudet J: The upper arm flap. J Microsurg 1:162, 1979.

Franklin JD: The deltoid flap: Anatomy and clinical applications. In: Buncke HJ, Furnas DW (eds): *Symposium on Clinical Frontiers in Reconstructive Microsurgery*, vol. 24. St. Louis: CV Mosby, 1984.

Gao X-S, Mao Z-R, Yang Z-N, Wang B-B: Medial upper arm skin flap: Vascular anatomy and clinical applications. Ann Plast Surg 15:348, 1985.

Iwahira Y, Muruyama Y: Medial arm fasciocutaneous island flap coverage of an electrical burn of the upper extremity. Ann Plast Surg 20:120, 1988.

Kaplan EN, Pearl RM: An arterial medial arm flap—vascular anatomy and clinical applications. Ann Plast Surg 4:205, 1980.

Katsaros J, Schusterman M, Beppu M, Banis JC, Acland RD: The lateral upper arm flap: Anatomy and clinical applications. Ann Plast Surg 12:489, 1984.

Maruyama Y, Onishi K, Iwahira Y: The ulnar recurrent fasciocutaneous island flap: Reverse medial arm flap. Plast Reconstr Surg 79:381, 1987.

Masquelet AC, Rinaldi S, Mouchet A, Gilbert A: The posterior arm free flap. Plast Reconstr Surg 76:908, 1985.

Murray KA, Rebot MT, Singh GB, Russell RC: The deltoid free flap: Anatomical studies and clinical experience. Br J Plast Surg 38:437, 1985.

Newsom HT: Medial arm free flap. Plast Reconstr Surg 67:63, 1981.

Russell RC, Guy RJ, Zook EG, Merrell JC: Extremity reconstruction using the free deltoid flap. Plast Reconstr Surg 76:586, 1985.

Sheker L, Lister G: The lateral arm fasciocutaneous flap. In: Strauch B, Vasconez LO, Hall-Findlay E (eds): *Grabb's Encyclopedia of Flaps*, vol. II. Boston: Little, Brown, 1990, p. 1127.

Shenaq SM, Dinh TA: Total penile and urethral reconstruction with an expanded sensate lateral arm flap: Case report. J Reconstr Microsurg 5:245, 1989.

Song R, Song Y, Yu Y, Song Y: The upper arm free flap. Clin Plast Surg 9:27, 1982.

Taylor GI, Daniel RK: The anatomy of several free flap donor sites. Plast Reconstr Surg 56:243, 1975.

2 FOREARM REGION

Forearm Flaps

Anatomy of the Radial Artery [1]
(Fig. 2-1)

After passing under the bicipital aponeurosis [11], the brachial artery divides into radial and ulnar arteries [1,2] about 1 cm below the bend of the elbow. The radial artery [1] passes deeply between the brachioradialis [6] and pronator teres [7] muscles in the upper third of its course, and between the tendons of the brachioradialis and flexor carpi radialis [8] in the lower two thirds of its course. Growing gradually superficial, it is covered only by skin and fascia at the wrist. It then winds backward, around the lateral side of the carpus, beneath the tendons of the abductor pollicis longus and extensor pollicis brevis. Passing through the "snuff box" and the interspace between the first and second metacarpal bones, it forms the deep palmar arch by uniting with the deep branch of the ulnar artery.

Beside the radial recurrent artery [4] branching near its origin and the superficial palmar branch arising just above the wrist, the radial artery gives off 9 to 17 fasciocutaneous branches. In the proximal half of its course that is covered by the brachioradialis muscle, there are 4.2 branches on average (range, 0 to 10), and in the distal half that is directly under the skin and fascia, there are 9.6 branches on average (range, 4 to 14). All these branches, with an average diameter of 0.5 mm (range, 0.1 to 1.1 mm), form a rich vascular network in the subcutaneous layer, with fasciocutaneous branches from the ulnar, interosseous, and brachial arteries.

The most proximal branch sometimes arises from the recurrent radial artery. It has a diameter of 0.5 to 1.0 mm and is named the inferior cubital artery. It emerges from the septum between the brachioradialis and pronator teres, and about 4 cm below the bend of the elbow, where the cephalic vein gives off the median cubital vein and the deep cummunicating branch with the venae comitantes of the radial artery. It then runs distally and laterally along the radial side of the forearm in the subcutaneous layer. A constant branch arises from the artery about 7 cm above the wrist joint.

Generally, all of the forearm skin can be adequately supplied by the fasciocutaneous branches of the distal part of the radial artery.

Anatomy of the Ulnar Artery [2]

Beginning at the same point as the radial artery [1], the ulnar artery [2] passes distally and medially across and under the pronator teres [7], the median nerve, the flexor carpi radialis [8], and the flexor digitorum superficialis [10]. It reaches the medial side of the forearm at about midway between the elbow and the wrist. It then runs between the flexor carpi ulnaris [12] and the flexor digitorum superficialis [10] muscles or tendons. The ulnar nerve is adjacent and medial to the lower two thirds of the artery.

At the wrist, the ulnar artery crosses the flexor retinaculum lateral to the pisiform bone, and ends by dividing into the deep palmar branch and the superficial palmar branch.

Shortly after its origin, the artery immediately gives off the anterior and posterior ulnar recurrent arteries and the common interosseous artery [5]. Distal to the common interosseous artery, the ulnar artery gives off three to five fasciocutaneous branches between the flexor carpi ulnaris [12] and the flexor digitorum superficialis [10] that join the rich subcutaneous vascular network already described. The largest and most constant among these branches is that situated about 4 cm distal to the common interosseous artery [5].

Variations

On occasion, the radial and ulnar arteries originate higher than usual from the brachial artery in the arm, even occasionally from the axillary artery. When they arise higher, they are usually superficial to the flexor muscle, deep or superficial to the deep fascia. At the wrist, the radial artery turns around it, superficial to the extensor tendons of the thumb.

Rarely, the brachial artery divides into these two arteries at the middle portion of the forearm.

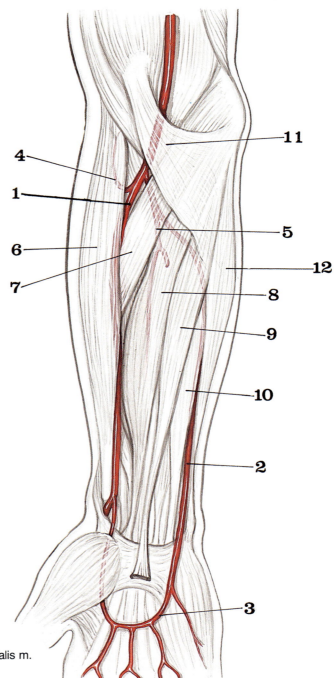

1. Radial a.
2. Ulnar a.
3. Superficial palmar arch
4. Recurrent radial a.
5. Common interosseous a.
6. Brachioradialis m.
7. Pronator teres m.
8. Flexor carpi radialis m.
9. Palmaris longus m.
10. Flexor digitorum superficialis m.
11. Bicipital aponeurosis
12. Flexor carpi ulnaris

Venous Drainage (Fig. 2-2)

Both the superficial and deep systems are equally capable of draining the forearm flap. In the superficial system, the cephalic vein [1] from the dorsal venous network ascends around the radial border of the forearm to its anterior surface, receiving tributaries from both surfaces. Below the front of the elbow, it gives off the median cubital vein [3], which receives a communicating branch from the deep vein, and passes medially to join the basilic vein [2]. Then, the cephalic vein ascends to the anterolateral aspect of the arm, superficial to the groove between the brachioradialis and the biceps at the elbow.

The basilic vein [2], receiving the dorsal venous network of the hand, ascends for about two thirds of its extent along the posterior ulnar border of the forearm. It then inclines forward to the medial bicipital groove.

The median vein of the forearm [4], draining

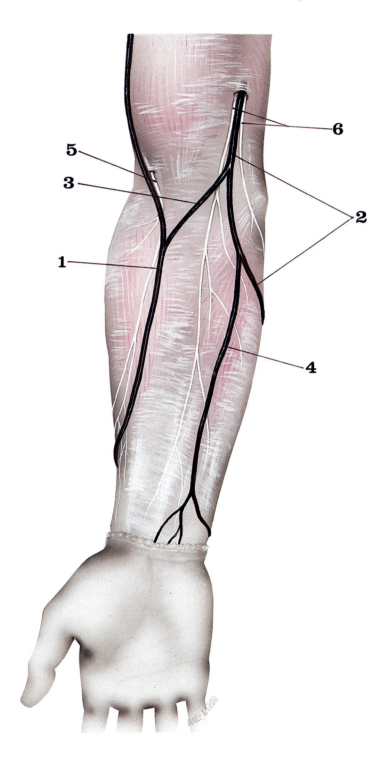

1. Cephalic v.
2. Basilic v.
3. Median cubital v.
4. Median V. of forearm
5. Lateral cutaneous n. of forearm
6. Medial cutaneous n. of forearm

the palmar venous plexus, ascends on the front of the forearm and ends in the basilic or median cubital vein.

Innervation

The lateral cutaneous nerve of the forearm [5] is a continuation of the musculocutaneous nerve. It passes deep to the cephalic vein [1] at the elbow and then descends along the radial border of the forearm to the wrist. It supplies the skin over the lateral half of the anterior surface of the forearm. The medial cutaneous nerve of the forearm [6] pierces the deep fascia with the basilic vein at about the middle of the arm and divides into anterior and posterior branches. The anterior branch descends anterior to the basilic vein at the elbow and supplies the skin over the medial half of the anterior surface of the forearm. The posterior branch lies anterior to the medial epicondyle of the humerus and supplies the skin over the medial third of the posterior surface of the forearm.

Measurements

		Diameter (mm)
Radial	Artery	2.5
	Vein	1.3
Ulnar	Artery	2.5
	Vein	2.3
Cephalic	Vein	2.8
Basilic	Vein	2.6

Retrograde Deep Venous System (Fig. 2-3)

The radial or ulnar artery is accompanied by a pair of venae comitantes. Even though some valves do exist in these deep veins (average: 3.6 valves for each), reverse forearm flaps are widely and successfully reported for reconstructions of the hand. In this type of flap, a retrograde venous drainage is accomplished by a "crossover" pattern through several communicating branches [2] between the two venae comitantes [1], and by a "bypass" pattern through the collateral branches.
   A. Antegrade venous flow
   B. Retrograde venous flow

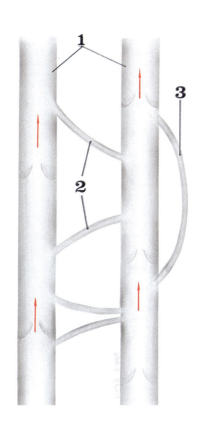
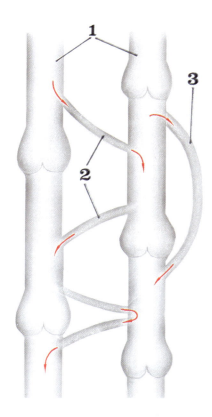

1. Venae comitantes
2. Communicating branch
3. Collateral branch

        A   B

COMMENT AND INSIGHTS

A number of fasciocutaneous branches constantly arise from the radial and ulnar arteries through the intermuscular septa to form a very rich vascular network in the subcutaneous and deep fascial layers of the forearm. Therefore the forearm flap based on the radial vessels is remarkably hardy and robust. Also, it is able to provide a large territory, including almost all the forearm skin and the lower third of the arm, on which the shape, size, and location of the flap can be designed very freely.

The quite superficial and constant anatomy of the radial artery and its large caliber and long vascular pedicle facilitate easy harvesting, dissection, and microsurgical transfer of the flap. This donor site provides thin and pliable skin, with fine texture and scanty subcutaneous tissue. However, the lateral forearm skin is relatively hairy, especially in white males.

This flap can be combined with a segment of the radius bone, the brachioradialis, flexor carpi radialis, and palmaris longus muscles or tendons, and the superficial branch of the radial nerve. Medial and lateral cutaneous nerves of the forearm provide sensibility for the skin flap.

Since it has the excellent properties described herein, the radial forearm flap is very versatile and widely applied in reconstructive microsurgery: (1) for facial reconstruction involving soft tissue defects, with or without mandibular bone loss; (2) in intraoral reconstruction for oral lining in mucosal defects, with or without mandibular bone loss; (3) for repair of defects in the lower limb, especially because the sensory forearm flap may be suitable for resurfacing weight-bearing areas; (4) for penile reconstruction with a fabricated sensory forearm flap; and (5) for reconstructing pharyngoesophageal defects, using a tubed forearm flap.

The radial artery of the flap can be anastomosed at both ends as an artery graft to save an acutely ischemic extremity that has resulted from a segmental defect of its main artery, with wide loss of soft tissue.

The osteocutaneous flap provides a limited segment of cortex bone of radius, useful in reconstruction of nonweight-bearing areas, such as in mandibular defects. The flap can also be a tendinocutaneous one. The reversed island flap is very useful in hand surgery to reconstruct soft tissue, tendon, or bone defects; also, a thumb can be reconstructed with a fabricated reversed osteocutaneous flap. If cosmesis of the forearm is very important, a purely fascial flap can be used to cover a wound; this requires the use of a split-thickness skin graft to cover the fascial flap.

The donor defect is usually covered with a split-thickness skin graft, except in cases of narrow flaps or purely fascial flaps. Results may include some cosmetic problems, especially if the defect is on the lateral aspect of the forearm. Medial deviations in flap design may obviate this problem to some extent and provide a less hairy flap.

It is not mandatory to repair the radial artery when the hand has good circulation after flap harvesting. However, in order to prevent postoperative fracture of the radius when creating an osteocutaneous flap, taking the bone with the flap should not include more than 40% of the cross-section, and the arm should be immobilized in an above-elbow plaster cast for at least 3 weeks.

Compared with the radial forearm flap, the ulnar forearm flap possesses similar properties. However the ulnar forearm flap and its axis are located on the medial aspect of the forearm; therefore it may produce better cosmetic results and avoid a hairy flap. However, the proximal arterial pedicle is limited distal to the takeoff of the common interosseous artery, and fewer case reports would seem to require further clinical experience before freely recommending this flap. Nonetheless, the ulnar forearm flap might be a real alternative to the radial forearm flap.

RADIAL FOREARM FLAP

(Fig. 2-4) The territory of this flap may be extended from the lower third of the anterior aspect of the arm proximally to the wrist flexion crease distally. Distal width is from the extensor hallucis longus tendon radially to the extensor carpi ulnaris tendon ulnarly. Proximal width is from the lateral to medial humeral epicondyles.

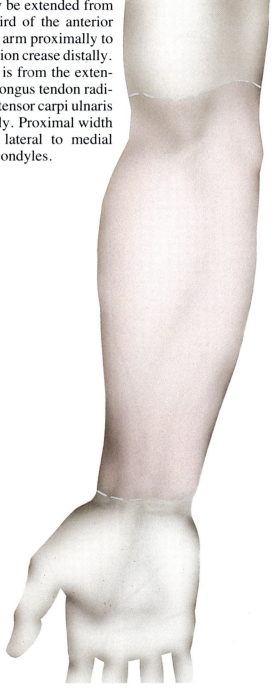
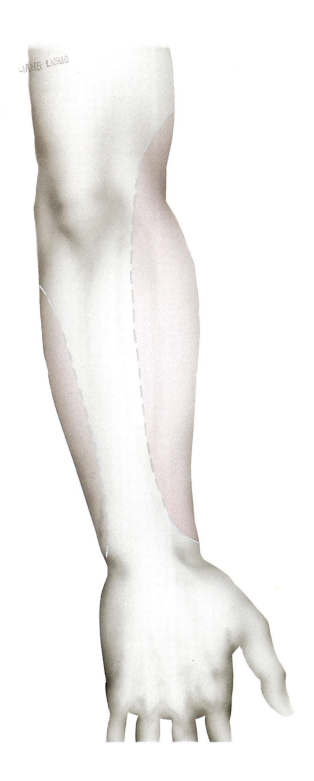

1. Radial a. and its venae comitantes
2. Brachioradialis m.
3. Cephalic v.
4. Flexor carpi radialis m.
5. Flexor digitorum superficialis m.
6. Palmaris longus m.
7. Flexor carpi ulnaris m.
8. Basilic v.
9. Medial cutaneous n. of forearm
10. Median v. of forearm
11. Median cubital v.
12. Superficial branch of radial n.
13. Pronator quadratus m.
14. Lateral cutaneous n. of forearm
15. Supinator m.
16. Pronator teres m.
17. Median n.
18. Flexor pollicis longus m.

Flap Design (Fig. 2-5)

A line is drawn from a point 1 cm below the center of the antecubital fossa to the tubercle of the scaphoid, corresponding to the surface anatomy of the radial artery and the anterolateral intermuscular septum. The radial forearm flap is usually designed along this line as an axis, although the flap can be somewhat deviated medially for hairless skin. Along the axis, any part—distal, middle, or proximal—can be used for the flap, depending on requirements at the recipient site.

Preoperatively, it is imperative that the patency of the ulnar artery be confirmed with an Allen's test, by ultrasonic Doppler flowmeter testing, or arteriography.

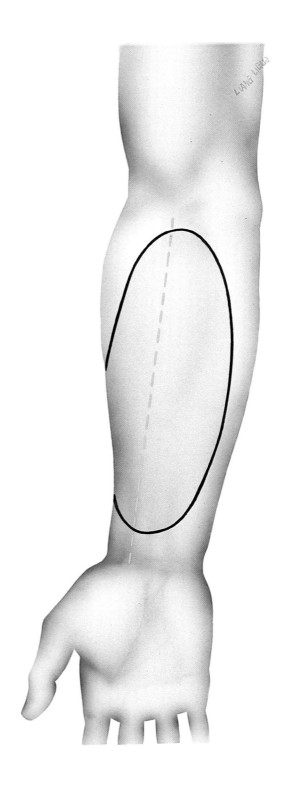

(**Fig. 2-6**) A pneumatic tourniquet is applied only with elevation exsanguination.

At the distal border of the flap, the radial vascular bundle [1] is identified at the lateral edge of the flexor carpi radialis tendon [4] and dissected out. The cephalic vein [3] is isolated on the distal lateral edge of the flap and ligated.

1. Radial a. and its venae comitantes
2. Brachioradialis m.
3. Cephalic v.
4. Flexor carpi radialis m.
5. Flexor digitorum superficialis m.
6. Palmaris longus m.
7. Flexor carpi ulnaris m.
17. Median n.

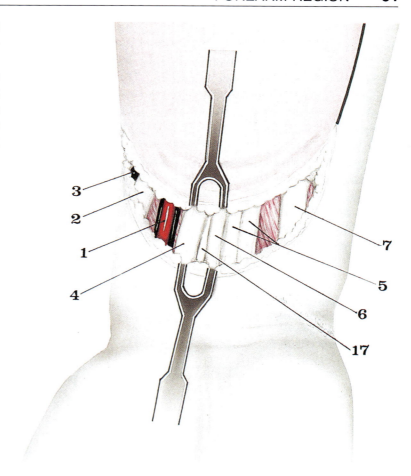

(**Fig. 2-7**) The distal ulnar portion of the flap, including the deep fascia, is elevated from the flexor muscles and tendons, toward the lateral edge of the flexor carpi radialis [4]. This procedure is usually carried out gradually from distal to proximal, tracing the exposed radial vascular bundle. Although the palmaris longus [6] is not required in the flap, the deep fascia that encircles it should be divided, preserving the palmaris longus on the forearm. Special attention should be paid to preserve paratenons on all the tendons, and not to damage the fasciocutaneous branches emerging from the intermuscular septum.

4. Flexor carpi radialis m.
5. Flexor digitorum superficialis m.
6. Palmaris longus m.
7. Flexor carpi ulnaris m.

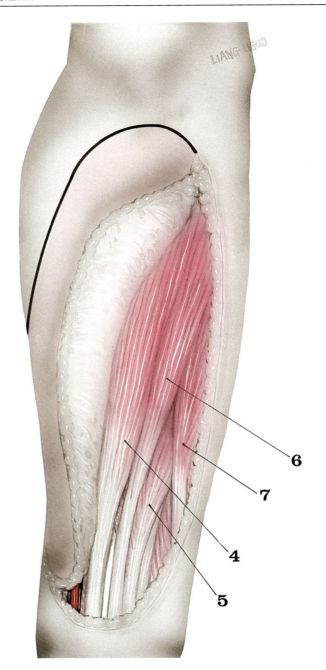

(**Fig. 2-8**) At the proximal medial border of the flap, the basilic vein [8] is dissected out, and the medial cutaneous nerve of the forearm [9] can be identified near the vein; it may be included with the flap, if a sensory flap is required.

8. Basilic v.
9. Median cutaneous n. of forearm
10. Median v. of forearm
11. Median cubital v.
16. Pronator teres m.

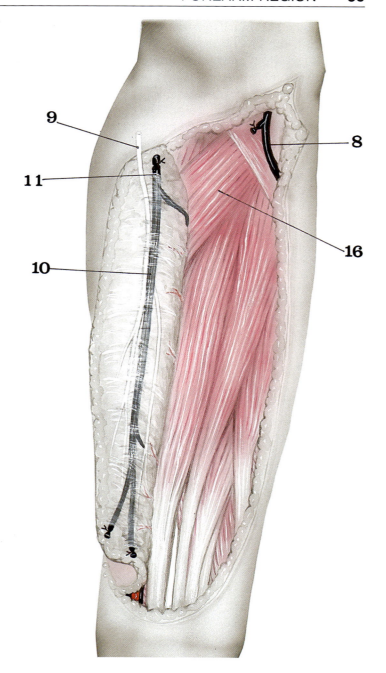

54 ATLAS OF MICROVASCULAR SURGERY

(Fig. 2-9) The radial portion of the flap is raised from the brachioradialis [2] toward its medial edge. Retracting the muscle laterally, the radial vascular bundle [1] connecting with the flap is dissected from its base up to its takeoff from the brachial artery. The fasciocutaneous perforators arising from the radial artery are visualized. During the dissection, the superficial branch of the radial nerve [12] should be identified and preserved.

1. Radial a. and its venae comitantes
2. Brachioradialis m.
3. Cephalic v.
12. Superficial branch of radial n.
13. Pronator quadratus m.
18. Flexor pollicis longus m.

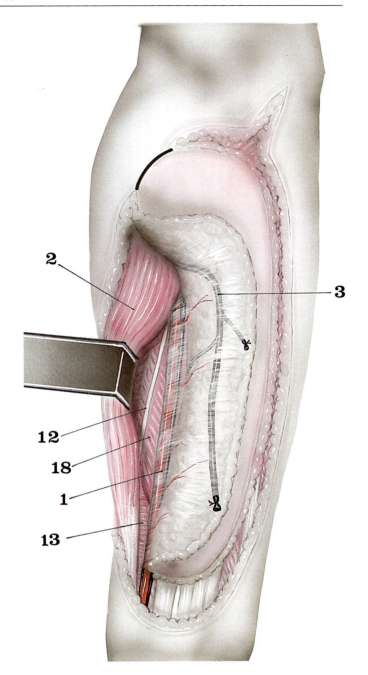

(Fig. 2-10) At the proximal lateral edge of the flap, the cephalic vein [3] is isolated, and the lateral cutaneous nerve of the forearm [14] is identified near the vein over the groove between the brachioradialis [2] and biceps muscles. Generally, the cephalic vein [3] is selected for venous drainage of the flap. The proximal length of the cephalic vein [3] can be dissected to be as long as required. The basilic vein is preserved for the donor site, if possible.

Both ends of the radial artery can be selected as a pedicle for microvascular anastomosis. Before cutting the radial artery at either end, the circulation of the hand should be carefully assessed after releasing the tourniquet and clamping the artery at its distal end.

2. Brachioradialis m.
3. Cephalic v.
14. Lateral cutaneous n. of forearm
15. Supinator m.

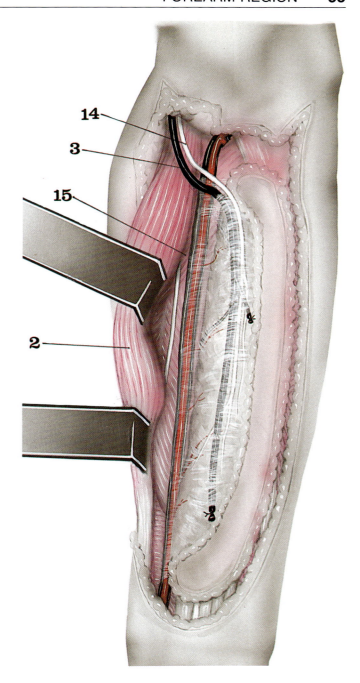

(Fig. 2-11) The radial forearm flap with an antegrade blood flow is ready for transfer, after the distal end of the radial vascular bundle [1] is divided and ligated.

1. Radial a. and its venae comitantes
3. Cephalic v.
9. Medial cutaneous n. of forearm
11. Median cubital v.
14. Lateral cutaneous n. of forearm

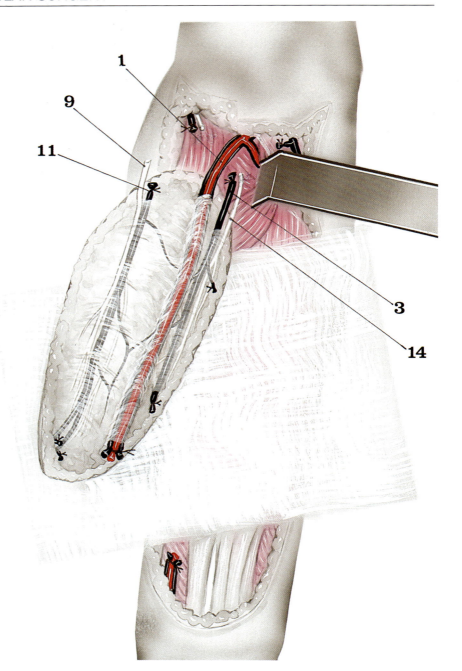

RADIAL FOREARM FLAP FOR PENILE RECONSTRUCTION

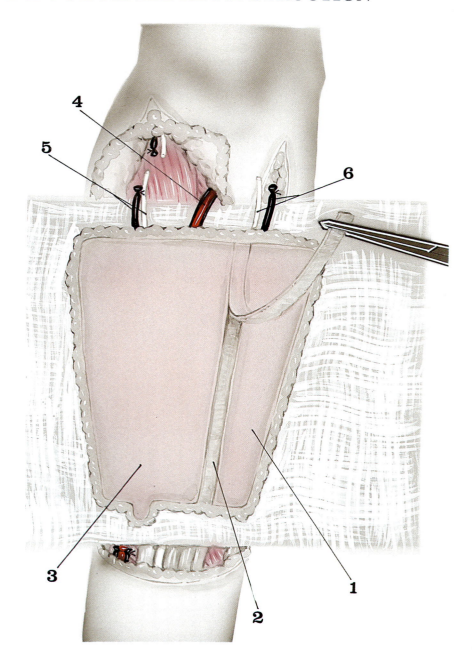

(Fig. 2-12) A radial forearm flap with a width of about 13 cm and a length of about 12 cm is raised with its sensory nerves. The outer surface of the flap is divided into areas A [1], B [2], and C [3]. Area A [1] is to be the inner surface of the urethra, 2.0 to 3.0 cm in width. Area B [2] is 0.5 to 1.0 cm in width and is deepithelialized. Area C [3] is to be the outer surface of the penis and is 8 to 10 cm in width. A small skin tongue flap is designed on the middle of its distal edge to form the orifice of the urethra.

1. Area A
2. Area B
3. Area C
4. Radial a. and v.
5. Cephalic v. and lateral cutaneous n. of forearm
6. Basilic v. and medial cutaneous n. of forearm

(Fig. 2-13) Area A [1] is sutured to roll around a catheter with its skin surface inside.

1. Area A
2. Area B
3. Area C
4. Radial a. and v.
5. Cephalic v. and lateral cutaneous n. of forearm
6. Basilic v. and medial cutaneous n. of forearm

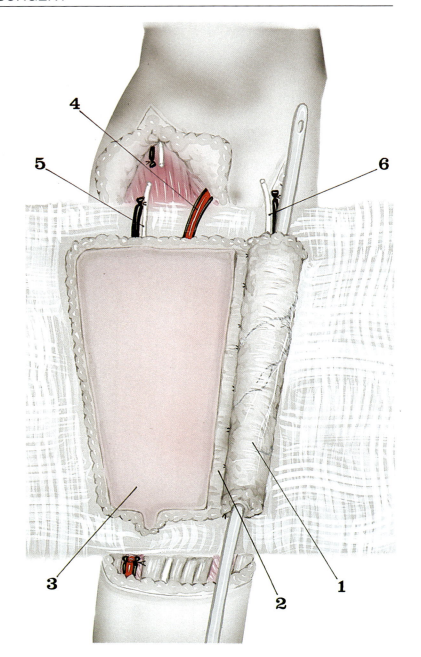

(Fig. 2-14) Area C [3] is overwrapped around with its skin surface outside. The distal edges of areas A and C are sutured to each other to create the orifice of the urethra.

1. Area A
3. Area C
4. Radial a. and v.
5. Cephalic v. and lateral cutaneous n. of forearm
6. Basilic v. and medial cutaneous n. of forearm

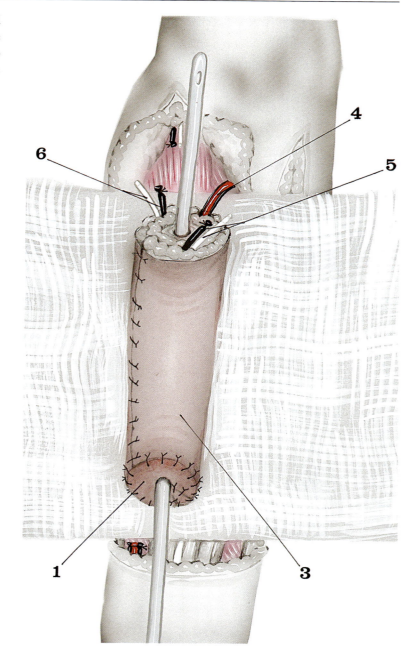

(Fig. 2-15) A constructed penis is illustrated in cross-section.

1. Area A
2. Area B
3. Area C
4. Radial a. and v.
5. Cephalic v. and lateral cutaneous n. of forearm
6. Basilic v. and medial cutaneous n. of forearm

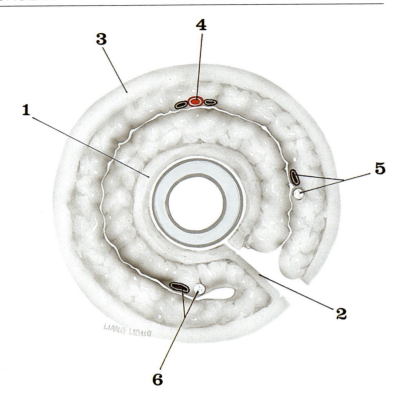

REVERSED RADIAL FOREARM ISLAND FLAP

Flap Design (Fig. 2-16)

A point of pulsation of the radial artery [2] at the wrist is chosen as a rotation axis. The pedicle length of the reversed flap [3] should be equal to or 1 cm more than the distance between the defect [1] on the hand and this axial point. Flap elevation is similar to the procedure described previously.

1. Wound defect debrided
2. Rotation axis
3. Skin flap
4. Radial a. and v.

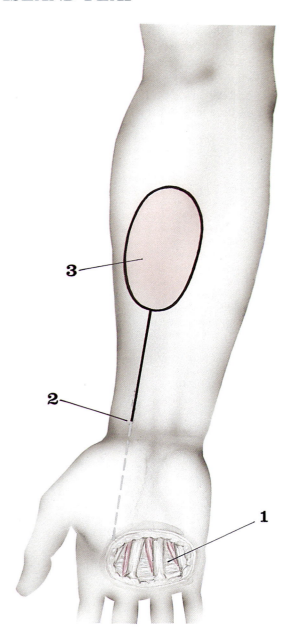

Note: This type of flap is widely applied in hand reconstructions. The retrograde arterial blood flow comes from the ulnar artery through the deep palmar arch, while the venae comitantes are responsible for venous drainage in a retrograde direction. At the outset, engorgement of the veins with progressive swelling of the flap occurs after ligating the proximal vascular pedicle; however, venous drainage will improve in a few days through the communicating and collateral branches described before.

(**Fig. 2-17**) The proximal radial vascular bundle is divided and ligated distal to the bifurcation of the brachial artery. Its distal pedicle [4] can be further dissected to the wrist, sometimes even to the snuff box, passing the flap with its pedicle underneath the abductor pollicis longus and extensor pollicis brevis, to obtain a longer pedicle length for transfer to the hand.

1. Wound defect debrided
4. Radial a. and n.

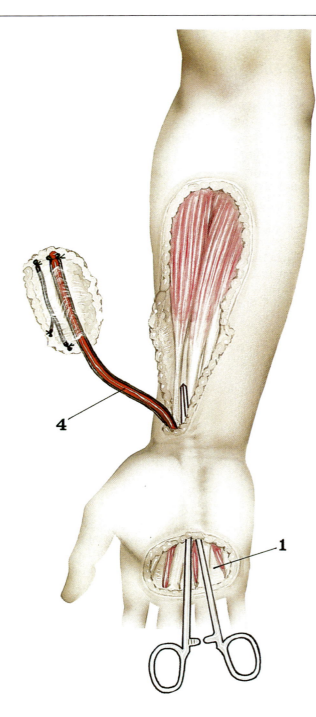

RADIAL FOREARM OSTEOCUTANEOUS FLAP

(Fig. 2-18) An anterolateral segment of the radial bone that lies between the insertions of the pronator teres [1] and the brachioradialis [2] can be included in a radial forearm flap. A length of up to 10 cm and 40% of the cross-section of the radius may be safely removed. The radius must be splinted with an above-elbow cast for 3 to 4 weeks, since fractures have been reported.

The segment of the radius is nourished by two fascioperiosteal branches through the intermuscular septum and musculoperiosteal branches, through the flexor pollicis longus and pronator quadratus from the radial artery.

1. Pronator m. or its insertion
2. Brachioradialis m. or its insertion
3. Superficial branch of radial n.
4. Periosteum and intermuscular septum
5. Radius bone
6. Radial a. and v.
7. Flexor pollicis longus m.
8. Pronator quadratum m.
9. Cephalic v. and lateral cutaneous n. of forearm

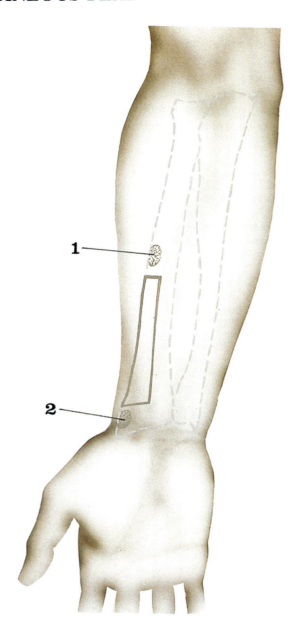

(Fig. 2-19) The flap is raised from both the radial and ulnar sides, as already described, until the anterolateral intermuscular septum [4] containing the radial vessels is reached. Laterally retracting the brachioradialis [2], the superficial branch of the radial nerve [3] is protected, and the periosteum [4] is incised longitudinally beyond the attachment of the septum to the radius bone [5].

2. Brachioradialis m. or its insertion
3. Superficial branch of radial n.
4. Periosteum and intermuscular septum
5. Radius bone
6. Radial a. and v.
9. Cephalic v. and lateral cutaneous n. of forearm

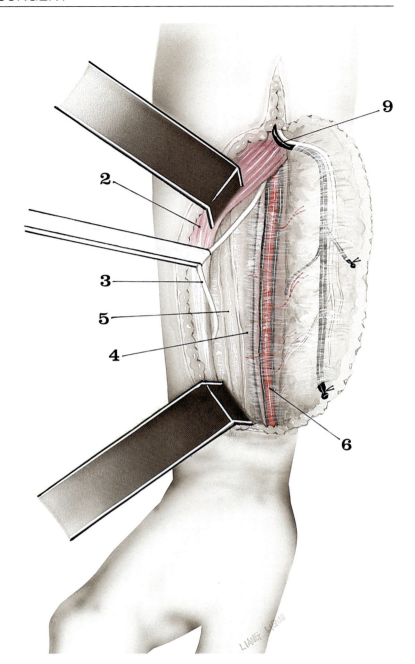

(**Fig. 2-20**) Medially retracting the flexor carpi radialis, the muscle bellies of the flexor pollicis longus [7] and pronator quadratus [8] are divided and elevated, to reach the periosteum of the radius [5] and to incise it.

1. Pronator m. or its insertion
5. Radius bone
7. Flexor pollicis longus m.
8. Pronator quadratum m.

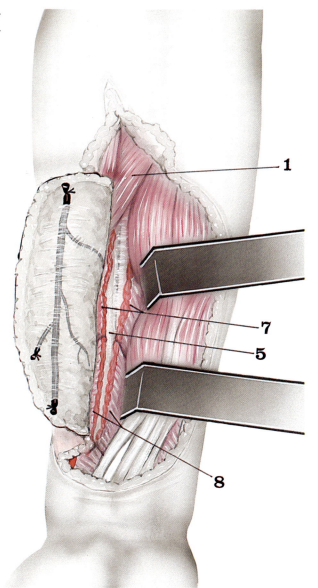

(Fig. 2-21) The radius bone segment [5] is divided with a Gigli saw, and the osteocutaneous flap is elevated, with attention paid to preserve the intermuscular septum with the flap and an intact segment of the radius.

5. Radius bone
6. Radial a. and v.
9. Cephalic v. and lateral cutaneous n. of forearm

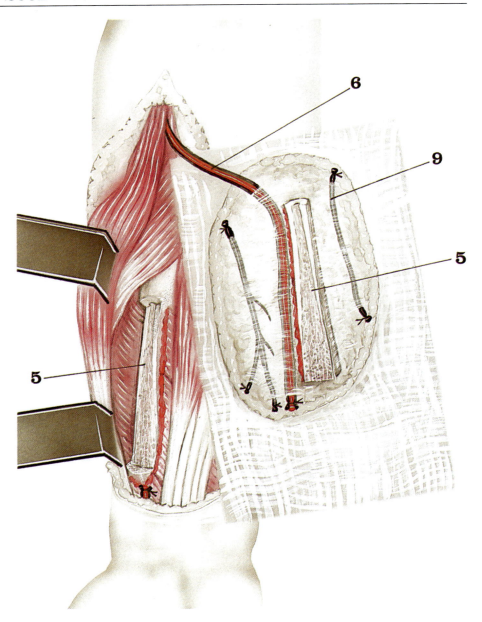

RADIAL FOREARM TENDINOCUTANEOUS FLAP

(**Fig. 2-22**) The brachioradialis [1], flexor carpi radialis [3], and palmaris longus [2] tendons are available, singly or in combination, for a vascularized transfer with the forearm flap. These tendons are nourished by a series of small transverse branches from the radial artery communicating with the subfascial plexus.

1. Brachioradialis m.
2. Palmaris longus m.
3. Flexor carpi radialis m.
4. Radial a. and v.
5. Median n.
6. Pronator teres m.
7. Cephalic v.
8. Flexor pollicis longus m.
9. Pronator quadratus m.

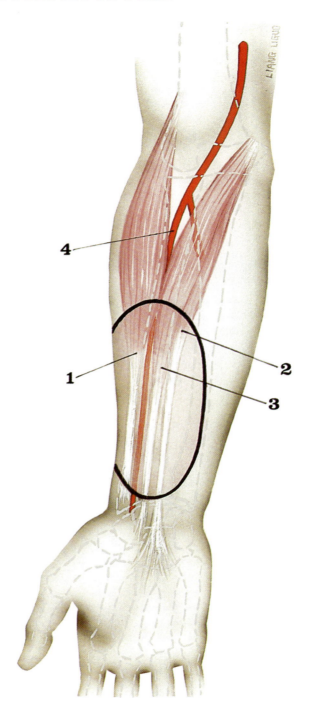

68 ATLAS OF MICROVASCULAR SURGERY

(**Fig. 2-23**) The radial forearm flap, with the brachioradialis [1], flexor carpi radialis [3], and palmari longus [2] tendons, is shown elevated, with the dissection underneath these tendons keeping them intact with the flap.

1. Brachioradialis m.
2. Palmaris longus m.
3. Flexor carpi radialis m.
4. Radial a. and v.
5. Median n.
6. Pronator teres m.
7. Cephalic v.
8. Flexor pollicis longus m.
9. Pronator quadratus m.

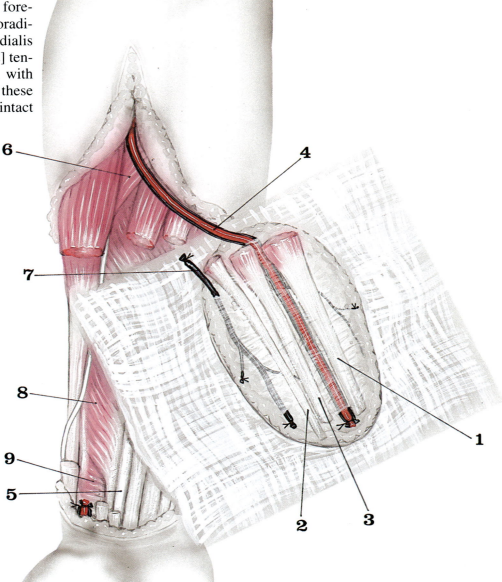

ULNAR FOREARM FLAP

(Fig. 2-24) A line is drawn from the medial epicondyle of the humerus to the lateral edge of the pisiform bone. The surface anatomy of the ulnar artery commences at a point 1 cm below the center of the antecubital fossa via the junction of the upper and middle thirds of the line, running distally along the line. The upper third of the artery runs deep to the pronator teres, the flexor carpi radialis, the palmaris longus, and the flexor digitorum superficialis. The flap is therefore outlined on the medial aspect of the forearm along the middle and lower thirds of the surface line of the ulnar artery, used as an axis for the flap.

1. Basilic v. and medial cutaneous n. of forearm
2. Ulnar a., v., and n.
3. Flexor carpi ulnaris m.
4. Flexor digitorum superficialis m.
5. Common interosseous a.
6. Flexor digitorum profunda m.
7. Median n.

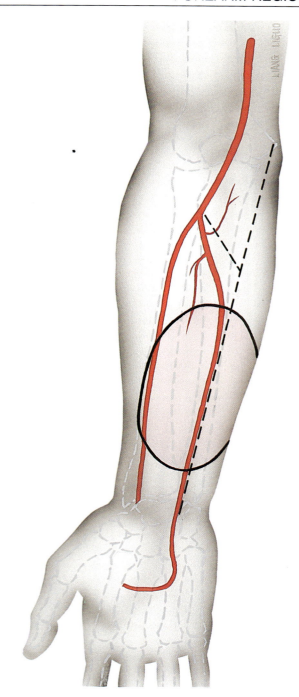

(**Fig. 2-25**) Distally, the ulnar vascular bundle [2] is dissected out and separated from the ulnar nerve in the anterior medial intermuscular septum between the flexor carpi ulnaris and flexor digitorum superficialis tendons. Proximally, the basilic vein and the medial cutaneous nerve of the forearm [1] are isolated.

1. Basilic v. and medial cutaneous n. of forearm
2. Ulnar a., v., and n.

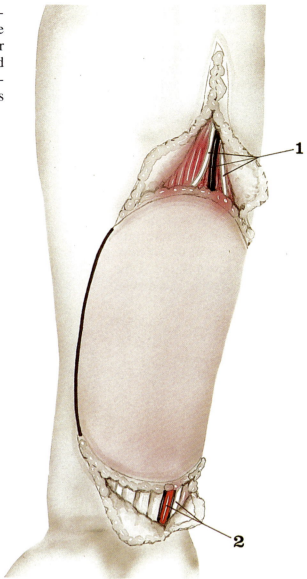

(**Fig. 2-26**) The medial portion of the flap, with the deep fascia, is raised from the flexor carpi ulnaris [3] toward the intermuscular septum at the lateral edge of this muscle. Preserving the fascia and branches in the septum, the flexor carpi ulnaris is retracted medially to expose the ulnar vessels [2].

1. Basilic v. and medial cutaneous n. of forearm
2. Ulnar a., v., and n.
3. Flexor carpi ulnaris m.

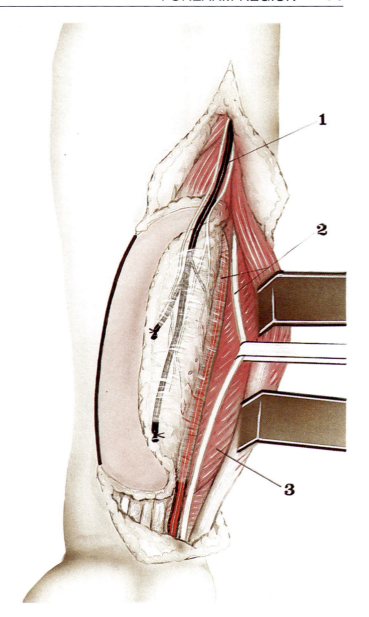

(Fig. 2-27) The lateral portion of the flap with the deep fascia is elevated from the flexor muscles toward the septum. The ulnar vascular bundle is separated from its base and the ulnar nerve. Retracting the flexor digitorum superficialis [4] laterally, the ulnar vessels [2] are dissected proximally up to the takeoff of the common interosseous artery [5].

2. Ulnar a., v., and n.
4. Flexor digitorum superficialis m.
5. Common interosseous a.
6. Flexor digitorum profunda m.
7. Median n.

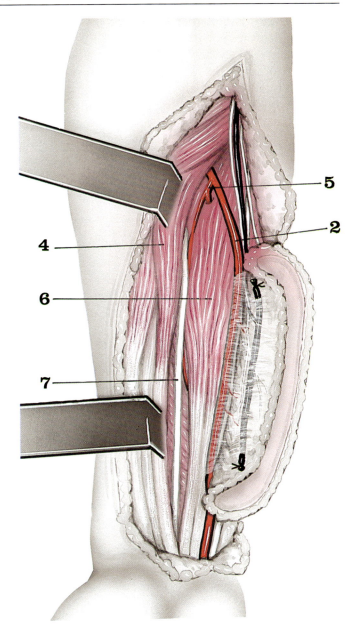

(**Fig. 2-28**) At this point, the circulation of the hand should be assessed by clamping the ulnar artery. Then, the ulnar vessels [2] are divided proximally, just distal to the common interosseous artery. The basilic vein [1] can be dissected proximally for a sufficient length. If it is required, a longer length for the arterial pedicle can be obtained with the distal dissection of the ulnar vascular bundle.

1. Basilic v. and median cutaneous n. of forearm
2. Ulnar a., v., and n.
3. Flexor carpi ulnaris m.
6. Flexor digitorum profunda m.

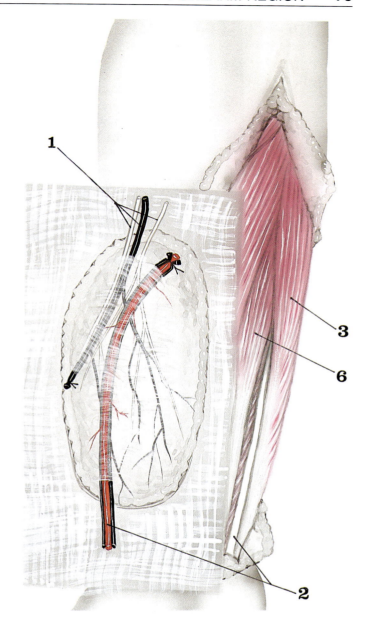

Note: The ulnar forearm flap can include the flexor carpi ulnaris and palmaris longus muscles as a myocutaneous flap and a segment of the ulnar bone as an osteocutaneous flap. It can also be used as a reversed island flap similar to the radial forearm flap.

74 ATLAS OF MICROVASCULAR SURGERY

RECIPIENT SITE EXPOSURES

Bifurcation of the Radial and Ulnar Arteries

(**Fig. 2-29**) An S-shaped incision is made from the medial bicipital groove, via the flexion crease, to the medial border of the brachioradialis muscle.

1. Brachial a. and v.
2. Median n.
3. Biceps m.
4. Brachioradialis m.
5. Pronator teres m.
6. Brachialis m.
7. Triceps m.
8. Bicipital aponeurosis
9. Tendon of biceps m.
10. Supinator m.
11. Ulnar a. and v.
12. Radial a. and v.
13. Recurrent radial a.

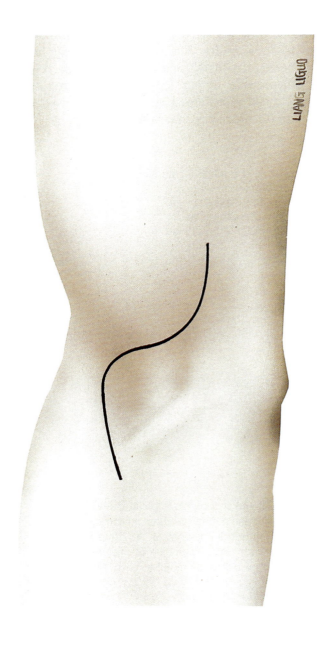

(Fig. 2-30) The superficial veins, including the median cubital vein, are ligated. The deep fascia and bicipital aponeurosis [8] are divided vertically along the medial side of the biceps muscle [3] and tendon, and the biceps tendon is retracted laterally, to display the contents of the fossa where the brachial artery lies between the biceps tendon and the median nerve [2].

1. Brachial a. and v.
2. Median n.
3. Biceps m.
4. Brachioradialis m.
5. Pronator teres m.
6. Brachialis m.
7. Triceps m.
8. Bicipital aponeurosis

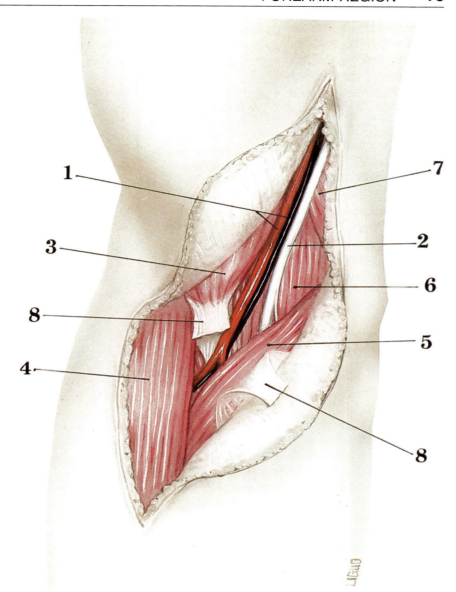

(Fig. 2-31) The brachioradialis [4] is retracted laterally. Tracing the brachial artery, the bifurcation is identified, and the radial artery [12] can be dissected further along the lateral border of the pronator teres [5]. Using care to protect the median nerve [2], the pronator teres is retracted to expose the ulnar artery [11]. The radial recurrent artery [13] arises from the radial artery near its origin.

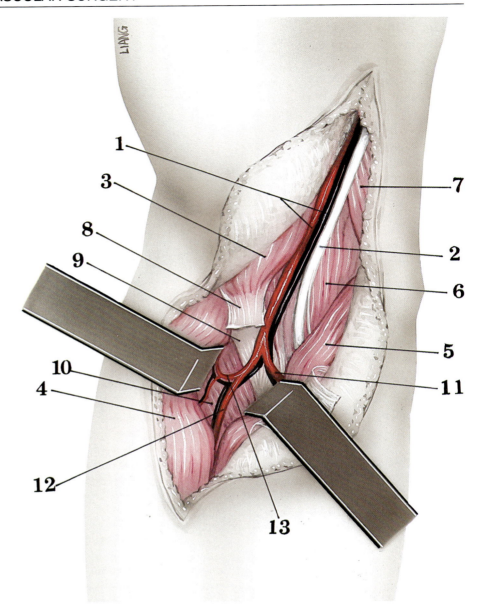

1. Brachial a. and v.
2. Median n.
3. Biceps m.
4. Brachioradialis m.
5. Pronator teres m.
6. Brachialis m.
7. Triceps m.
8. Bicipital aponeurosis
9. Tendon of biceps m.
10. Supinator m.
11. Ulnar a. and v.
12. Radial a. and v.
13. Recurrent radial a.

The ulnar artery gives off anterior and posterior ulnar recurrent arteries and the common interosseous artery, after its origination.

Radial Artery in the Forearm

(**Fig. 2-32**) A line is drawn from the antecubital fossa to the tubercle of the scaphoid. A skin incision can be made on the line at its proximal, middle, or distal portion, depending on the level of recipient artery required.

1. Radial a. and v.
2. Superficial branch of radial n.
3. Recurrent radial a.
4. Brachioradialis m.
5. Flexor carpi radialis m.
6. Pronator teres m.
7. Supinator m.
8. Bicipital aponeurosis
9. Flexor pollicis longus m.

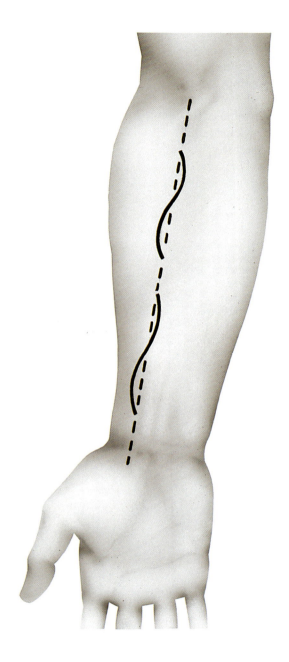

(Fig. 2-33) If the *proximal part* of the radial artery [1] is required, the incision is deepened to identify and enter the intermuscular septum between the brachioradialis [4] and the flexor carpi radialis [5] muscles. Retracting the brachioradial [4] muscle laterally, the radial artery [1] can be exposed and dissected out.

1. Radial a. and v.
2. Superficial branch of radial n.
3. Recurrent radial a.
4. Brachioradialis m.
5. Flexor carpi radialis m.
6. Pronator teres m.
7. Supinator m.
8. Bicipital aponeurosis

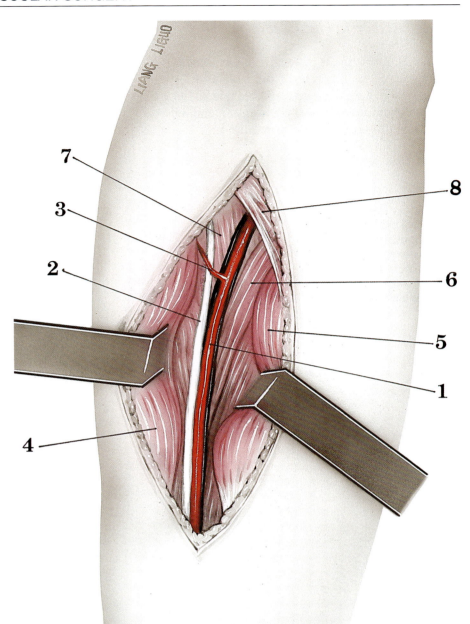

(**Fig. 2-34**) If the *distal part* of the radial artery [1] is required, the deep fascia is divided and the radial artery can be easily isolated between the tendons of the brachioradialis [4] and flexor carpi radialis [5]. The cephalic vein is available near the incision, lying in the superficial fascia at the radial side of the wrist.

1. Radial a. and v.
2. Superficial branch of radial n.
4. Brachioradialis m.
5. Flexor carpi radialis m.
9. Flexor pollicis longus m.

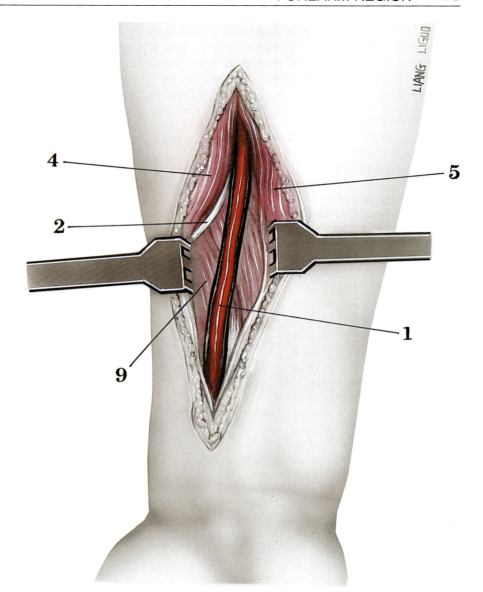

Ulnar Artery in the Forearm

(Fig. 2-35) A line is drawn from the medial epicondyle of the humerus to the lateral edge of the pisiform bone. The incision can be made on the middle or distal third of the line.

1. Ulnar a. and v.
2. Ulnar n.
3. Flexor carpi ulnaris m.
4. Flexor digitorum superficialis m.
5. Flexor digitorum profundus m.
6. Dorsal cutaneous branch of ulnar n.
7. Pronator quadratum m.

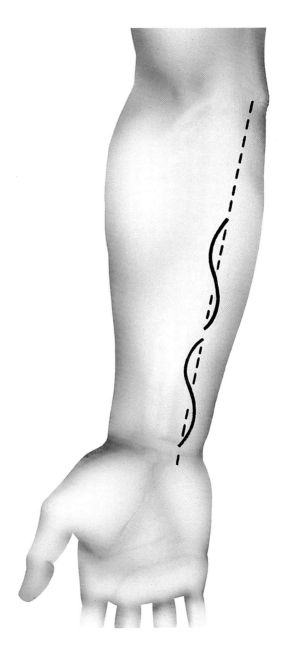

(**Fig. 2-36**) In the *middle third*, by deepening the incision and dividing the deep fascia, the intermuscular septum between the flexor carpi ulnaris [3] and flexor digitorum superficialis [4] muscles is identified and entered. Retracting the flexor carpi ulnaris muscle medially and the flexor digitorum superficialis muscle laterally, the ulnar artery [1] is located on the radial side of the ulnar nerve [2] and then isolated.

1. Ulnar a. and v.
2. Ulnar n.
3. Flexor carpi ulnaris m.
4. Flexor digitorum superficialis m.
5. Flexor digitorum profundus m.

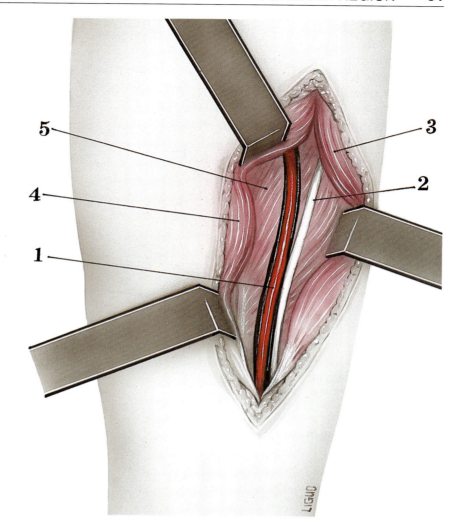

(Fig. 2-37) In the *distal third*, the deep fascia is incised. While retracting the flexor carpi ulnaris tendon [3], care should be taken to protect the dorsal cutaneous branch of the ulnar nerve [6] that is given off about 5 cm above the wrist and then passes under the flexor carpi ulnaris tendon via the ulnar side of the wrist, to reach the back of the hand. The ulnar artery [1] can be identified and isolated between the tendons of the flexor carpi ulnaris [3] and flexor digitorum [4] on the radial side of the ulnar nerve [2].

1. Ulnar a. and v.
2. Ulnar n.
3. Flexor carpi ulnaris m.
4. Flexor digitorum superficialis m.
6. Dorsal cutaneous branch of ulnar n.
7. Pronator quadratum m.

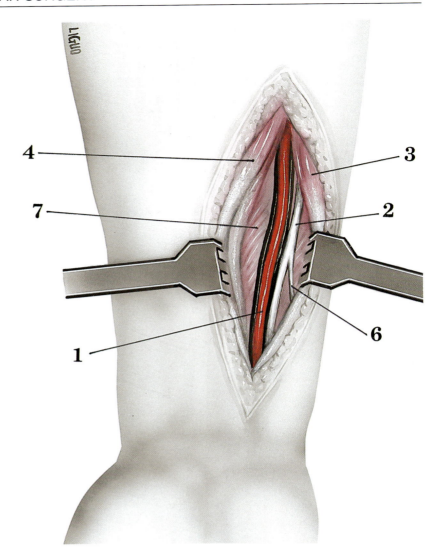

BIBLIOGRAPHY

Biemer E, Stock W: Microneurovascular skin and osteocutaneous free radial artery flap. In: Strauch B, Vasconez LO, Hall-Findlay E (eds): *Grabb's Encyclopedia of Flaps*, vol 3. Boston: Little, Brown, 1990, p 1801.

Biemer E, Stock W: Total thumb reconstruction: A one-stage reconstruction using an osteo-cutaneous forearm flap. Br J Plast Surg 36:52, 1983.

Boorman JG, Green MF: A split Chinese forearm flap for simultaneous oral lining and skin cover. Br J Plast Surg 39:179, 1986.

Chang T-S, Hwang W-Y: Forearm flap in one-stage reconstruction of the penis. Plast Reconstr Surg 74:251, 1984.

Cherup LL, Zachary LS, Gottlieb LJ, Petti CA: The radial forearm skin graft: Fascial flap. Plast Reconstr Surg 85:898, 1990.

Chicarilli ZN, Ariyan S, Cuono CB: Single-stage repair of complex scalp and cranial defects with the free radial forearm flap. Plast Reconstr Surg 77:577, 1986.

Chicarilli ZN, Price GJ: Complete plantar foot coverage with the free neurosensory radial forearm flap: Case report. Plast Reconstr Surg 78:94, 1986.

Cormack GC, Duncan MJ, Lamberty BGH: The blood supply of the bone component of the compound osteo-cutaneous radial artery forearm flap: An anatomical study. Br J Plast Surg 39:173, 1986.

Emerson DJM, Sprigg A, Page RE: Some observations on the radial artery island flap. Br J Plast Surg 38:107, 1985.

Fatah MF, Nancarrow JD, Murray DS: Raising the radial artery forearm flap: The superficial ulnar artery "trap." Br J Plast Surg 38:394, 1985.

Fenton OM, Roberts JO: Improving the donor site of the radial forearm flap. Br J Plast Surg 38:504, 1985.

Foucher G, van Genechten F, Merle N, Michon J: A compound radial artery forearm flap in hand surgery: An original modification of the Chinese forearm flap. Br J Plast Surg 37:139, 1984.

Glasson DW, Lovie MJ, Duncan GM: The ulnar forearm free flap in penile reconstruction. Aust NZ J Surg 56:477, 1986.

Groenevelt F, Schoorl R: The reversed forearm flap using scarred skin in hand reconstruction. Br J Plast Surg 38:398, 1985.

Hallock GG: Soft tissue coverage of the upper extremity using the ipsilateral radial forearm flap. Contemp Orthopaed 15:15, 1987.

Hallock GG: Island forearm flap for coverage of the antecubital fossa. Br J Plast Surg 39:533, 1986.

Harii K, Ebihara S, Ono I, et al: Pharyngoesophageal reconstruction using a fabricated forearm free flap. Plast Reconstr Surg 75:463, 1985.

Jin Y-T, Guan W-X, Shi T-M, et al: Reversed island forearm fascial flap in hand surgery. Ann Plast Surg 15:340, 1985.

Jones BM, O'Brien CJ: Acute ischaemia of the hand resulting from elevation of a radial forearm flap. Br J Plast Surg 38:396, 1985.

Khashaba AA, McGregor IA: Haemodynamics of the radial forearm flap. Br J Plast Surg 39:441, 1986.

Lamberty BGH, Cormack GC: The antecubital fasciocutaneous flap. Br J Plast Surg 36:428, 1983.

Lamberty BGH, Cormack GC: The forearm angiotomes. Br J Plast Surg 35:420, 1982.

Lin S-D, Lai C-S, Chiu C-C: Venous drainage in the reverse forearm flap. Plast Reconstr Surg 74:508, 1984.

Lovie MJ, Duncan GM, Glasson DW: The ulnar artery forearm free flap. Br J Plast Surg 37:486, 1984.

Mahaffey PJ, Tanner NSB, Evans HB, McGrouther DA: The degloved hand: Immediate complete restoration of skin cover with a contralateral forearm free flap. Br J Plast Surg 38:101, 1985.

Marty FM, Dontandon D, Gumener R, Zbrodowski A: The use of subcutaneous tissue flaps in the repair of soft tissue defects of the forearm and hand: An experimental and clinical study of a new technique. Br J Plast Surg 37:95, 1984.

Maruyama Y, Takeuchi S: The radial recurrent fasciocutaneous flap: Reverse upper arm flap. Br J Plast Surg 39:458, 1986.

Mixter RC, Wood MB: Closure of a defect of the femur with a compound free forearm transfer including both the radius and the ulna. Br J Plast Surg 36:470, 1983.

Moore MH, Sinclair SW, Blake G: The hairless osteotomized radial forearm flap. Plast Reconstr Surg 76:301, 1985.

Muehlbauer W, Herndl E, Stock W: The forearm flap. Plast Reconstr Surg 70:336, 1982.

Nakayama Y, Soeda S, Iino T: A radial forearm flap based on an extended dissection of the cephalic vein. The longest venous pedicle?: Case report. Br J Plast Surg 39:454, 1986.

Reid CD, Moss ALH: One-stage flap repair with vascularised tendon grafts in a dorsal hand injury using the "Chinese" forearm flap. Br J Plast Surg 36:473, 1983.

Small JO, Millar R: The radial artery forearm flap: An anomaly of the radial artery. Br J Plast Surg 38:501, 1985.

Song R, Gao Y, Song Y, et al: The forearm flap. Clin Plast Surg 9:21, 1982.

Soutar DS, McGregor IA: The radial forearm flap in intraoral reconstruction: The experience of 60 consecutive cases. Plast Reconstr Surg 78:1, 1986.

Soutar DS, Scheker LR, Tanner NSB, McGregor IA: The radial forearm flap: A versatile method for intra-oral reconstruction. Br J Plast Surg 36:1, 1983.

Swanson E, Boyd JB, Manktelow RT: The radial forearm flap: Reconstructive applications and donor-site defects in 35 consecutive patients. Plast Reconstr Surg 85:258, 1990.

Swanson E, Boyd JB, Mulholland RS: The radial forearm flap: A biomechanical study of the osteotomized radius. Plast Reconstr Surg 85:267, 1990.

Thomas A: Storage of a free forearm flap for 55 hours. Plast Reconstr Surg 78:91, 1986.

Timmons MJ: The vascular basis of the radial forearm flap. Plast Reconstr Surg 77:80, 1986.

Timmons MJ, Missotten FEM, Poole MD, Davies DM: Complications of radial forearm flap donor sites. Br J Plast Surg 39:176, 1986.

3 HAND AND WRIST

Anatomy of the Radial Artery—Deep Palmar Arch System (Fig. 3-1)

The *radial artery* [1] turns to the dorsal aspect of the carpus between the lateral ligament of the wrist and the tendons of the abductor pollicis longus and extensor pollicis brevis at the wrist. It then runs on the scaphoid and trapezium bones in the "snuff box," where it is crossed by the origin of the cephalic vein and superficial branch of the radial nerve. Having passed through the proximal end of the first interosseous space between the heads of the first dorsal interosseous, the artery goes between the oblique and transverse head of the adductor pollicis [12,13] and runs transversely across the palm.

At the base of the fifth metacarpal, it anasto-

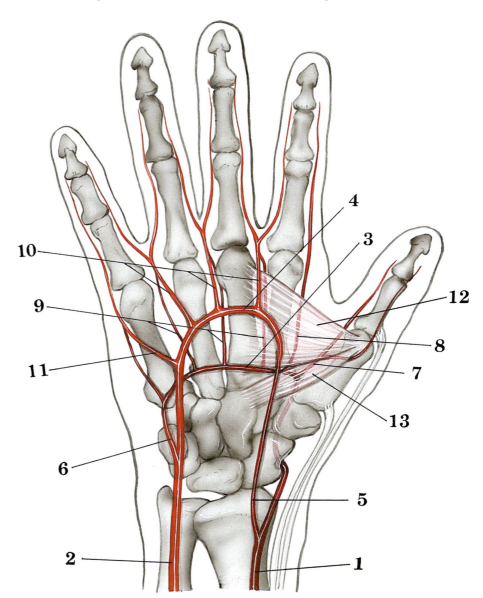

1. Radial a.
2. Ulnar a.
3. Deep palmar arch
4. Superficial palmar arch
5. Superficial palmar branch
6. Deep palmar branch
7. Princeps pollicis a.
8. Radial indicis a.
9. Palmar metacarpal a.
10. Common palmar digital a.
11. Ulnar palmar digital a. of little finger
12. Transverse head of adductor pollicis m.
13. Oblique head of adductor pollicis m.

moses with the deep palmar branch of the ulnar artery [6] to form the *deep palmar arch* [3], which lies on the bases of the metacarpal bones and the interossei and is covered by the oblique head of the aductor pollicis, the flexor tendons of the fingers, and the lumbricals.

The *princeps pollicis artery* [7] is given off from the radial artery just as it curves medially into the palm. It runs under the oblique head of the adductor pollicis and lateral to the first palmar interosseous muscle. At the base of the proximal phalanx of the thumb, it lies deep to the flexor pollicis longus tendon, and divides into a pair of digital arteries, running along the radial and ulnar sides of the tendon.

The *radialis indicis artery* [8] usually springs from the proximal part of the princeps pollicis artery [7], passing between the first dorsal interosseous and transverse head of the adductor pollicis [12] and running along the radial side of the index.

The *three palmar metacarpal arteries* [9] arise from the deep palmar arch and join the common digital arteries of the superficial palmar arch at the web of the finger.

Anatomy of the Ulnar Artery—Superficial Palmar Arch System

The *ulnar artery* [2] goes into the hand with the ulnar nerve superficial to the flexor retinaculum, and lateral to the pisiform bone. It then runs medial to the hook of the hamate and curves in the palm at the level of the palmar midpoint to form the superficial palmar arch [4], anastomosing with the superficial palmar branch of the radial artery [5]. The superficial palmar arch lies deep to the palmar fascia and in front of the flexor tendons and digital branches of the medial nerve.

Three common palmar digital arteries [10] are given off from the convexity of the superficial palmar arch [4] and travel distally on the second, third, and fourth lumbricals. Each merges with the palmar metacarpal artery from the deep palmar arch [9] and then divides into two proper palmar digital arteries, about 1 cm proximal to the web.

Each *proper palmar digital artery* travels along the side of the flexor tendon, dorsal to the digital nerve and deep to Cleland's ligament, which is a thin fibrous sheet attaching from the lateral side of the phalanx to the dermis of the volar skin in the finger. The palmar digital artery on the ulnar side of the little finger arises from the arch under the palmaris brevis.

Measurement

	Diameters (average; mm)
Radial a. (at anatomic snuff box)	1.8–2.0
Deep palmar arch	1.4
Princeps pollicis a.	1.3
Palmar metacarpal aa.	1.1
Ulnar a. (in front of flexor aponeurosis)	2.0–2.4
Superficial palmar arch	1.8
Common palmar digital aa.	1.5–1.7
Proper palmar digital aa.	
At web space	0.8–1.2
At distal interphalangeal joint	0.4–0.6

Variations of the Superficial Palmar Arch (Fig. 3-2)

A. Typical radioulnar communication of superficial palmar arch (35% of cases).
B. Superficial palmar arch formed only by ulnar artery (39% of cases).
C. Superficial palmar arch completed by ulnar and median artery; the latter, replacing the radial artery, accompanies the median nerve (4% of cases).
D. Three arteries (ulnar, median, and superficial branch of radial artery) join together to form the arch (1% of cases).
E. In this incomplete arch, the proper volar arteries are derived from the radial and ulnar arteries, without communication across the middle line of the hand at the superficial level (16% of cases).
F. Three arteries (ulnar, median, and superficial branch of radial artery) separately contribute to the digital vessels, without anastomosing with each other at the superficial level (5% of cases).

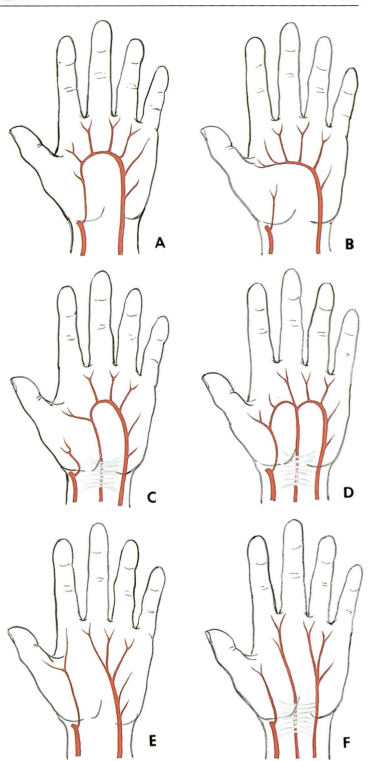

Variations of the Deep Palmar Arch (Fig. 3-3)

A. Typical radioulnar communication of deep palmar arch (35% of cases).
B. The deep palmar arch is complete, and it also supplies the ulnar side of the hand (13% of cases).
C. The deep palmar branch of the ulnar artery does not join the deep palmar arch, but the radioulnar communication is still complete, with connections between the palmar metacarpal arteries and the common palmar digital arteries (49% of cases).
D. The radial and ulnar arteries supply each side in the deep system; there may be poor communication, if the superficial palmar arch is incomplete (3% of cases).

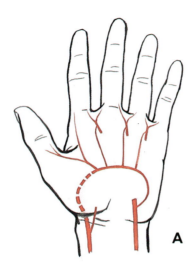
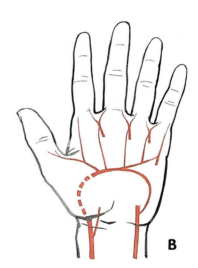
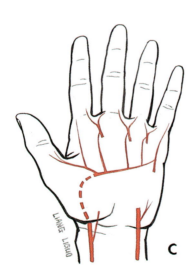
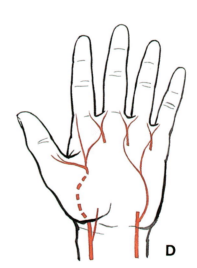

RECIPIENT SITE EXPOSURES

Radial Artery in the Anatomic Snuff Box

(Fig. 3-4) A curvilinear incision is made from the styloid process of the radius to a point between the bases of the first and second metacarpals.

1. Cephalic v.
2. Superficial branch of radial n.
3. Extensor pollicis longus tendon
4. Extensor pollicis brevis tendon
5. Radial a. and v.

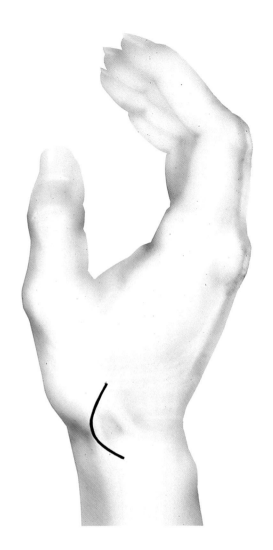

(**Fig. 3-5**) The cephalic vein [1] and superficial branch of the radial nerve [2] are identified in the subcutaneous tissue and retracted dorsally.

1. Cephalic v.
2. Superficial branch of radial n.
3. Extensor pollicis longus tendon
4. Extensor pollicis brevis tendon

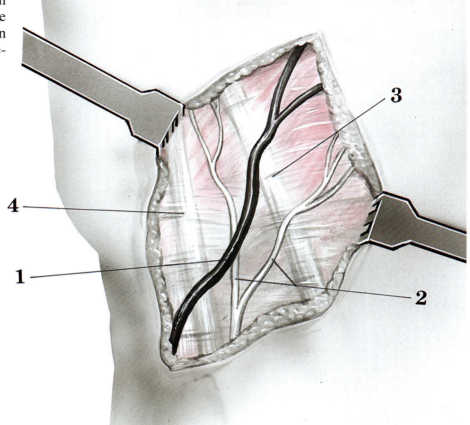

(**Fig. 3-6**) The deep fascia is divided longitudinally between the tendons of the extensors pollicis longus and brevis [3,4], which are then retracted dorsally and volarly.

The radial artery [5], accompanied by two venae comitantes, is identified and exposed as it emerges under the tendons of the abductor pollicis longus and flexor pollicis brevis, running distally to the interspace of the first and second metacarpals.

1. Cephalic v.
2. Superficial branch of radial n.
3. Extensor pollicis longus tendon
4. Extensor pollicis brevis tendon
5. Radial a. and v.

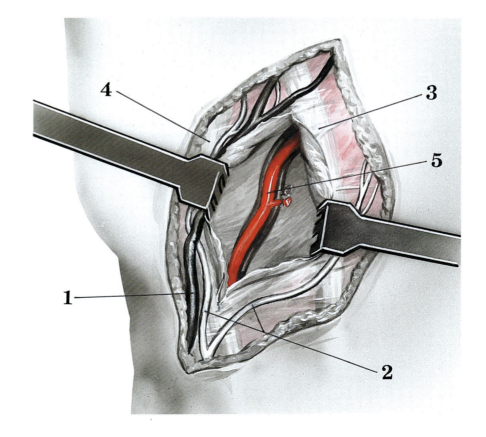

Ulnar Artery at the Wrist

(Fig. 3-7) A skin incision is made along the hypothenar crease. At the flexion crease of the wrist, it curves medially and then turns upward for a short distance along the radial side of the flexor carpi ulnaris tendon.

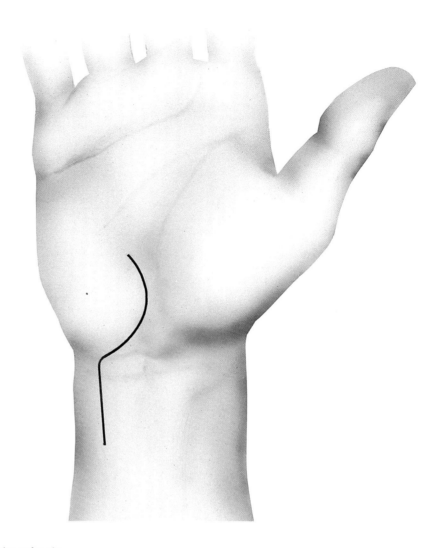

1. Flexor carpi ulnaris m.
2. Flexor digitorum superficialis tendons
3. Pisiform
4. Superficial part of the flexor retinaculum
5. Palmaris brevis m.
6. Palmar fascia
7. Hypothenar m.
8. Ulnar a.
9. Ulnar n.
10. Deep branch of the ulnar n.
11. Ulnar palmar digital a. of little finger

(Fig. 3-8) The palmar and deep fascia are incised along the line with a skin incision to identify the pisiform bone [3], the flexor carpi ulnaris tendon [1], and the palmaris brevis [5]. The latter runs transversely from the flexor retinaculum [4] and the palmar fascia [6] to the dermis on the ulnar side of the hand.

1. Flexor carpi ulnaris m.
2. Flexor digitorum superficialis tendons
3. Pisiform
4. Superficial part of the flexor retinaculum
5. Palmaris brevis m.
6. Palmar fascia
7. Hypothenar m.

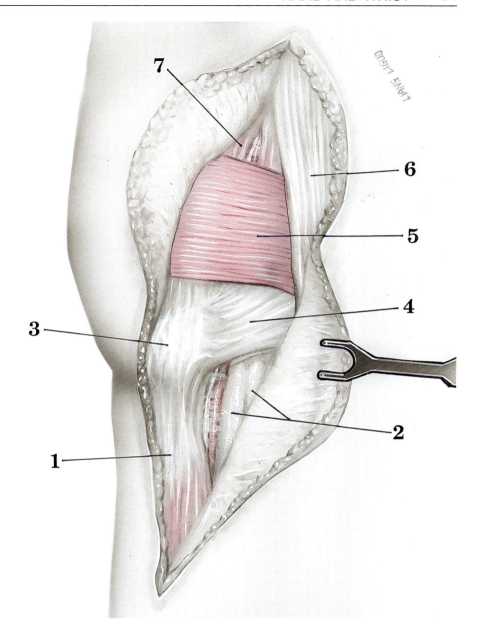

(Fig. 3-9) The palmaris brevis muscle [5] and the superficial part of the flexor retinaculum [4] are divided lateral to the pisiform bone [3]. Then, the ulnar artery [8] can be identified lateral to the ulnar nerve [9], between the pisiform bone and the flexor retinaculum. Retracting the flexor carpi ulnaris tendon [1] medially, the dissection proceeds proximally, to expose the ulnar artery and nerve. Although the ulnar nerve needs to be mobilized, care should be taken not to injure the deep branch of the nerve [10], which disappears between the flexor and abductor digiti minimi to reach the deeper layer of the palm.

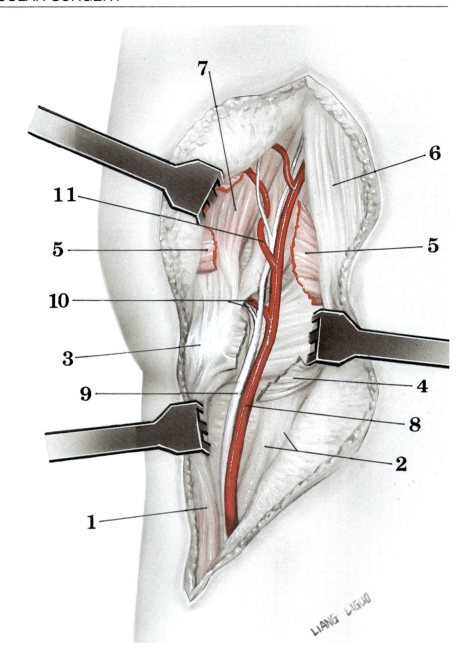

1. Flexor carpi ulnaris m.
2. Flexor digitorum superficialis tendons
3. Pisiform
4. Superficial part of the flexor retinaculum
5. Palmaris brevis m.
6. Palmar fascia
7. Hypothenar m.
8. Ulnar a.
9. Ulnar n.
10. Deep branch of the ulnar n.
11. Ulnar palmar digital a. of little finger

HAND AND WRIST

Princeps Pollicis Artery and the Origin of the Deep Palmar Arch

This artery is a dominant blood supply to the thumb, and it is located deeply under the thenar muscle. Both volar and dorsal approaches to the artery are possible.

Volar Approach

(Fig. 3-10) A curved incision is made from the ulnar side of the base of the thumb at the first web, along the thenar crease to the wrist between the thenar and hypothenar eminences.

1. Median n.
2. Flexor retinaculum divided
3. Flexor pollicis longus tendon
4. Transverse and oblique heads of adductor pollicis m.
5. Thenar m.
6. Recurrent branch of median n.
7. Palmar fascia
8. Flexor digitorum superficialis tendons
9. Lumbrical m.
10. First dorsal interosseous m.
11. Princeps pollicis a.
12. Radial indicis a.
13. Deep palmar arch

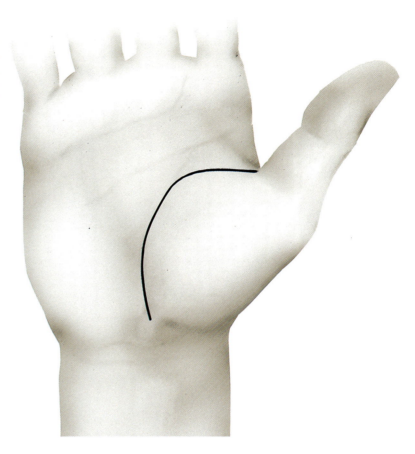

94 ATLAS OF MICROVASCULAR SURGERY

(**Fig. 3-11**) The palmar fascia [7] and flexor retinaculum [2] are divided, and the motor branch (sometimes called the recurrent branch) and sensory branches to the thumb and index of the median nerve [1] are then identified and carefully protected.

1. Median n.
2. Flexor retinaculum divided
3. Flexor pollicis longus tendon
4. Transverse and oblique heads of adductor pollicis m.
5. Thenar m.
6. Recurrent branch of median n.
7. Palmar fascia
8. Flexor digitorum superficialis tendons
9. Lumbrical m.

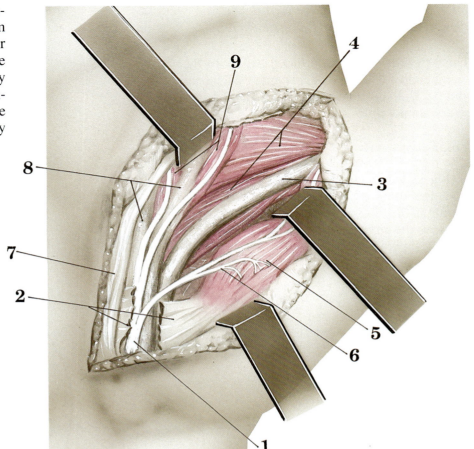

(Fig. 3-12) Retracting the thenar muscles [5] with the motor and sensory branches of the thumb radially, and the flexor pollicis longus tendon [3] and oblique head of the adductor pollicis [4] ulnarly, the princeps pollicis artery [11] is identified on the palmar aspect of the first metacarpal bone, under the oblique head of the adductor pollicis [4]. If a wider exposure is required, the lateral insertion of the oblique head of the adductor pollicis can be divided, and the radial indicis artery [12] and origin of the deep palmar arch [13] can be exposed.

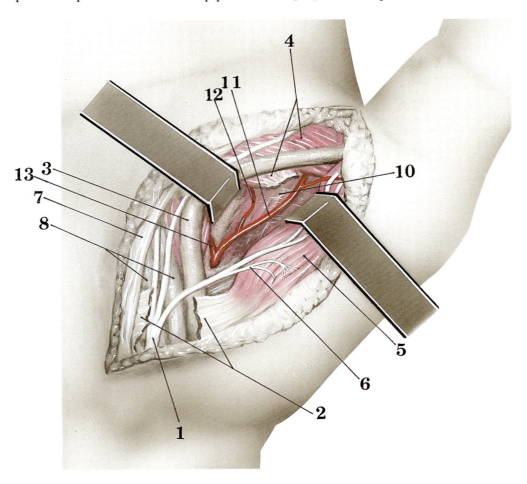

1. Median n.
2. Flexor retinaculum civided
3. Flexor pollicis longus tendon
4. Transverse and oblique heads of adductor pollicis m.
5. Thenar m.
6. Recurrent branch of median n.
7. Palmar fascia
8. Flexor digitorum superficialis tendons
9. Lumbrical m.
10. First dorsal interosseous m.
11. Princeps pollicis a.
12. Radial indicis a.
13. Deep palmar arch

Dorsal Approach

(Fig. 3-13) An incision is made from the ulnar side of the metacarpophalangeal joint of the thumb to the anatomic snuff box.

1. Adductor pollicis m.
2. Extensor pollicis longus tendon
3. First dorsal interosseous m.
4. First metacarpal
5. Radial a.
6. Princeps pollicis a.
7. Radial indicis a.
8. Deep palmar arch

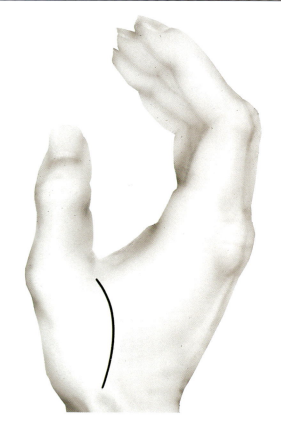

(Fig. 3-14) The extensor pollicis longus tendon [2] is isolated and retracted radially. The radial artery [5] is identified over the junction of the bases of the first and second metacarpal bones.

1. Adductor pollicis m.
2. Extensor pollicis longus tendon
3. First dorsal interosseous m.
4. First metacarpal
5. Radial a.

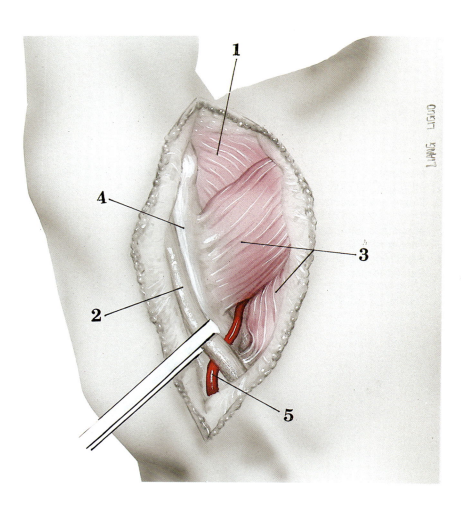

(**Fig. 3-15**) Tracing the radial artery [5] distally, the first dorsal interosseous muscle [3] is divided, and the origins of the princeps pollicis and radialis indicis arteries [6,7], as well as the origin of the deep palmar arch [8], are then identified. Along the palmar aspect of the first metacarpal bone [4], the dissection proceeds to isolate the princeps pollicis artery [6]. If greater exposure is needed, the insertion of the transverse head of the adductor pollicis [1] can be detached.

1. Adductor pollicis m.
2. Extensor pollicis longus tendon
3. First dorsal interosseous m.
4. First metacarpal
5. Radial a.
6. Princeps pollicis a.
7. Radial indicis a.
8. Deep palmar arch

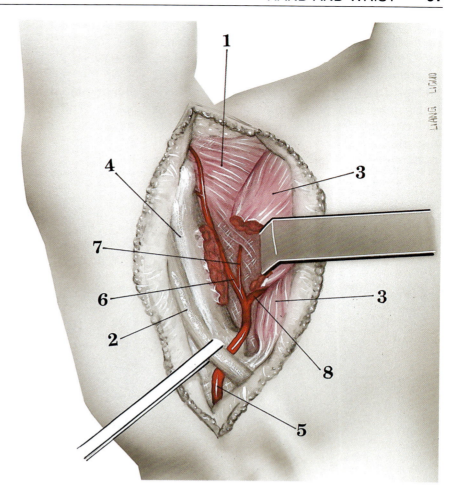

Superficial Palmar Arch

(**Fig. 3-16**) A skin incision is made along the proximal palmar and hypothenar creases, ending at the wrist between the thenar and hypothenar eminences.

1. Ulnar a. and n.
2. Flexor tendon
3. Common palmar digital a.
4. Flexor retinaculum
5. Median n.
6. Thenar m.
7. Palmar fascia
8. Common digital n.
9. Superficial palmar arch

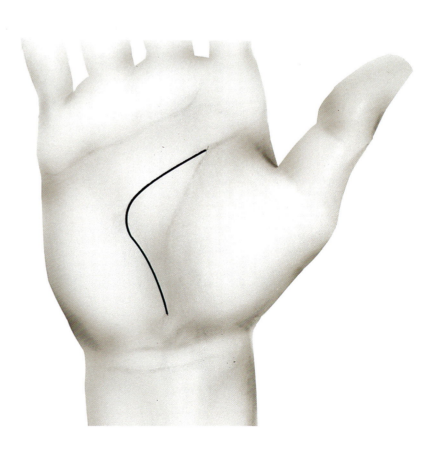

(Fig. 3-17) Deepening the skin incision, the palmar fascia [7] is divided and the dissection is then carried out under the fascia. The skin flap, together with the palmar fascia, is mobilized and turned over to the radial side. The superficial palmar arch [9] is exposed superficial to and crossing the flexor tendons [2] and the common digital nerve of the medial nerve [8]. At that point, it gives off three common palmar digital arteries [3] and then anastomoses with the superficial palmar branch of the radial artery.

At the proximal portion of the incision, dividing the palmaris brevis facilitates the exposure of the origin of the superficial palmar arch, that is, the distal continuation of the ulnar artery [1].

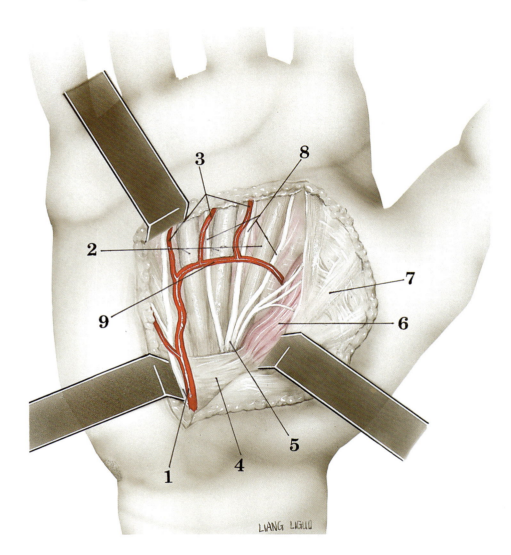

1. Ulnar a. and n.
2. Flexor tendon
3. Common palmar digital a.
4. Flexor retinaculum
5. Median n.
6. Thenar m.
7. Palmar fascia
8. Common digital n.
9. Superficial palmar arch

Digital Artery and Nerve

(Fig. 3-18) A longitudinal skin incision is made on the line of the junction of the volar and dorsal skin of the finger.

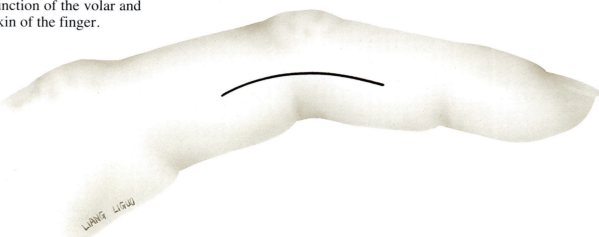

1. Digital a.
2. Digital n.
3. Flexor tendons
4. Articular capsule and lateral ligament of proximal interphalangeal joint
5. Phalanx
6. Cleland's ligament
7. Extensor tendon

(Fig. 3-19) Cleland's ligament [6] is divided longitudinally, and the neurovascular bundle [1,2] is then exposed. Generally, the digital nerve [2] may be identified first; the digital artery [1] is located dorsal and lateral to the nerve.

1. Digital a.
2. Digital n.
3. Flexor tendons
4. Articular capsule and lateral ligament of proximal interphalangeal joint
6. Cleland's ligament

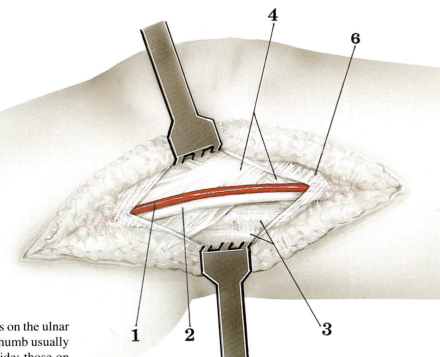

Note. The proper palmar digital arteries on the ulnar side of the index and middle fingers and thumb usually are somewhat larger than on the radial side; those on the radial side of the ring and little fingers are larger than on the ulnar side.

(Fig. 3-20) Approach to the digital artery and nerve in cross-section.

1. Digital a.
2. Digital n.
3. Flexor tendons
5. Phalanx
6. Cleland's ligament
7. Extensor tendon

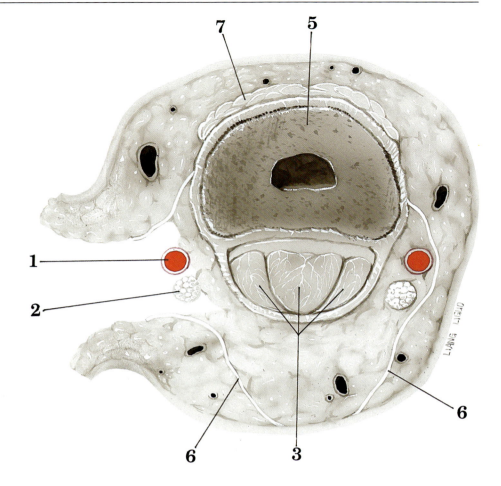

Part Two
LOWER EXTREMITY

4 GLUTEAL REGION

Gluteus Maximus Flap

Anatomy (Fig. 4-1)

The origins of the muscle involve the posterior gluteal line of the ilium, the aponeurosis of the erector spinae, the dorsal surface of the lower part of the sacrum, the side of the coccyx, and the sacrotuberous ligament. The upper part and the superficial fibers of the lower part are attached to the iliotibial tract of the fasciae latae and the deep fiber of the lower part to the gluteal tuberosity of the femur.

The muscle functions to extend the hip and to rotate the thigh laterally. In shape, it is broad, flat, thick, and quadrilateral. Muscle dimensions are 150 mm in length, 147 mm in width, and 22 mm in thickness at the midpoint.

Blood Supply

Both superior and inferior gluteal arteries [4,5] are the terminal branches of the internal iliac artery. They pass out of the pelvis above and below the piriformis muscle [2], supplying the upper half and lower half of the gluteus maximus [1], respectively.

Past the greater sciatic foramen, the *superior gluteal artery* [4] divides into a superficial branch to the gluteus maximus and a deep branch between the gluteus medius and iliac bone. The *inferior gluteal artery* [5] descends between the greater trochanter and the ischial tuberosity as a small direct cutaneous branch and accompanies the posterior femoral cutaneous nerve of the thigh to the popliteal fossa. It supplies the gluteus maximus and the skin of the buttock, as well as the back of the thigh, and anastomoses with the perforators of the deep femoral artery and circumflex femoral arteries.

Innervation

The *inferior gluteal nerve* leaves the pelvis below the piriformis and divides into branches entering the deep surface of the gluteus maximus, along with the inferior gluteal artery. The *posterior femoral cutaneous nerve* issues from the pelvis through the greater sciatic foramen below the piriformis, with the inferior gluteal vascular bundle. It descends deep to the fasciae latae with the direct cutaneous branch of the inferior gluteal artery. Its branches are distributed to the gluteal region, the perineum, and the flexor aspect of the thigh and leg.

Dimensions of Vessels

	Superior Gluteal		Inferior Gluteal	
	Artery	*Vein*	*Artery*	*Vein*
Diameter	2.0–3.0 mm	2.0–4.0 mm	2.5–3.5 mm	2.5–4.0 mm
Pedicle length	2–3 cm		2–3 cm	

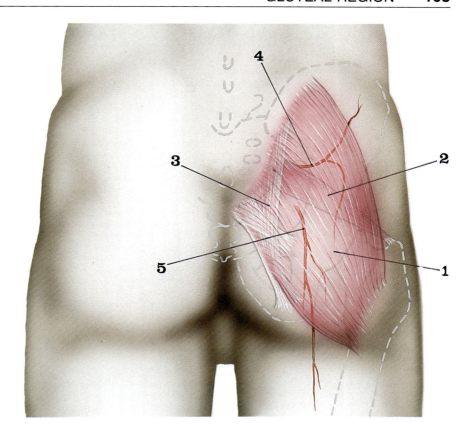

1. Gluteus maximus m.
2. Piriformis m.
3. Sacrotuberous ligament
4. Superior gluteal a.
5. Inferior gluteal a.

COMMENT AND INSIGHTS

The superior gluteal free flap provides a large amount of fat and muscle tissue from the buttock, and it is especially useful for reconstructing the breast. In such reconstructions, due to the short length of the vascular pedicle, the internal mammary vessels under the fifth costal cartilage are commonly used as recipient vessels for direct anastomoses; otherwise, vein grafts would be advisable.

The donor defect can be closed directly and donor scar and contour are inconspicuous and acceptable. The gluteal thigh flap provides the possibility of a sensate flap from the buttock and back of the thigh.

The shortness of the vascular pedicle in both gluteal flaps does limit the extent of application.

SUPERIOR GLUTEUS MYOCUTANEOUS FLAP

(**Fig. 4-2**) The axis of the flap is a line from the posterior superior iliac spine to the apex of the greater trochanter of the femur. The emergence of the superior gluteal artery is at the junction of the upper and middle thirds of the line. The width of the flap can approach 13 cm and still allow for the direct closure of the donor defect. The usual shape of the flap is elliptical and the size generally about 10 cm in width and 30 cm in length.

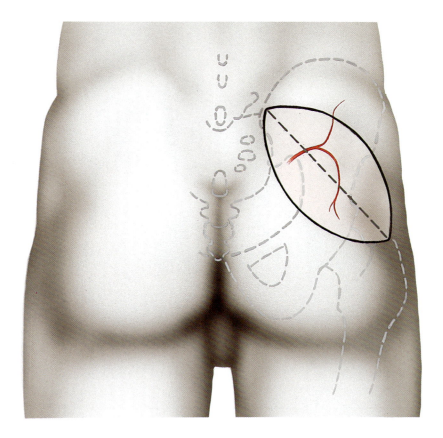

1. Gluteus maximus m.
2. Gluteus medius m.
3. Gluteus minimus m.
4. Piriformis m.
5. Superior gluteal a. and v.
6. Superficial branch
7. Deep branch

(**Fig. 4-3**) The first incision is begun along the superior and lateral borders, exposing the lateral edge of the gluteus maximus [1]. Then, blunt dissection proceeds between the muscle and the gluteus medius [2].

1. Gluteus maximus m.
2. Gluteus medius m.

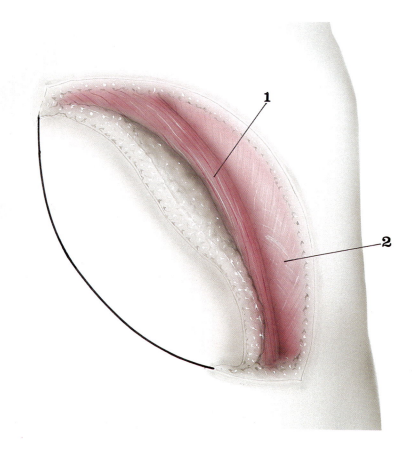

(Fig. 4-4) After the exposed portions of the muscle origin and insertion are divided, the superior gluteal vessels can be exposed between the gluteus medius [2] and piriformis [4] muscles, approximately 5 cm lateral to the sacral edge. The deep branch of the superior gluteal artery [7] is divided. The gluteus minimus [3] is seen at the depth of the wound.

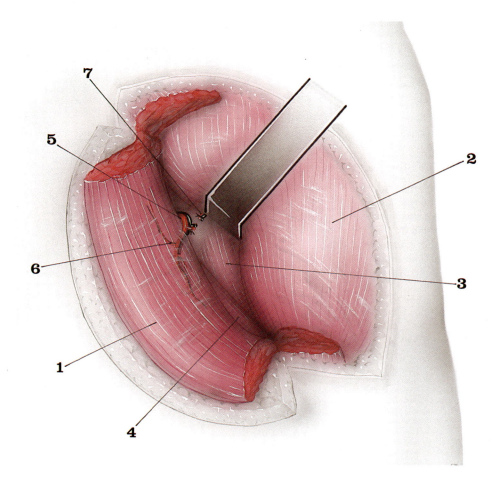

1. Gluteus maximus m.
2. Gluteus medius m.
3. Gluteus minimus m.
4. Piriformis m.
5. Superior gluteal a. and v.
6. Superficial branch
7. Deep branch

(Fig. 4-5) The rest of the elliptical skin incision is completed; then, the upper third of the gluteus maximus [1] is used in the flap and the muscle is separated at a line beyond the entrance of the superior gluteal vessels [5]. The myocutaneous flap is isolated on its vascular pedicle, which can be dissected proximally up to 2 or 3 cm, separating the superior gluteal nerve from it.

1. Gluteus maximus m.
2. Gluteus medius m.
3. Gluteus minimus m.
4. Piriformis m.
5. Superior gluteal a. and v.
6. Superficial branch

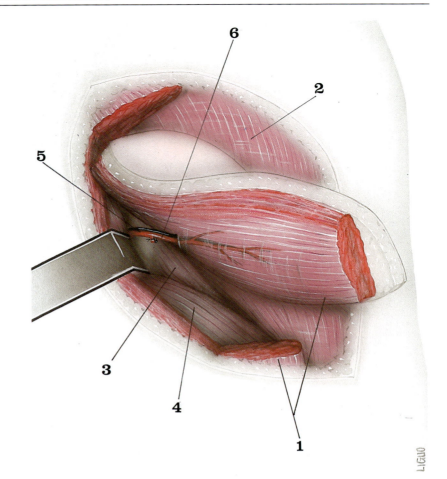

GLUTEAL THIGH FLAP (Based on the Inferior Gluteal Vessels)

(Fig. 4-6) The central axis of this flap is midway between the greater trochanter and the ischial tuberosity and perpendicular to the gluteal crease, whereas the inferior gluteal artery leaves the pelvis at about the midpoint of a line joining the posterior superior iliac spine and the ischial tuberosity. To permit direct closure, flap width should be less than 12 cm; flap length can range from 12 to 34 cm.

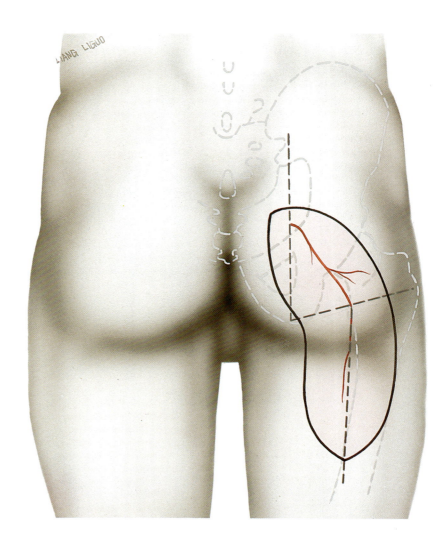

1. Gluteus maximus m.
2. Direct cutaneous branch of inferior gluteal a. and v.
3. Hamstring m.
4. Sciatic n.
5. Piriformis m.
6. Inferior gluteal a., v., and n.
7. Ischial tuberosity
8. Superior gemellus m., internal obturator m, and inferior gemellus m.
9. Quadratus femoris
10. Adductor brevis and magnus m.
11. Posterior femoral cutaneous n.

(Fig. 4-7) The distal part of the flap, including the fasciae latae of the thigh, is raised over the hamstring muscles [3] and the caudal edge of the muscle [1] is exposed.

1. Gluteus maximus m.
2. Direct cutaneous branch of inferior gluteal a. and v.
3. Hamstring m.

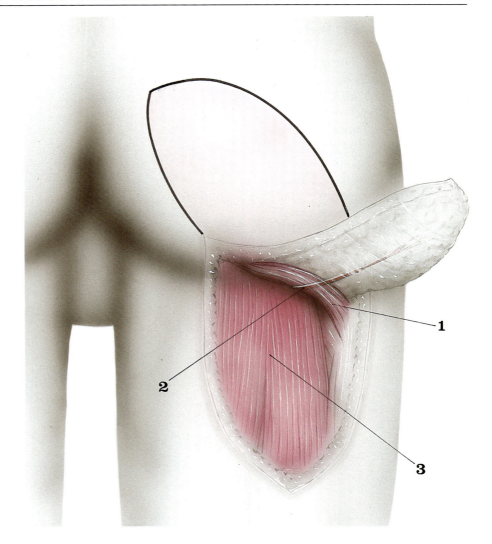

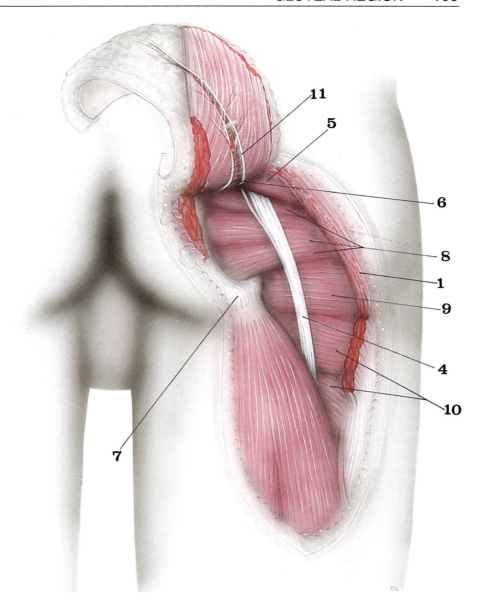

(Fig. 4-8) The insertions of the gluteus maximus are incised to the degree necessary for flap mobility, but no higher than the greater trochanter. The sciatic nerve [4], the posterior femoral cutaneous nerve [11], and the inferior gluteal neurovascular bundle [6] are identified below the piriformis [5].

1. Gluteus maximus m.
4. Sciatic n.
5. Piriformis m.
6. Inferior gluteal a., v., and n.
7. Ischial tuberosity
8. Superior gemellus m., internal obturator m., and inferior gemellus m.
9. Quadratus femoris
10. Abductor brevis and magnus m.
11. Posterior femoral cutaneous n.

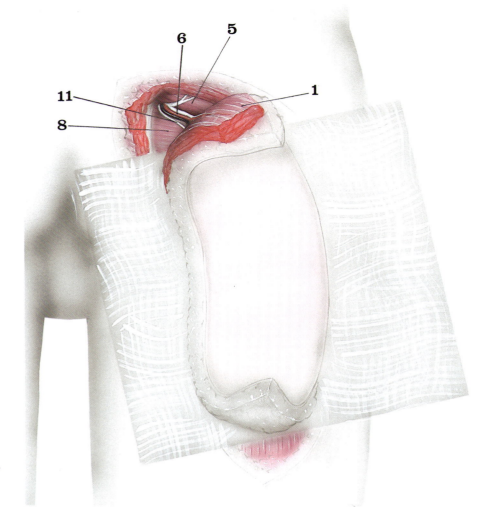

(Fig. 4-9) The upper portion of the incision is completed, and the gluteus maximus muscle [1] is divided, keeping a distance from the entrance of the neurovascular pedicle. The gluteal thigh flap is isolated on the inferior gluteal neurovascular bundle [6] and posterior femoral cutaneous nerve [11]. While harvesting the flap, the perineal branch of the posterior femoral cutaneous nerve and superior muscular branches of the inferior gluteal nerve should be left intact, if possible.

1. Gluteus maximus m.
5. Piriformis m.
6. Inferior gluteal a., v., and n.
8. Superior gemellus m., internal obturator m., and inferior gemellus m.
11. Posterior femoral cutaneous n.

VASCULARIZED ILIAC BONE GRAFT (Based on the Superior Gluteal Vessels)

Anatomy of the Deep Branch of the Superior Gluteal Artery (Fig. 4-10)

Regarding this artery [1], see this chapter, p. 102 on the gluteus maximus flap.

The deep branch [3] of the superior gluteal artery lies between the gluteus medius and bone, branching quickly into a superior [4] and inferior [5] division.

The superior division [4] runs along the upper border of the gluteus minimus [6] to the anterior superior iliac spine, anastomosing with the deep circumflex iliac artery and the lateral circumflex femoral artery. The average diameters of the deep superior branch and its venae comitantes are 2.9 mm, ranging from 1.7 to 5 mm, and 3.7 mm, ranging from 1.0 to 6.5 mm, respectively. The length of the pedicle is approximately 2 cm. The inferior division [5] enters the gluteus minimus obliquely.

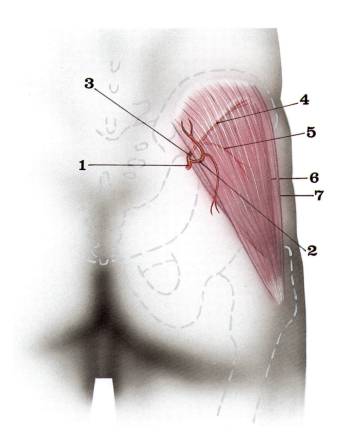

1. Superior gluteal a.
2. Superficial branch
3. Deep branch
4. Superior division
5. Inferior division
6. Gluteus minimus m.
7. Gluteus medius m.

COMMENT AND INSIGHTS

There have been only a few cases reported, and reliability might be clarified by further anatomic investigation and clinical application.

The pedicle length is so short that anastomosis must be performed under difficult conditions. Usually, an additional vein graft is necessary.

For these reasons, if a vascularized iliac bone graft is needed, one based on the deep circumflex iliac artery should be recommended as the first choice.

Harvesting Technique

(Fig. 4-11) The incision is made from the point between the posterior and middle thirds of the iliac crest, running along the crest anteriorly. At a point 4 cm posterior to the anterior superior iliac spine, it turns inferiorly to the greater trochanter of the femur.

1. Gluteus maximus m.
2. Gluteus medius m.
3. Tensor fasciae latae m.
4. Iliac crest
5. Deep superior branches of superior gluteal a., v., and n.
6. Gluteus minimus m.
7. Iliacus m.
8. Three layers of muscles of abdominal wall
9. Inner table of iliac bone

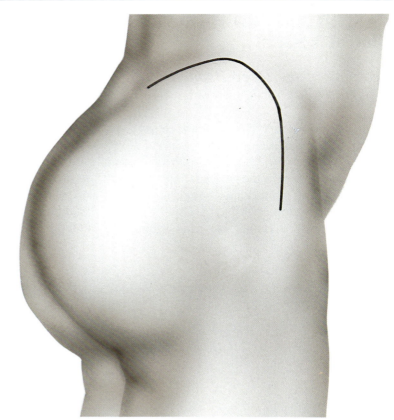

(Fig. 4-12) The skin flap is elevated to expose the gluteus medius [2]. The interspaces between the gluteus maximus [1], medius [2], and tensor fasciae latae [3] are identified.

1. Gluteus maximus m.
2. Gluteus medius m.
3. Tensor fasciae latae m.

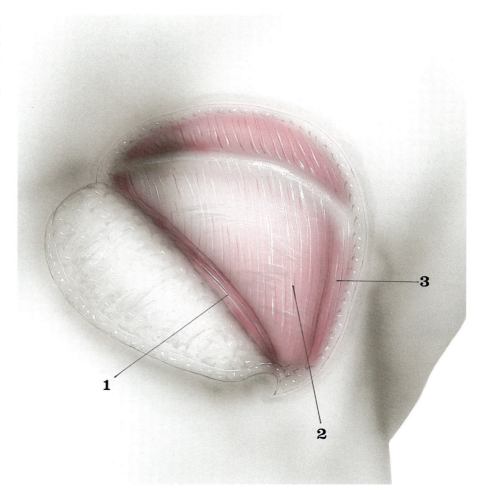

(Fig. 4-13) The gluteus medius muscle [2] is divided, leaving a 1 to 2 cm fringe on the iliac bone. Then, the deep superior branches of the superior gluteal vessels [5] and the superior gluteal nerve [5] are identified, just above the attachment of the gluteus minimus [6]. The vascular bundle is carefully dissected to separate the nerve from it and the origins of the gluteus maximus [1] and tensor fasciae latae can be partially detached to expose the gluteus medius widely.

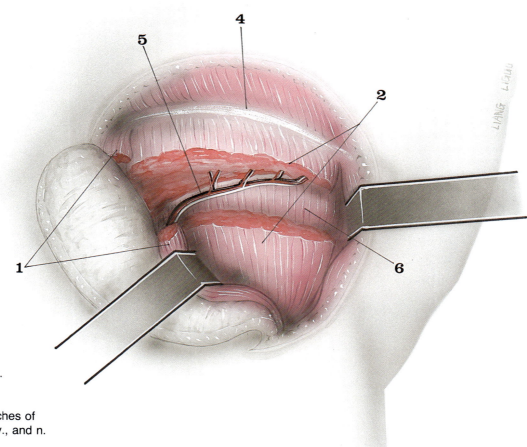

1. Gluteus maximus m.
2. Gluteus medius m.
4. Iliac crest
5. Deep superior branches of superior gluteal a., v., and n.
6. Gluteus minimus m.

(Fig. 4-14) The origins of the three layers of the abdominal muscle [8] are sharply divided from the iliac crest, and the iliacus muscle [7] is detached subperiosteally to expose the inner surface of the ilium [9].

4. Iliac crest
7. Iliacus m.
8. Three layers of muscles of abdominal wall
9. Inner table of iliac bone

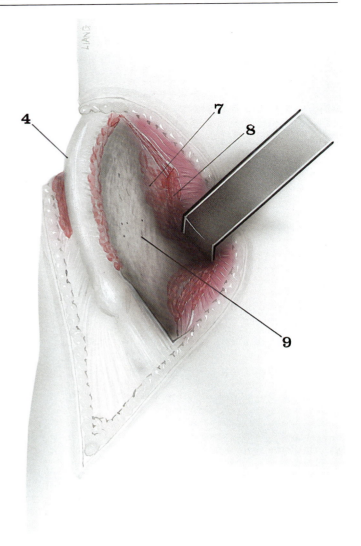

(**Fig. 4-15**) The required segment of the ilium is divided with care not to damage the vascular pedicle. Then, the vascularized iliac bone based on the deep superior branch of the superior gluteal vessels [5] is raised. Alternatively, only the outer table may be harvested for nonweight-bearing indications.

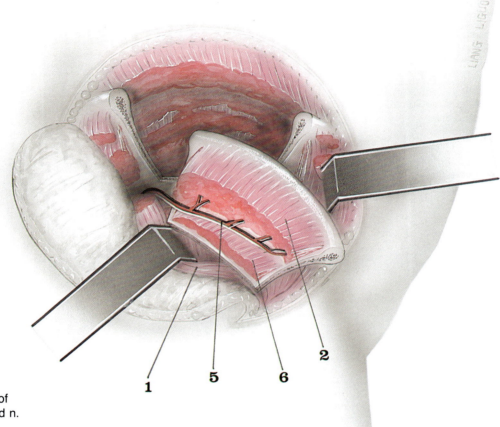

1. Gluteus maximus m.
2. Gluteus medius m.
5. Deep superior branches of superior gluteal a., v., and n.
6. Gluteus minimus m.

RECIPIENT SITE EXPOSURE

Superior Gluteal Artery

(Fig. 4-16) An incision is made from the posterior superior iliac spine, along the iliac crest for about 7 cm, turning downward toward the apex of the greater trochanter of the femur.

1. Gluteus maximus m.
2. Gluteus medius m.
3. Iliac crest
4. Gluteal a.
5. Superficial branch
6. Deep branch
7. Gluteal n.
8. Gluteus minimus m.
9. Piriformis m.

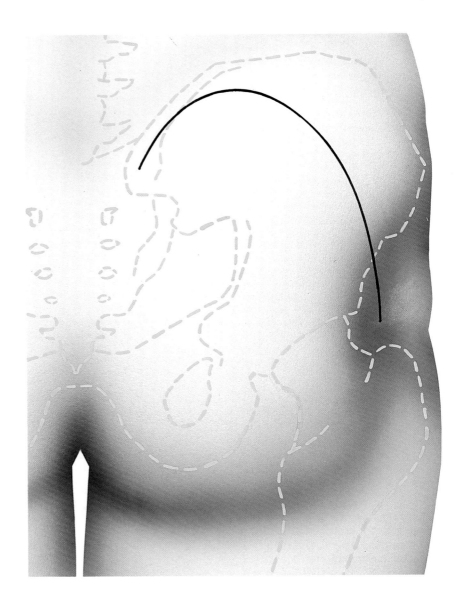

(Fig. 4-17) The upper lateral edge of the gluteus maximus [1] is identified, and its origin on the posterior gluteal line of the ilium is then detached.

1. Gluteus maximus m.
2. Gluteus medius m.
3. Iliac crest

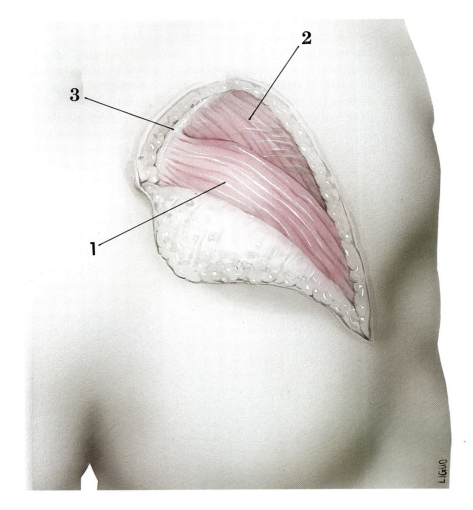

(Fig. 4-18) Dissection proceeds between the glutei maximus [1] and medius [2] muscles. The muscle flap is turned over and down; the superficial branch of the superior gluteal artery [5] is visible on its deep surface. Retracting the muscle flap inferiorly, the emergence of the superficial branch can be identified between the gluteus medius [2] and the piriformis [9], near the junction of the upper and middle thirds of the line joining the posterior superior iliac spine to the apex of the greater trochanter of the femur.

Retracting the gluteus medius superiorly, further dissection is carried out to expose the main trunk of the superior gluteal artery [4] and its bifurcation with the deep branch [6] above the piriformis [9]. The superior gluteal nerve [7] accompanies the deep branch of the superior gluteal artery [6] to supply the gluteus medius [2] and minimus [8] muscles.

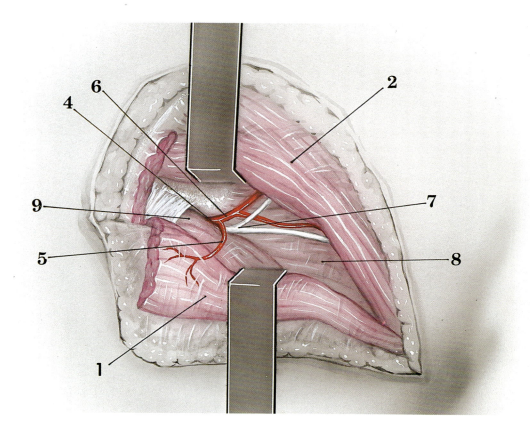

1. Gluteus maximus m.
2. Gluteus medius m.
4. Gluteal a.
5. Superficial branch
6. Deep branch
7. Gluteal n.
8. Gluteus minimus m.
9. Piriformis m.

BIBLIOGRAPHY

Buchanan DL, Agris J: Gluteal plication closure of sacral pressure ulcers. Plast Reconstr Surg 72:49, 1983.

Fujino T: Microvascular free transfer of a gluteal musculocutaneous flap. In: Strauch B, Vasconez LO, Hall-Findlay E (eds): *Grabb's Encyclopedia of Flaps*, vol. 2. Boston: Little, Brown, 1990, pp 1319ff.

Fujino T, Harashina T, Aoyagi F: Reconstruction for aplasia of the breast and pectoral region by microvascular transfer of a free flap from the buttock. Plast Reconstr Surg 56:178, 1975.

Huang G-K, Hu R-Q, Hua M, et al: Microvascular free transfer of iliac bone based on the deep superior branches of the superior gluteal vessels. Plast Reconstr Surg 75:68, 1985.

Hurwitz DJ: Closure of a large defect of the pelvic cavity by an extended compound myocutaneous flap based on the inferior gluteal artery. Br J Plast Surg 33:256, 1980.

Hurwitz DJ, Swartz WM, Mathes SJ: The gluteal thigh flap: A reliable, sensate flap for the closure of buttock and perineal wounds. Plast Reconstr Surg 68:521, 1981.

Le-Quang C: Two new free flaps developed from aesthetic surgery. II. The inferior gluteal flap. Aesthetic Plast Surg 4:159, 1980.

Mathes SJ, Nahai F: *Clinical Atlas of Muscle and*

Musculocutaneous Flaps. St. Louis: CV Mosby, 1979, pp. 94–98.

Mialhe C, Brice M: A new compound osteo-myocutaneous free flap: The posterior iliac artery flap. Br J Plast Surg 38:30, 1985.

Orgel MG, Kucan JO: A double-split gluteus maximus muscle flap for reconstruction of the rectal sphincter. Plast Reconstr Surg 75:62, 1985.

Ramirez OM, Hurwitz DJ, Futrell JW: The expansive gluteus maximus flap. Plast Reconstr Surg 74:757, 1984.

Ramirez OM, Orlando JC, Hurwitz DJ: The sliding gluteus maximus myocutaneous flap: Its relevance in ambulatory patients. Plast Reconstr Surg 74:68, 1984.

Scheflan M, Nahai F, Bostwick J III: Gluteus maximus island musculocutaneous flap for closure of sacral and ischial ulcers. Plast Reconstr Surg 68:533, 1981.

Shaw WW: Breast reconstruction by superior gluteal microvascular free flaps without silicone implants. Plast Reconstr Surg 72:490, 1983.

Walton RL, Hurwitz DJ, Bunkis J: Gluteal thigh flap for reconstruction of perineal defects. In: Strauch B, Vasconez LO, Hall-Findlay E (eds:) *Grabb's Encyclopedia of Flaps,* vol. 3. Boston: Little, Brown, 1990, pp. 1455ff.

5 GROIN REGION

Groin Flaps

ILIAC FLAP AND INFERIOR EPIGASTRIC FLAP

Anatomy (**Fig. 5-1**)

The skin territory of the groin flaps consists of the upper portion of the thigh, the lower portion of the abdomen, and the iliac area. The blood supply is provided by an arterial network that converges mainly from the following five arteries: superficial circumflex iliac artery (SCIA) [3], superficial epigastric artery (SEA) [6], fourth lumbar artery, deep circumflex iliac artery, and superior gluteal artery. The first three are discussed in this section and the latter two in the section on the vascularized iliac bone graft.

The SCIA [3] arises from the anterolateral aspect of the femoral artery [1], about 2.5 cm below the inguinal ligament, and runs toward the superior anterior iliac spine. It divides into two branches less than 1.5 cm after its origin.

The superficial branch [4] runs into the subcutaneous level immediately and parallel to the inguinal ligament 2 cm below it. This branch, with an average diameter of 0.8 mm, is absent in 14% of cases.

The deep branch [5] runs beneath the deep fascia parallel to the inguinal ligament and 1.5 cm below it. This branch crosses the lateral femoral cutaneous nerve [7], gives off branches to the sartorius, and then penetrates the deep fascia at the lateral border of the sartorius muscle, continuing subcutaneously and giving off small branches to the iliac crest. The deep branch with an average diameter of 1.0 mm appears in 100% of cases.

The superficial and deep branches are of about equal importance in supplying the flap. Their common stem averages about 1.5 cm in length and 1.5 mm in diameter.

The (SEA) [6] usually arises from the front of the femoral artery [1], about 1 cm below the inguinal ligament. Piercing the cribriform fascia, it ascends in front of the ligament and between the two layers of the superficial fascia of the abdominal wall toward the umbilicus. The average diameter of this artery is about 1.4 mm.

Venous Drainage

There are two drainage systems in this area. The dominant venous system is the superficial cutaneous veins involving the superficial circumflex iliac vein (SCIV) [9] and the superficial epigastric vein (SEV) [10]. The deep veins, such as the venae comitantes of these arteries, serve as an additional drainage system. The average diameter of the venae comitantes is about 1.1 mm.

Regarding the superficial venous system, in 50 to 60% of cases, the SCIV and SEV form a saphenous bulb (common trunks) with an average diameter of 2.5 mm, ranging from 1.2 to 5.0 mm. Although they drain into the saphenous vein separately, their average diameter is approximately 2.0 mm.

GROIN REGION

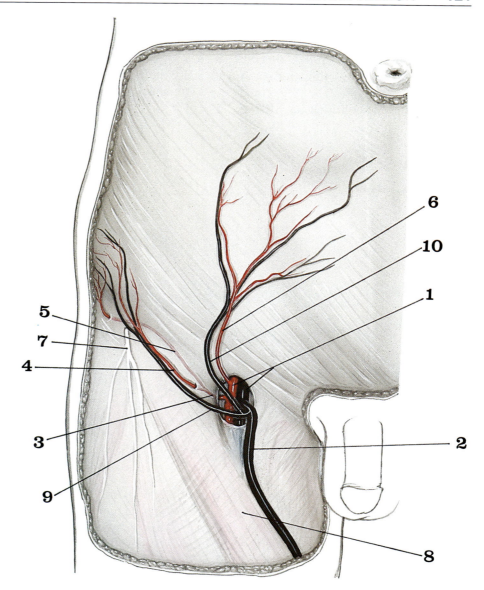

1. Femoral a. and v.
2. Saphenous v.
3. Superficial circumflex iliac a. (SCIA)
4. Superficial branch of SCIA
5. Deep branch of SCIA
6. Superficial epigastric a. (SEA)
7. Lateral femoral cutaneous n.
8. Sartorius m.
9. Superficial circumflex iliac v. (SCIV)
10. Superficial epigastric v. (SEV)

(Fig. 5-2) Variations of the SCIA and SEA are illustrated.

A. A common origin in 48% of cases, with a mean diameter of 1.4 mm (range, 0.8 to 3.0 mm).

B. A large SCIA without an SEA in 35% of cases, with a mean diameter of 1.4 mm (range, 0.8 to 3.0 mm).

C. Separate origins in 17% of cases, with a mean diameter of 1.1 mm (range, 0.8 to 1.8 mm).

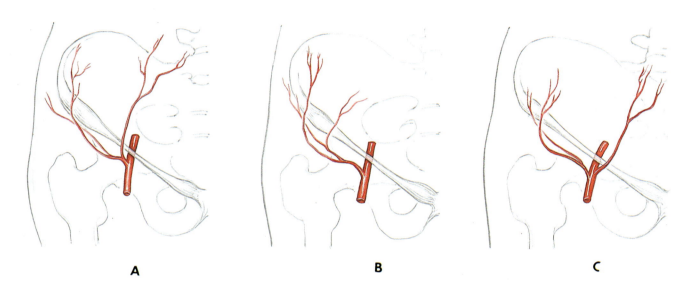

COMMENT AND INSIGHTS

The groin flap was one of the earliest flaps used in microsurgical tissue transplantation. There have been many cases reported in the literature. However, as a result of variation in vasculature, small caliber, and short length of arterial pedicle, difficulty in harvesting the flap, and an awkward and cramped position for microvascular anastomoses, the dominant position of the groin flap has gradually given way to subsequent and more currently used donor sites.

This donor site can provide a greater amount of skin coverage. The defect can usually be closed primarily with minimal morbidity and the donor scar is quite inconspicuous. Therefore groin flaps still have a place in reconstructive microsurgery.

The medial portion of the flap is rather bulky and hairy. The modified groin flap provides somewhat thinner and more hairless tissue and a longer vascular pedicle. But the procedure becomes more complicated and risky, and the available area for the flap decreases.

For a reliable vascularized iliac bone graft, the osteocutaneous flap based on the deep circumflex iliac artery (DCIA) is recommended, rather than one based on the SCIA.

There are only a few reports of cases of iliac skin flap based on the fourth lumbar vessels; reliability is a problem.

Innervation of the cutaneous portion of these flaps comes segmentally from the cutaneous branches of the XIIth thoracic nerve and one iliohypogastric nerve. A truly sensible flap in this area is therefore difficult to achieve.

ILIOFEMORAL FLAP

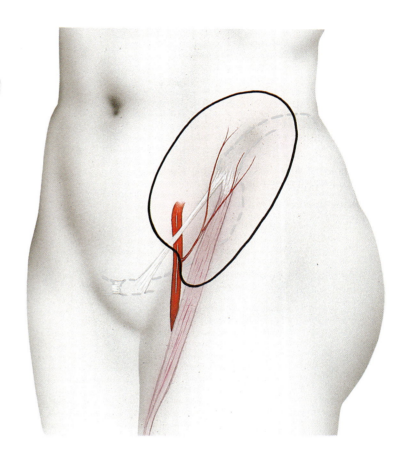

(Fig. 5-3) The surface anatomy of the SCIA is determined by a line drawn from a point on the femoral artery 2.5 cm below the inguinal ligament to the anterosuperior iliac spine. Although it is advised that the central axis of the flap be designed a little higher than this line, it can be expanded to the angle of the scapula.

The inferior border of the flap is drawn 5 cm below and parallel to the inguinal ligament, and an S-shaped median border lies just over the femoral artery or 1 to 2 cm lateral to it. Superior and lateral borders are designed to meet the requisite dimensions. The common size of this flap is 10 × 20 cm, and the largest size reported is up to 22 × 31 cm.

1. Deep branch of SCIA
2. Anterosuperior iliac spine
3. Sartorius m.
4. Lateral femoral cutaneous n.
5. Femoral a. and v.
6. Saphenous v.
7. SCIV
8. SCIA
9. Superficial branch of SCIA
10. SEV

124   ATLAS OF MICROVASCULAR SURGERY

Two techniques can be employed in flap elevation.

Lateral-to-Medial Procedure

(Fig. 5-4) The lateral portion of the flap is elevated superficially to the deep fascia until the anterosuperior iliac spine [2] is reached. Meticulous dissection is necessary at the lateral border of the sartorius muscle to ensure inclusion of the SCIA [1].

1. Deep branch of SCIA
2. Anterosuperior iliac spine

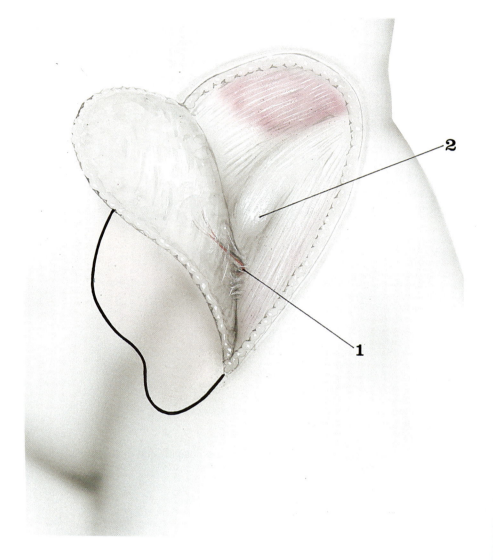

(Fig. 5-5) A branch to the muscle should be ligated to allow the superficial circumflex iliac vessel and a patch of the fascia of sartorius [3] to be attached to the flap. Dissection then proceeds through areolar tissue over the fascia of the iliacus muscle along the pulsative course of the SCIA [1], to the origin of the femoral vessels. The origin of the SCIA is followed, and the SEA can also be found and dissected.

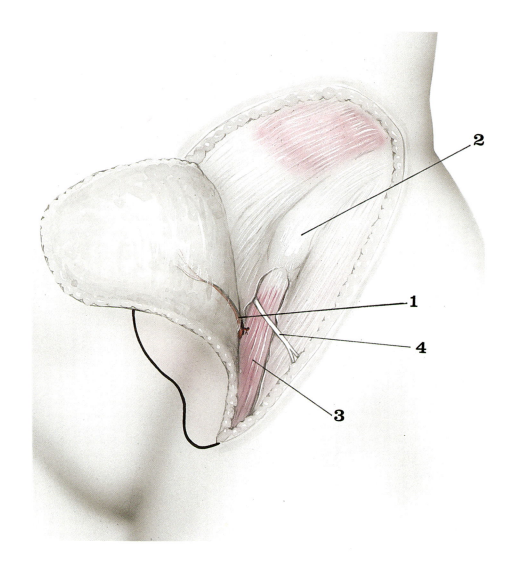

1. Deep branch of SCIA
2. Anterosuperior iliac spine
3. Sartorius m.
4. Lateral femoral cutaneous n.

(Fig. 5-6) After the procedures just described have been performed, the medial border of the flap is incised to expose the superficial cutaneous vein. The SEV and SCIV [7] are identified and preserved.

The groin flap may be isolated on two arteries and several veins. However, one artery and one vein that appear optimal for microvascular anastomoses are finally selected.

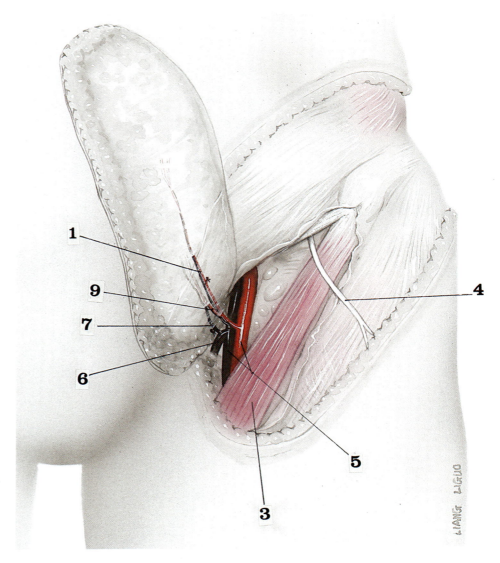

1. Deep branch of SCIA
3. Sartorius m.
4. Lateral femoral cutaneous n.
5. Femoral a. and v.
6. Saphenous v.
7. SCIV
9. Superficial branch of SCIA

Medial-to-Lateral Procedure

(Fig. 5-7) Dissection is started in the medial S-shaped incision, the base of the flap. The saphenous vein [6] and femoral artery and vein [5] are identified and dissected from below and medially. Further dissection reveals the variations of the SCIV [7] and SEV [10].

3. Sartorius m.
5. Femoral a. and v.
6. Saphenous v.
7. SCIV
10. SEV

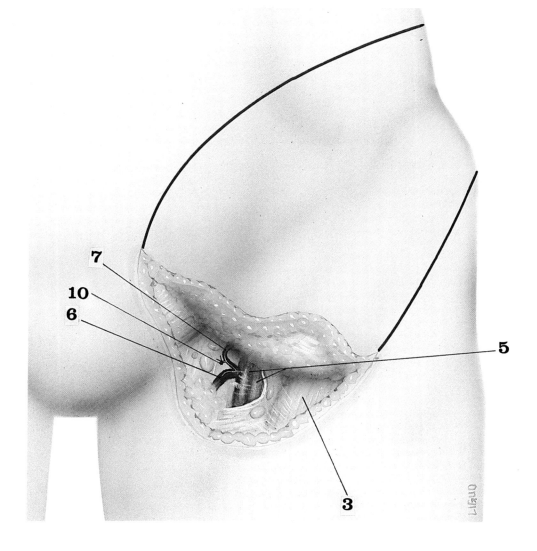

(Fig. 5-8) The origins of the SCIA [8] and SEA are identified following the course of the femoral vessels [5]. After the dissection of the medial aspect of the flap, the lateral portion is then elevated until the lateral border of the sartorius [3] is reached. Here, the deep fascia should be divided and turned medially with the flap, thus avoiding damage to the SCIA [8]. The groin flap is isolated.

The obtained vascular pedicle length in both procedures just described can be less than 1 cm for the arteries and 2 to 3 cm for the superficial veins.

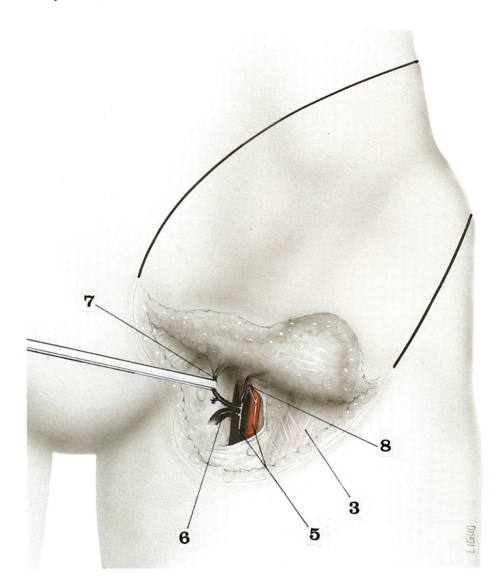

3. Sartorius m.
5. Femoral a. and v.
6. Saphenous v.
7. SCIV
8. Superficial branch of SCIA

ILIAC FLAP

The iliac flap is a modified groin flap and is designed for the purpose of increasing vascular pedicle length and for decreasing the thickness of the medial portion of the flap.

(**Fig. 5-9**) The medial margin of the flap lies lateral to the femoral triangle (the medial border of the sartorius). To explore the vessels, the medial incision is T-shaped, lying on its side. The cross limb and stem of the T correspond to the medial margin of the flap and the surface anatomy of the SCIA.

1. Femoral a. and v.
2. SCIA
3. SCIV
4. Saphenous v.

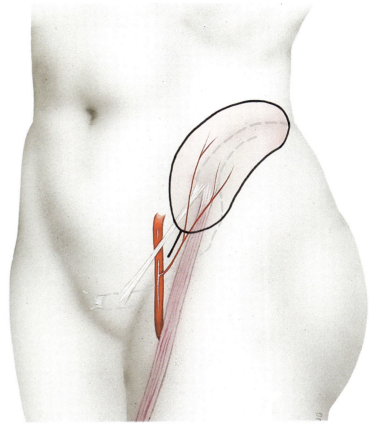

(Fig. 5-10) The technique of elevating this flap is similar to the medial-to-lateral procedure. Both the superficial and deep branches of the SCIA [2] are preserved in this flap as much as possible. The vascular pedicle can reach a length of approximately 4 cm.

1. Femoral a. and v.
2. SCIA
3. SCIV
4. Saphenous v.

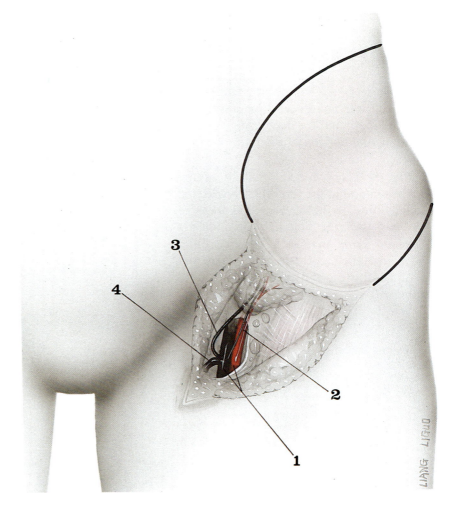

OSTEOCUTANEOUS GROIN FLAP (Based on the SCIA)

(Fig. 5-11) The skin flap is designed as the groin flap already described, and the proposed segment of bone is drawn on the iliac crest.

1. Femoral a. and v.
2. Saphenous v.
3. SCIA
4. SCIV
5. Sartorius m.
6. Iliac bone

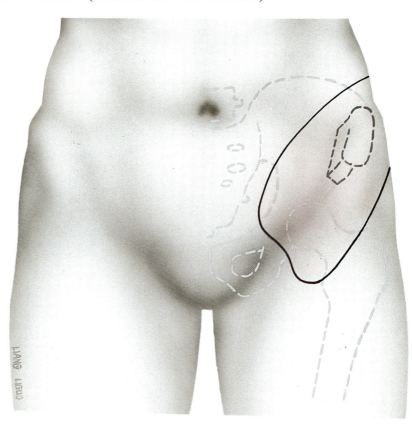

GROIN REGION 131

(**Fig. 5-12**) The lateral-to-medial procedure is used. The flap is raised around the proposed iliac bone [6] segment, keeping the skin flap, fascia, and iliac crest intact. The bony attachment of the external and internal oblique above and of the tensor fascia lata below are divided, leaving a 1 cm fringe of muscle attached to the bone. If the bone segment includes the anterosuperior iliac spine, 1 cm of sartorius muscle [5] and the inguinal ligament should be included in the graft.

During this procedure, attention must be paid to identifying and preserving the SCIA [3] in the flap at the lateral border of the sartorius, before dividing the bone. Bone segments have been reported with sizes of 6 × 1 cm and 8 × 3 cm.

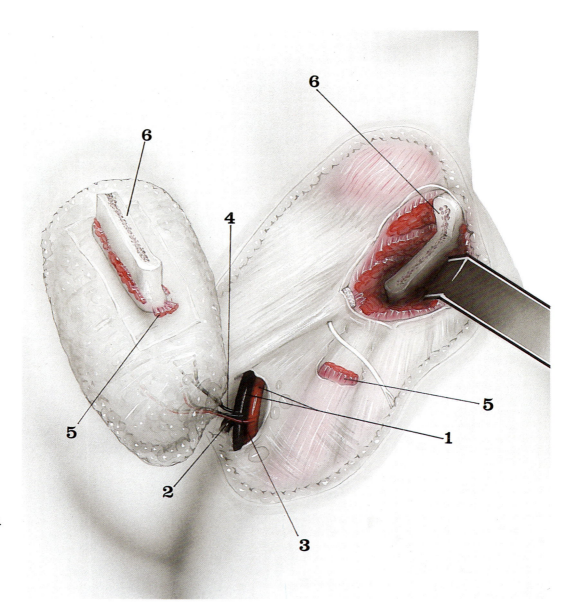

1. Femoral a. and v.
2. Saphenous v.
3. SCIA
4. SCIV
5. Sartorius m.
6. Iliac bone

COMPOSITE GROIN FLAP WITH "TENDON" TRANSFER

(**Fig. 5-13**) The external oblique aponeurosis is nourished from the SCIA through the loose areolar tissue on its surface where there is one of the anastomotic zones between the deep and superficial systems of vessels.

1. External oblique m. or aponeurosis
2. Internal oblique m.
3. Areolar tissue
4. Inguinal ligament
5. Femoral a. and v.
6. SCIA
7. SCIV

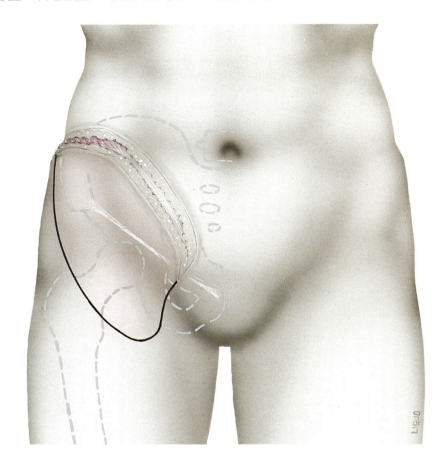

GROIN REGION 133

(Fig. 5-14) The lateral and superior edges of the groin flap are incised and the filmy, mobile layer of areolar tissue is identified on the surface of the external oblique aponeurosis [1].

1. External oblique m. or aponeurosis
2. Internal oblique m.

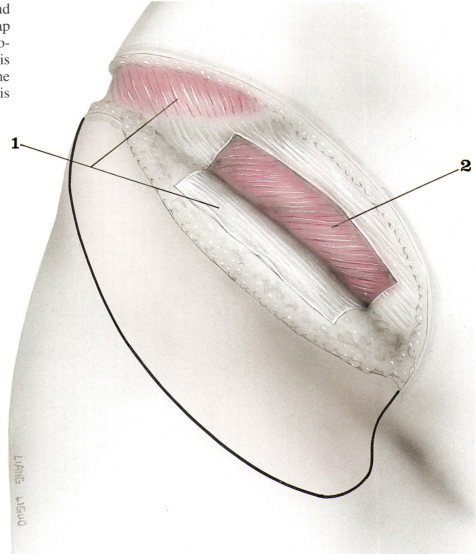

(Fig. 5-15) The areolar layer is incised 6 cm above and parallel to the inguinal ligament and gently peeled downward from the aponeurosis for a short distance. Then, the aponeurosis is divided in the direction of its fibers along the upper border of the intended graft. Vertical cuts are made at both ends for a distance and shape following the tendon caliber and length needed at the recipient site. Usually, repair of an ordinary extensor tendon needs an incision of 1.5 cm, repair of a tibialis anterior tendon, 2.0 cm, and of an Achilles tendon, 4 to 5 cm.

The strip of the aponeurosis is separated from the underlying internal oblique muscle and its lower border is incised from its deep surface. Then, the areolar tissue is carefully dissected with this tendinous portion from the other part of the aponeurosis, until the inguinal ligament is reached. The graft is attached along its length to the undersurface of the flap by a 4 to 5 cm "keel" of areolar tissue.

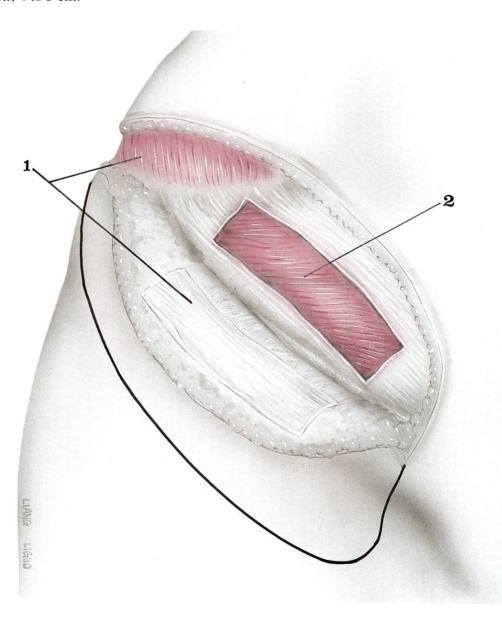

1. External oblique m. or aponeurosis
2. Internal oblique m.

(Fig. 5-16) The groin flap with the "tendon" graft [1] is isolated on the SCIA [6], following either the lateral-to-medial or medial-to-lateral approach already described. The aponeurosis strip is then tubed along its length with invagination of the cut edge.

1. External oblique m. or aponeurosis
2. Internal oblique m.
3. Areolar tissue
4. Inguinal ligament
5. Femoral a. and v.
6. SCIA
7. SCIV

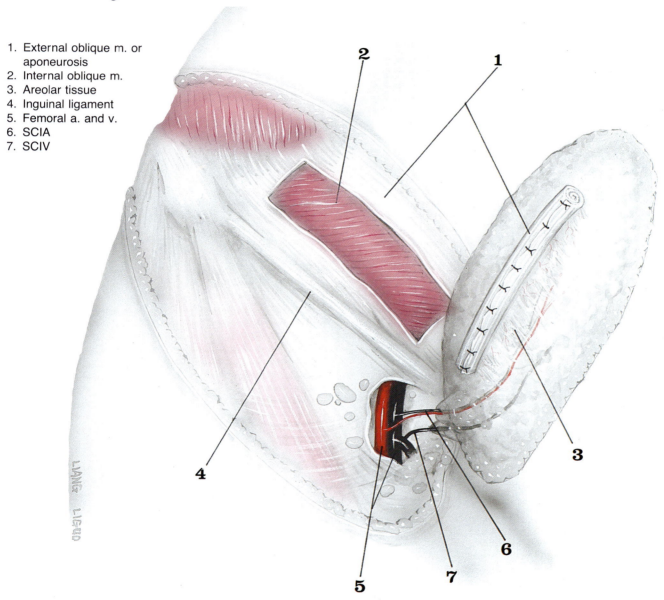

LOWER ABDOMINAL FLAP

Superficial Inferior Epigastric Flap (Fig. 5-17)

The axis of this flap is the line between the umbilicus and the femoral artery. The upper limit of the flap is at the level of the umbilicus; the lower limit, approximately 2 to 4 cm below the inguinal ligament; medially, to the midline of the abdomen; laterally, up to the anterosuperior iliac spine.

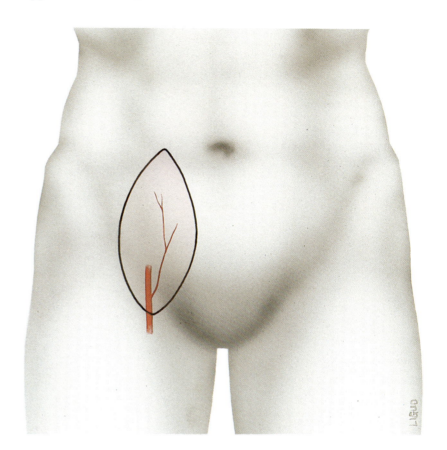

1. Femoral a. and v.
2. Saphenous v.
3. SEA
4. SEV
5. SCIA

(Fig. 5-18) The lower-to-upper procedure is applied to raise the flap. Using a Y-shaped incision on the lower part of the flap, the SEV [4] and SCIV are exposed and then, following the femoral artery [1], the SEA [3] and SCIA [5] are identified.

1. Femoral a. and v.
2. Saphenous v.
3. SEA
4. SEV
5. SCIA

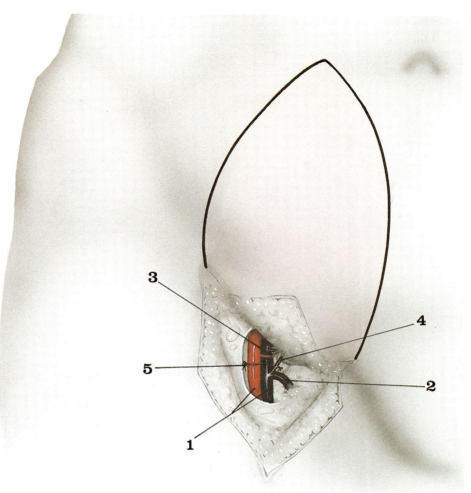

138　ATLAS OF MICROVASCULAR SURGERY

(Fig. 5-19) The upper part of the flap is elevated at the level superficial to the aponeurosis of the external oblique abdominis.

1. Femoral a. and v.
2. Saphenous v.
3. SEA
4. SEV
5. SCIA

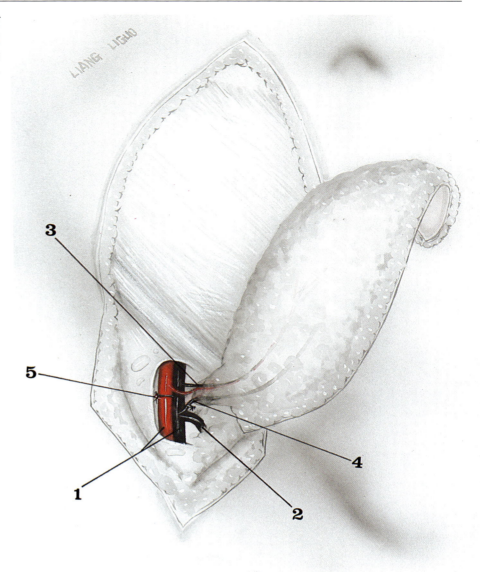

ILIAC FLAP (Based on the Fourth Lumbar Artery)

Anatomy (Fig. 5-20)

The fourth lumbar artery [4] arises from the posterolateral aspect of the abdominal aorta and runs behind the psoas major muscle. At its medial border, the artery divides into dorsal and ventral branches [5,6]. The dorsal branch passes between the sacrospinal and quadrate lumbar muscles, emerging in the inferior lumbar trigone [3] that is formed by the lateral margin of the latissimus dorsi [1], the posterior free border of the external oblique [2], and the iliac crest [7]. It runs lateroinferiorly in the subcutaneous tissue to supply the skin and bone of the iliac area.

The emerging point is located about 6.5 cm lateral to the back midline and 0.8 cm above the iliac crest. The diameter of the fourth lumbar artery is about 0.8 to 1.8 mm, and the diameter of the venae comitantes is 0.8 to 2.4 mm at the inferior lumbar trigone.

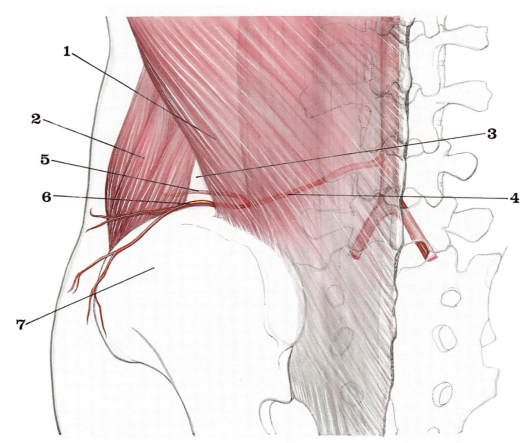

1. Latissimus dorsi m.
2. External oblique m.
3. Inferior lumbar trigone
4. Fourth lumbar a.
5. Ventral branch
6. Dorsal branch
7. Iliac bone

Harvesting Technique

(Fig. 5-21) The emerging point of the dorsal branch of the fourth lumbar vessel is marked on the lateral border of the sacrospinal muscle and just above the iliac crest. The axis of the flap goes along the iliac crest. The underlying iliac crest can be raised with the flap as an osteocutaneous flap.

Maximum flap size has been reported with an area of 9 × 11 cm and bone of 8 × 3 × 1 cm.

1. Latissimus dorsi m.
2. External oblique m.
3. Inferior lumbar trigone
4. Fourth lumbar a.
5. Ventral branch
6. Dorsal branch
7. Iliac bone

(Fig. 5-22) Making an 8 cm long incision 1 cm medial to the lateral border of the sacrospinal muscle [1], the dorsal branch of the fourth lumbar vessel [6] is identified in the inferior lumbar trigone.

1. Latissimus dorsi m.
6. Dorsal branch
7. Iliac bone

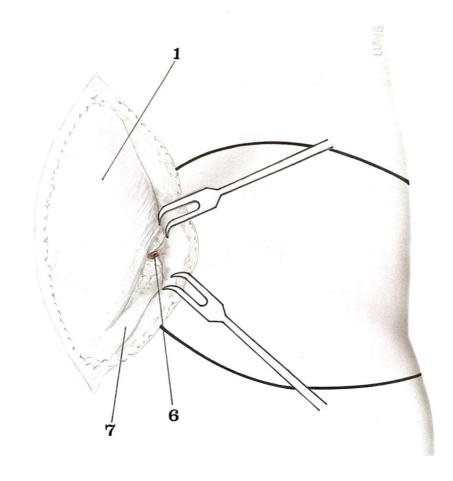

(Fig. 5-23) The osteocutaneous flap is isolated on its vascular pedicle [6], the length of which can be further dissected to reach 4 to 6 cm.

1. Latissimus dorsi m.
2. External oblique m.
6. Dorsal branch
7. Iliac bone

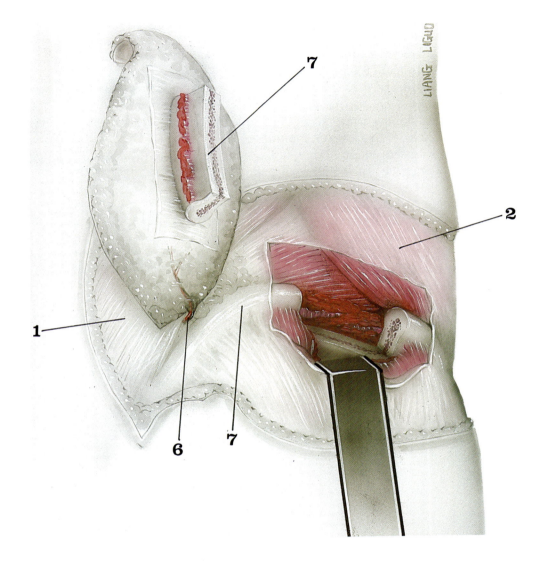

Vascularized Iliac Bone Graft

Anatomy of the Deep Circumflex Iliac Artery (Fig. 5-24)

The DCIA [2] arises from the posterolateral aspect of the external iliac artery [5], just above the inguinal ligament [3]. It runs parallel to the ligament toward the anterior superior iliac spine [7] in the fascial sheath formed by the junction of the transversalis and iliac fascia.

Approximately 1 cm medial to the anterior superior iliac spine, the artery gives off a large ascending branch [4] that pierces the transversus abdominis muscle and then runs superiorly along the undersurface of the internal oblique muscle.

After giving off the ascending branch, the DCIA penetrates the transversalis fascia and passes along the inner lip of the iliac crest, approximately 2 cm below the surface of the crest in the line of fusion between the iliacus and the transversalis fascia, ending at about the midpoint of the crest 6 to 9 cm beyond the anterosuperior iliac spine, where it reenters the transversus abdominis to anastomose with the iliolumbar and superior gluteus arteries. In its course along the iliac crest, the DCIA gives off perforators to the adjacent muscles and skin.

Venous Drainage

A vena comitans accompanies the artery. Usually, it diverges upward from the artery before draining into the external iliac vein.

Measurements of the DCIA System

	Diameter (mm)	Length of Pedicle (cm)
DCIA	Range: 1.5–30 Average: 2.0	5–6
Deep circumflex iliac vein	Range: 2.0–4.0 Average: 3.0	5–6
Ascending branch	Approximately 1.0	

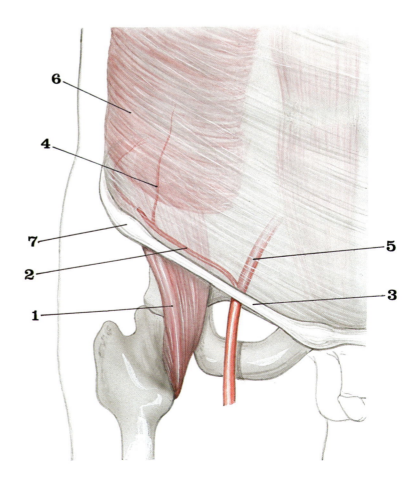

1. Iliacus m.
2. DCIA
3. Inguinal ligament
4. Ascending branch of DCIA
5. External iliac a.
6. External oblique m.
7. Anterior superior iliac spine

Variations in the Ascending Branch of the Deep Circumflex Iliac Artery (Fig. 5-25)

Type A. The branch originates within 1 cm medial to the anterior superior iliac spine (ASIS) (65%).

Type B. The branch originates 2 to 4 cm from the ASIS (15%).

Type C. There is no single vessel but 2 to 3 small branches near the ASIS (20%).

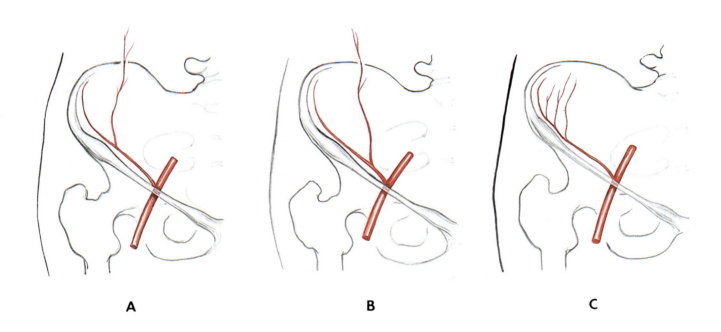

A B C

Anatomy of the Iliac Bone (Fig. 5-26)

The iliac crest, the upper border of the ilium, is convex above but sinuously curved and concave inward in its front part; it is concave outward in its posterior part. The entire length of the crest is 23 cm; the anterior 14 cm can usually be applied clinically for bone graft. The average thickness of the iliac crest is indicated below:

	Anterior Superior Iliac Spine	Tubercle of the Crest	Midpoint of Crest	Postero-superior Iliac Spine
Thick (cm)	1.4	1.7	0.8	2.2

A. Lateral view of ilium
B. Medial view of ilium

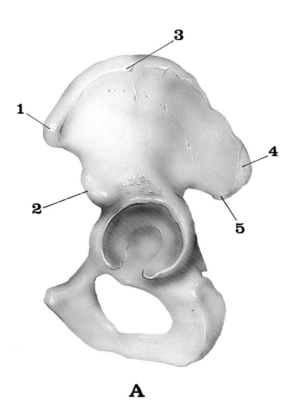
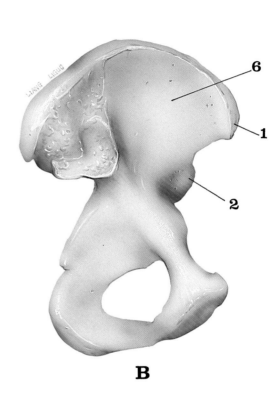

A **B**

1. Anterior superior iliac spine
2. Anterior inferior iliac spine
3. Tubercle of crest
4. Posterior superior iliac spine
5. Posterior inferior iliac spine
6. Iliac fossa

COMMENT AND INSIGHTS

This has been one of the most common donor sites for vascularized bone graft because the consistent vascular anatomy, long pedicle length, and adequate vessel diameter make the procedure reliable and safe. A good quality of iliac bone is provided in sufficient amounts. The natural curvature of the iliac bone is ideally suited for mandibular reconstruction, using the ipsilateral or contralateral crest, depending on which segment of the mandible needs rebuilding. The bone can also be used for certain bone defects in the extremities. However, for large, long bone defects, a vascularized fibula graft would be the better choice.

The donor defect should be carefully closed, since a potential for abdominal herniation still remains.

The DCIA dominantly supplies the inner lip and cortex of the iliac crest and body; the SCIA supplies the overlying skin; the superior gluteal artery supplies the outer lip and cortex of the iliac crest and body.

Among the vessels, the DCIA is the most reliable in supplying the iliac bone; it is therefore the preferred choice in vascularized iliac bone graft procedures.

VASCULARIZED ILIAC BONE GRAFT (Based on the Deep Circumflex Iliac Artery)

(Fig. 5-27) The patient is placed in a supine position with a sandbag under the buttock. The incision runs along the upper border of the inguinal ligament and iliac crest, extending for the required distance.

1. External iliac a. and v.
2. External oblique aponeurosis
3. Inguinal ligament
4. Internal oblique m.
5. DCIA
6. Transversus abdominis m.
7. Lateral cutaneous n. of thigh
8. Iliac crest
9. Iliacus m.
10. Ascending branch
11. Gluteus m. and tensor fasciae latae (TFL) m.

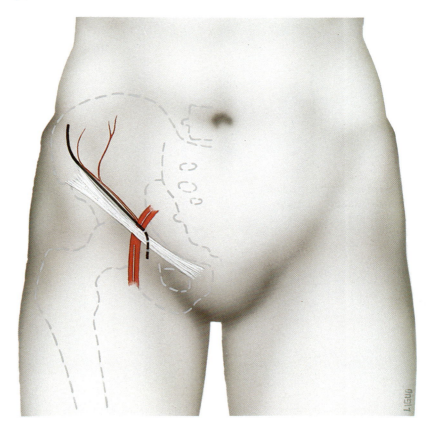

(Fig. 5-28) Through the medial incision, the external oblique aponeurosis [2] is split parallel with and 1 cm above the upper edge of the inguinal ligament [3] from the midpoint of the ligament to the anterior superior iliac spine. Retracting the spermatic cord or round ligament medially and upward, the posterior wall of the inguinal canal, consisting of the transversalis fascia at this point, is exposed and the external iliac artery [1] can then be palpated.

1. External iliac a. and v.
2. External oblique aponeurosis
3. Inguinal ligament
4. Internal oblique m.
5. DCIA

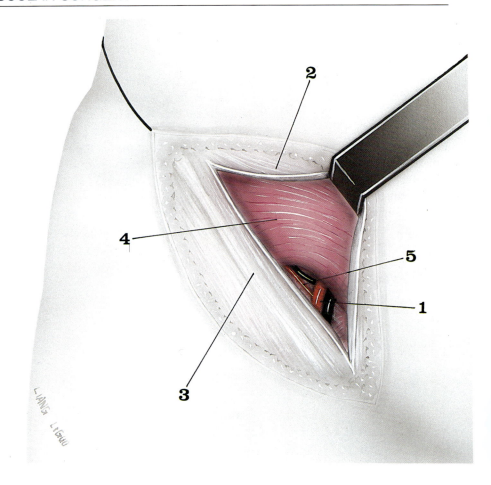

(Fig. 5-29) Following the dissection of the external iliac artery, the vascular bundle of the DCIA [5] is identified and dissected laterally in the sheath of the transversalis fascia, while the arching fibers of the internal oblique and transversus muscles [4.6] are detached from the inguinal ligament. Finding the ascending branch [10] at a point 1 cm above and medial to the anterior superior iliac spine between the internal oblique and transversus muscles and tracing it down usually makes identification and dissection of the vascular pedicle easier and faster.

Meanwhile, the lateral femoral cutaneous nerve [7] is found in this region, in some cases under the vessel; its continuity can be preserved. In other cases, it must be divided and repaired, if it is superficial to the vessels.

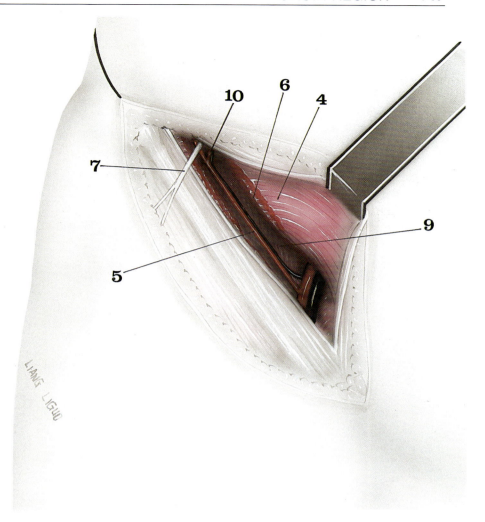

4. Internal oblique m.
5. DCIA
6. Transversus abdominis m.
7. Lateral cutaneous n. of thigh
9. Iliacus m.
10. Ascending branch

(Fig. 5-30) Following the dissection of the vascular pedicle, the incision is extended on the iliac crest [8]. In the upper lateral dissection, the three layers of abdominal muscles are detached from the crest. The ascending branch is ligated and the deep circumflex iliac artery [5] is traced laterally by dividing the transversalis fascia and separating extraperitoneal fat from the iliacus [9], keeping this vascular bundle intact with the iliacus muscle.

The iliacus fascia and muscle are divided at least 1 cm below the course of the DCIA [5] onto them, to expose the inner surface of the ilium. The distal end of this vessel is ligated.

5. DCIA
8. Iliac crest
9. Iliacus m.

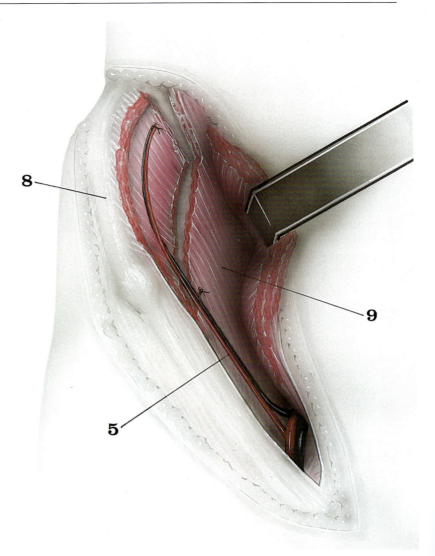

GROIN REGION 149

(**Fig. 5-31**) For flaps requiring the full thickness of iliac crest, the lower lateral dissection requires the TFL and gluteus medius [11] to be detached from the outer lip and cortex of the iliac crest and body subperiosteally.

8. Iliac crest
11. Gluteus m. and TFL m.

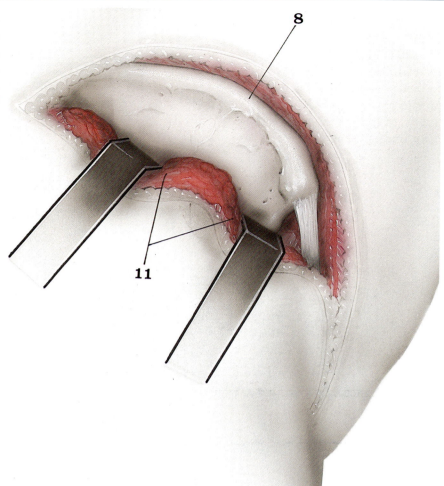

(Fig. 5-32) According to the requirements of size and shape, a segment of the iliac bone [8] is divided with an oscillating saw. For a better appearance at the donor site postoperatively, it is advisable to leave the anterior superior iliac spine in situ.

5. DCIA
8. Iliac crest
9. Iliacus m.

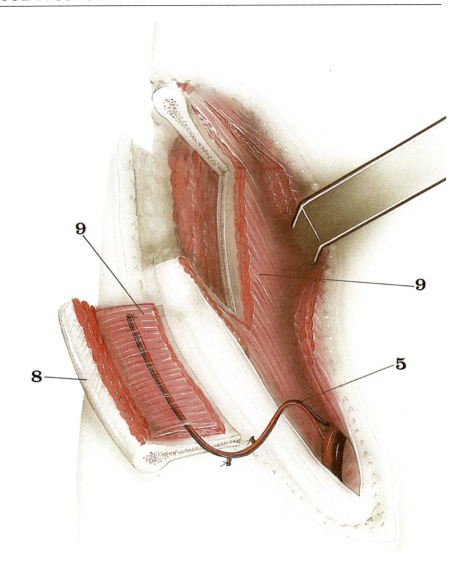

(**Fig. 5-33**) More commonly, the inner lip of the iliac crest alone is needed clinically. It can be isolated on the DCIA [5] independently, providing a less bulky flap and less deformity at the donor site.

5. DCIA
8. Iliac crest
9. Iliacus m.

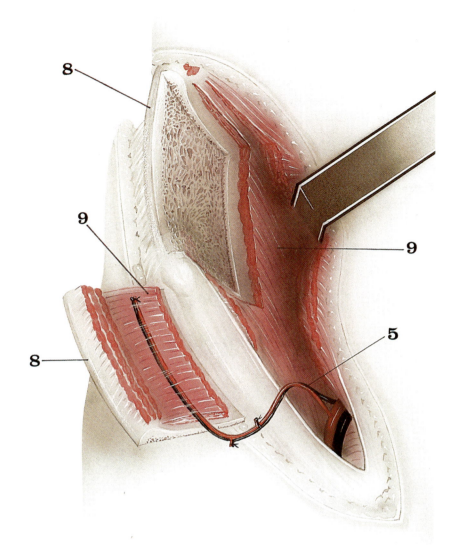

Donor Closure (Fig. 5-34)

The closure of this donor site must be carried out meticulously, in order to prevent postoperative herniation. The iliacus muscle [9] and fascia should be sutured to the transversalis muscle [6] and fascia.

2. External oblique aponeurosis
4. Internal oblique m.
6. Transverse abdominis m.
9. Iliacus m.

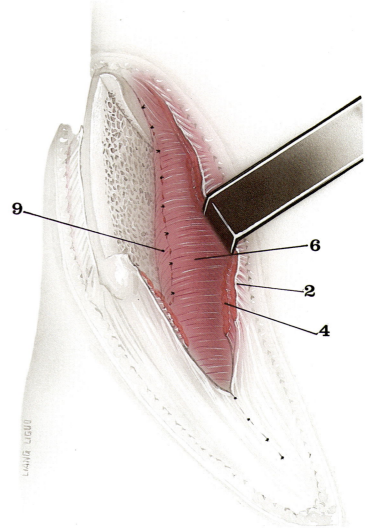

(**Fig. 5-35**) The internal and external oblique muscle [2] should be sutured to the gluteal and TFL muscles [11]. The inguinal canal and ligament should also be repaired if they have been divided.

2. External oblique aponeurosis
11. Gluteus m. and TFL m.

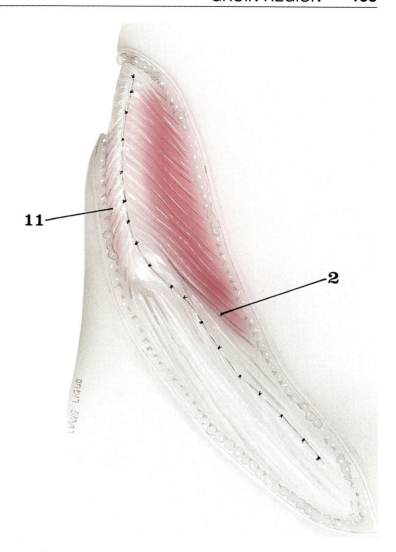

ILIAC OSTEOCUTANEOUS FLAP (Based on the Deep Circumflex Iliac Artery)

(Fig. 5-36) The axial line of the skin flap is placed along the upper border of the anterior part of the iliac crest. The largest skin area reported for this osteocutaneous flap is 20 × 16 cm.

1. External iliac a. and v.
2. DCIA
3. Inguinal ligament
4. Iliacus m.
5. Iliac bone
6. Glutei m. and TFL m.
7. Fringe of three layers of abdominal m.

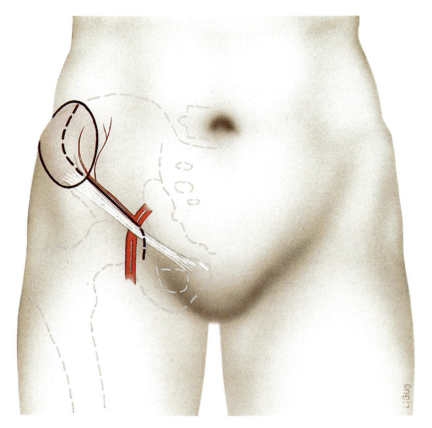

(Fig. 5-37) An anterolateral view of the flap design.

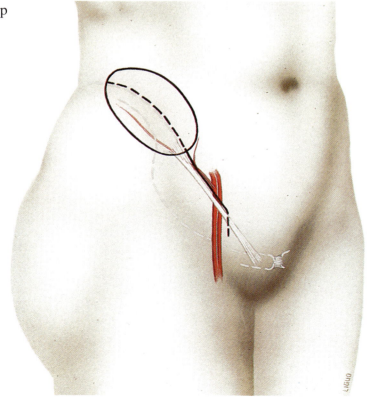

(Fig. 5-38) The vascular pedicle of the DCIA [2] in the inguinal region is dissected as previously described. The upper border of the skin flap is incised. The three layers of the abdominal muscle [7] are divided, leaving a 2 to 3 cm fringe with the skin flap to attach to the bone. Dividing the transversalis fascia, the continuation of the DCIA in the line of fusion between the iliacus and the transversalis fascia is identified.

1. External iliac a. and v.
2. DCIA
3. Inguinal ligament
4. Iliacus m.
5. Iliac bone
7. Fringe of three layers of abdominal m.

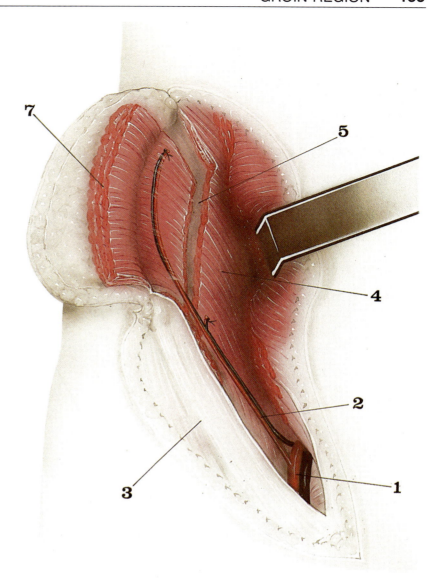

(Fig. 5-39) The lower border of the skin flap is incised. The TFL and gluteal muscles [6] are detached from the ilium [5].

5. Iliac bone
6. Glutei m. and TFL m.

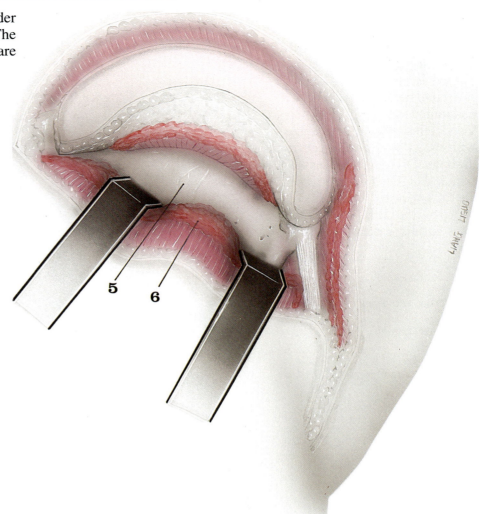

(Fig. 5-40) The required segment of the ilium [5] is divided and the osteocutaneous flap is raised.

2. DCIA
5. Iliac bone
7. Fringe of three layers of abdominal m.

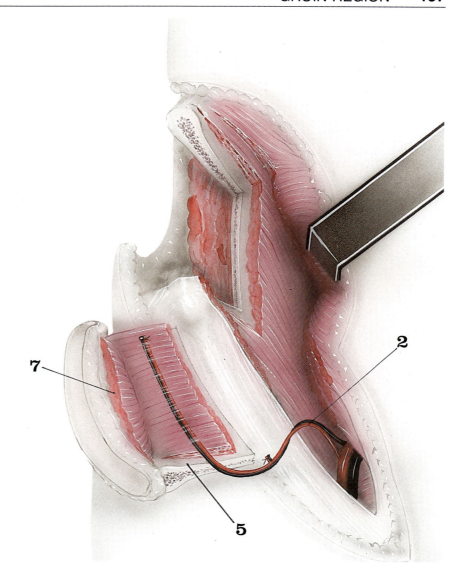

(**Fig. 5-41**) Clinically, the inner table alone is used for the iliac osteocutaneous flap.

1. External iliac a. and v.
2. DCIA
5. Iliac bone
7. Fringe of three layers of abdominal m.

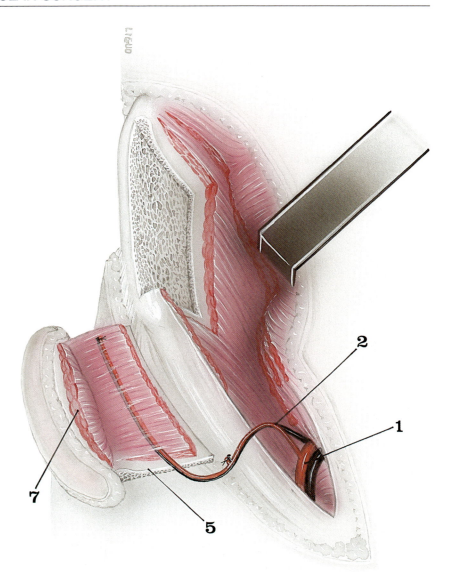

INTERNAL OBLIQUE FLAP

Anatomy (Fig. 5-42)

The origins of the muscle are the lateral half of the inguinal ligament, the anterior iliac crest, and the lumbodorsal fascia. Insertion includes the costal cartilage of the lower three or four ribs, the rectus sheath, and the pubis. The shape of the muscle is broad and flat, and its functions include compression of the abdominal contents. Innervation is segmentally from the VIIIth to XIIth intercostal, iliohypogastric, and ilioinguinal nerves.

Blood Supply

The DCIA [3] (see section on vascularized iliac bone graft) gives off an ascending branch [5], usually at a point 1 cm medial to the ASIS. After piercing the transversus muscle, the branch ascends between it and the internal oblique muscle [1], eventually to anastomose with the inferior epigastric artery. The ascending branch is often more than 1 mm in diameter. (For variations of this branch, also see the section on the vascularized iliac bone graft.)

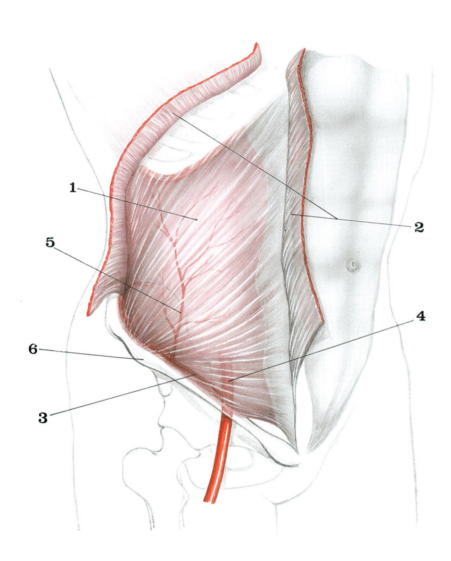

1. Internal oblique m.
2. External oblique m.
3. DCIA
4. External iliac a.
5. Ascending branch
6. Anterior superior iliac spine

COMMENT AND INSIGHTS

This flap provides a thin and broad muscle, with a thickness of 0.5 to 1.0 cm and a maximum dimension of 10 × 15 cm reported. Since the DCIA and its ascending branch are anatomically constant, length and diameter of the vascular pedicle are quite adequate for microvascular anastomosis. The procedure is thus very reliable and safe. The ascending branch has no cutaneous blood supply and cannot be used in a myocutaneous flap; however, by combining the DCIA vessels, the iliac bone can be combined with its overlying skin in an iliac osteocutaneous flap. All donor sites can be closed primarily, and the scar is inconspicuous and acceptable.

Sequelae to use of this flap include the potential for abdominal wall weakness or herniation. Also, this muscle flap cannot be transferred for functional repair, because of its segmental innervation.

Internal Oblique Muscle Flap

(**Fig. 5-43**) An incision is made above and parallel to the lateral two thirds of the inguinal ligament, extending for a short distance toward the tip of the scapula.

1. External oblique m.
2. Internal oblique m.
3. Transversus abdominis m.
4. DCIA
5. Ascending branch
6. Anterior superior iliac spine
7. External iliac a. and v.

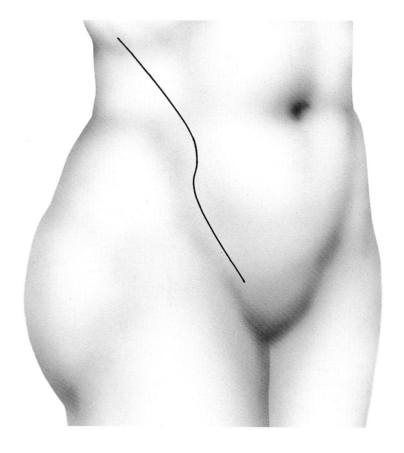

(Fig. 5-44) The external oblique aponeurosis and muscle [1] are incised to expose the internal oblique muscle [2].

1. External oblique m.
2. Internal oblique m.
6. Anterior superior iliac spine

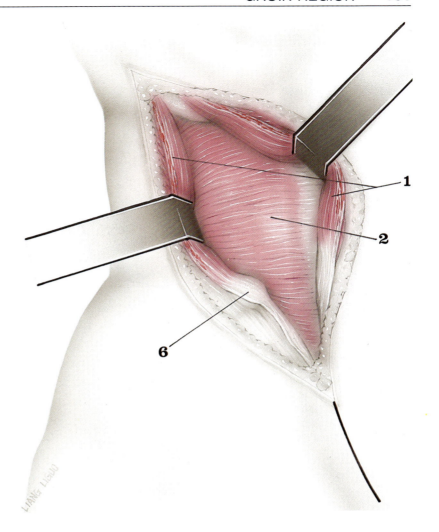

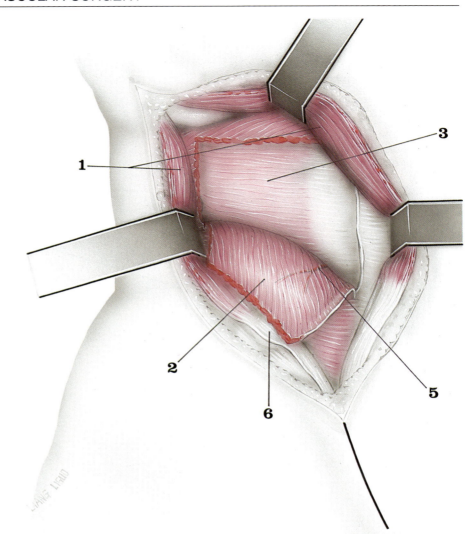

(Fig. 5-45) The internal oblique muscle [2] is divided transversely, just below the costal margin and elevated by dissection in a plane between it and the transversus abdominis muscle [3].

The ascending branch [5] is identified on the undersurface of the internal oblique muscle [2]; this is then detached from the rectus sheath, freeing the muscle from the transversus abdominis and leaving the ascending branch [5] attached to the undersurface of the muscle.

1. External oblique m.
2. Internal oblique m.
3. Transversus abdominis m.
5. Ascending branch
6. Anterior superior iliac spine

(**Fig. 5-46**) The internal oblique muscle is detached from the iliac crest, and the ascending branch [5] is traced to identify the DCIA [4] that lies in a sheath formed by the junction of the transversalis and iliacus fascia. (This can be dissected following the procedure described in the section on vascularized iliac bone graft.)

The distal continuation of the DCIA is ligated and the muscle flap is raised, with a pedicle length of 6 to 7 cm.

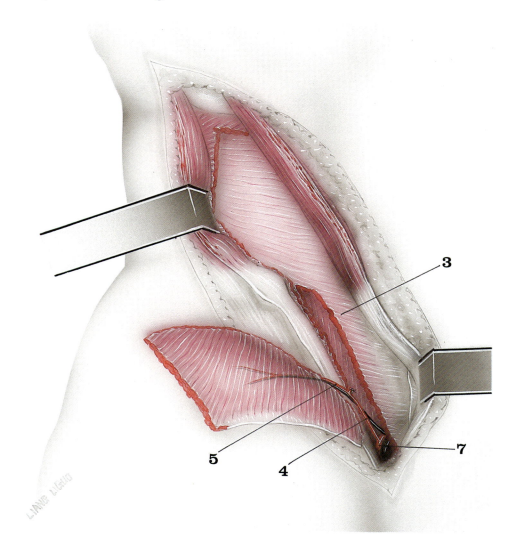

3. Transversus abdominis m.
4. DCIA
5. Ascending branch
7. External iliac a. and v.

Internal Oblique Osteomuscular Flap

(**Fig. 5-47**) A combination of muscle flap with vascularized iliac bone [6] can be designed for particular clinical purposes by utilizing the DCIA [4] and its supply, as well.

4. DCIA
5. Ascending branch
6. Anterior superior iliac spine
7. External iliac a. and v.

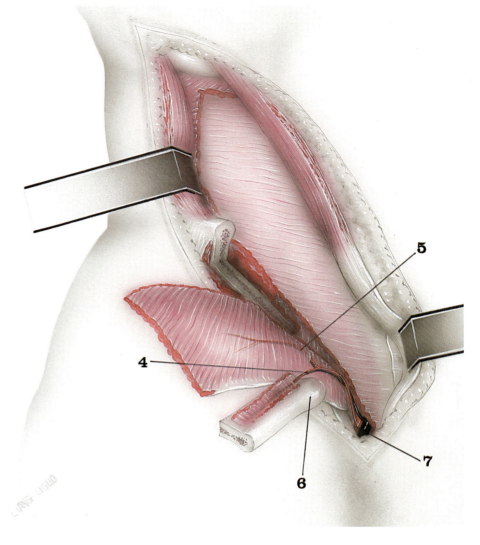

BIBLIOGRAPHY

Franklin JD, Shack RB, Stone JD, et al: Single-stage reconstruction of mandible and soft tissue defects using a free osteocutaneous groin flap. Am J Surg 140:492, 1980.

Huang G-K, Hu R-Q, Hua M, et al: Microvascular free transfer of iliac bone based on the deep superior branches of the superior gluteal vessels. Plast Reconstr Surg 75:68, 1985.

McCrabb DJ: The prevention of hernia and numbness of the thigh following deep circumflex iliac artery free groin flap. (Letter.) Plast Reconstr Surg 65:477, 1980.

Mialhe C, Brice M: A new compound osteo-myocutaneous free flap: The posterior iliac artery flap. Br J Plast Surg 38:30, 1985.

Ramasastry SS, Granick MS, Futrell JW: Clinical anatomy of the internal oblique muscle. J Reconstr Microsurg 2:117, 1986.

Ramasastry SS, Tucker JB, Swartz WM, Hurwitz DJ: The internal oblique muscle flap: An anatomic and clinical study. Plast Reconstr Surg 73:721, 1984.

Sattoh T, Tsuchiya M, Harii K: A vascularised iliac musculo-periosteal free flap transfer: A case report. Br J Plast Surg 36:109, 1983.

Taylor GI, Corlett RJ: Microvascular free transfer of a compound deep circumflex groin and iliac crest flap to the mandible. In: Strauch B, Vasconez LO, Hall-Findlay E (eds): *Grabb's Encyclopedia of Flaps*, vol. I. Boston: Little, Brown, 1990, p. 589.

Taylor GI, Corlett RJ: Microvascular free transfer of a compound deep circumflex groin and iliac crest flap to the upper extremity. In: Strauch B, Vasconez

LO, Hall-Findlay E (eds): *Grabb's Encyclopedia of Flaps,* vol. II. Boston: Little, Brown, 1990, p. 1197.

Taylor GI, Corlett RJ: Microvascular transfer of a compound deep circumflex groin and iliac crest flap. In: Strauch B, Vasconez LO, Hall-Findlay E: *Grabb's Encyclopedia of Flaps,* vol. III. Boston: Little, Brown, 1990, p. 1786.

Taylor GI, Townsend P, Corlett R: Superiority of the deep circumflex iliac vessels as the supply for free groin flaps. Plast Reconstr Surg 64:595, 1979.

Taylor GI, Townsend P, Corlett R: Superiority of the deep circumflex iliac vessels as the supply for free groin flaps: Clinical work. Plast Reconstr Surg 64:745, 1979.

Urken ML, Vickery C, Weinberg H, et al: The internal oblique-iliac crest osseomyocutaneous microvascular free flap in head and neck reconstruction. J Reconstr Microsurg 5:203, 1989.

6 THIGH REGION

Gracilis Flap

Anatomy (**Fig. 6-1**)

The origin of the gracilis muscle [1] is the body of the pubis and its inferior ramus, and the adjacent ramus of the ischium. Insertion is at the medial upper surface of the tibia below the condyle. The muscle functions as an accessory adductor of the thigh and flexor of the leg.

This is a thin, flat, strap-shaped muscle, broad above and narrow and tapering below. Its total length is 42 cm (muscle belly, 32 cm; tendon portion, 10 cm). Average width and thickness are 4 and 1 cm, respectively.

Blood Supply

The dominant nutrient vessels [8] arise mostly from the profunda femoris vessels [7], and occasionally from the medial circumflex femoris vessels. They pass inferomedially between the adductor longus [3] and brevis, and enter the upper third of the muscle, approximately 8 to 10 cm below the pubic tubercle.

Although there are several additional branches from the femoral vessels to the distal portion of the muscle, the dominant vessels alone can nourish the entire muscle belly, but they barely supply the distal third of overlying skin.

There are commonly two venae comitantes.

Innervation

The anterior branch of the obturator nerve runs between the adductor longus and brevis and divides into the motor and sensory nerves in the vicinity of the main vascular pedicle. The motor nerve enters the muscle with the vessels and bifurcates into two branches, while the sensory nerve descends, then crosses the gracilis muscle at its central part to serve the skin.

		Diameter (mm)	Length (cm) (from Origin to Entrance)
Dominant	A	1.2–1.8	6.0
	V	1.5–2.0	
Anterior branch of obturator nerve		1.0–2.0	5.0

THIGH REGION

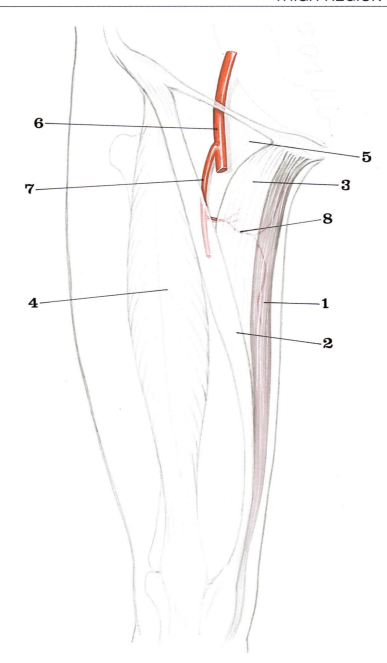

1. Gracilis m.
2. Sartorius m.
3. Adductor longus m.
4. Rectus femoris m.
5. Pectineus m.
6. Femoral a.
7. Deep femoral a.
8. Branch to the gracilis

COMMENT AND INSIGHTS

Despite the fact that the origin of the dominant artery varies occasionally, its course and entrance into the muscle are anatomically consistent. It can be easily elevated and reliably transferred, with adequate vessel diameter. The gracilis therefore remains one of the most useful muscles in microvascular repair.

The donor site provides a thin, strap-shaped functional muscle of medium size, especially suitable for functional reconstruction in the forearm.

The distal third of skin overlying the gracilis does not receive sufficient blood supply from the muscle. Only the upper two thirds of overlying skin can be used as a component in the musculocutaneous flap.

In addition to motor function, the anterior branch of the obturator nerve also supplies sensibility to the overlying skin and, a few months postoperatively, the musculocutaneous flap may have fair pressure and touch sensibility; however, sensation is not always good.

The donor defect can always be closed directly, and the linear scar on the medial aspect of the thigh does not present serious cosmetic problems. Nor does the loss of the gracilis produce any obvious morbidity.

Splitting the muscle longitudinally will allow for the possibility of differential contraction or the ability to harvest small segments for facial reanimation.

GRACILIS MUSCLE FLAP

(Fig. 6-2) The patient is placed in a supine position with the thigh abducted.

The anterior border of the gracilis muscle [1] corresponds to a line drawn between the posterior border of the tendon of the adductor longus [2] at the pubic tubercle, and the distal end of the incision *may* extend over the tendon of the semitendinosus muscle [9]. Usually, the incision is placed over the proximal 10 cm of the line; a second incision may be based distally, if the entire muscle is to be harvested. The position of the dominant vessels is marked 8 cm below the pubic tubercle.

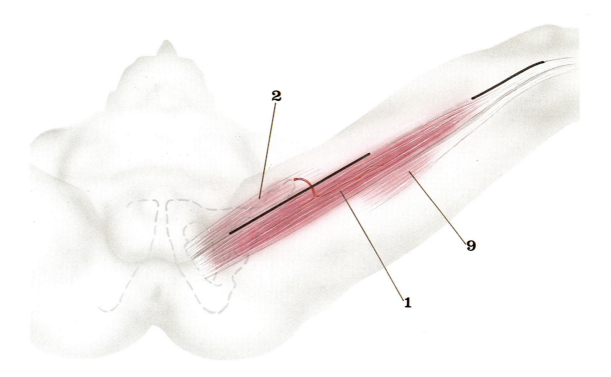

1. Gracilis m.
2. Adductor longus m.
3. Adductor brevis m.
4. Adductor magnus m.
5. Branch from deep femoral a. and v.
6. Anterior branch of obturator n.
7. Semimembranosus m.
8. Sartorius m.
9. Semitendinosus m.

(Fig. 6-3) At the first incision, the fascia over the adductor longus [2] and gracilis [1] is divided to identify its interspace. After retracting the adductor longus [2] laterally, the dominant vascular pedicle [5] and the anterior branch of the obturator nerve [6] can easily be found on the anterior surface of the adductor brevis [3], near the predicted point marked previously.

1. Gracilis m.
2. Adductor longus m.
3. Adductor brevis m.
4. Adductor magnus m.
5. Branch from deep femoral a. and v.
6. Anterior branch of obturator n.

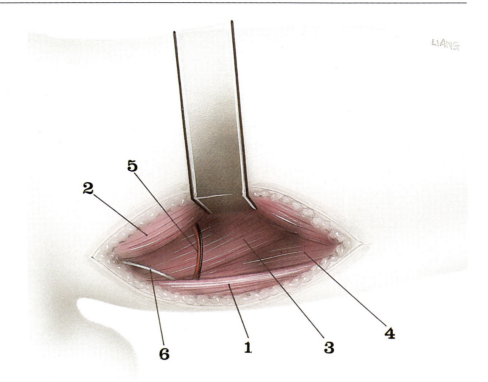

(**Fig. 6-4**) At the second incision, the distal musculotendinous portion of the gracilis muscle [1] will lie between the sartorius [8] anteriorly and the semimembranosus [7] posteriorly. After further verification by traction, the distal portion of the gracilis [1] is divided and bluntly dissected proximally from surrounding tissue, ligating the small branches from the femoral vessels.

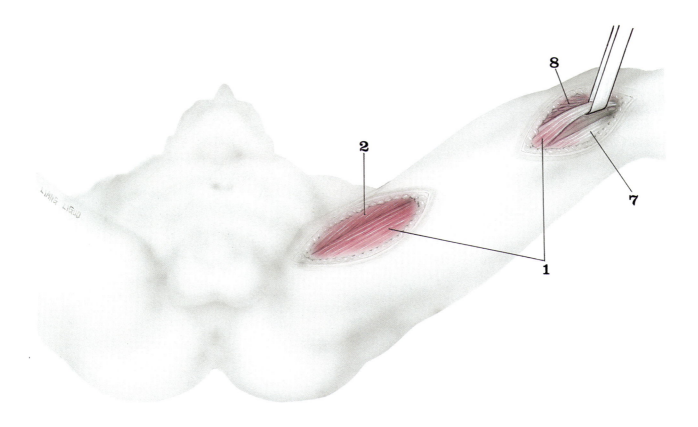

1. Gracilis m.
2. Adductor longus m.
7. Semimembranosus m.
8. Sartorius m.

(**Fig. 6-5**) The distal portion of the gracilis [1] is drawn into the proximal incision through a subcutaneous tunnel, and the origin of the gracilis is detached. The dominant pedicle [5] can be dissected toward its origin, to obtain as long a pedicle as possible.

1. Gracilis m.
2. Adductor longus m.
3. Adductor brevis m.
4. Adductor magnus m.
5. Branch from deep femoral a. and v.
6. Anterior branch of obturator n.

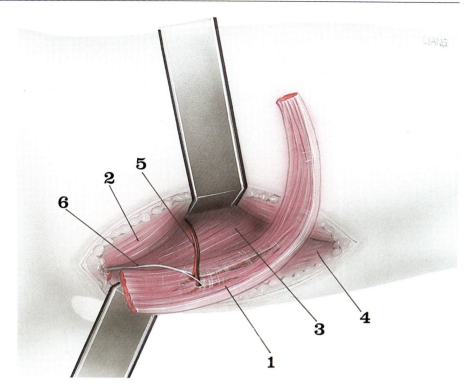

GRACILIS MYOCUTANEOUS FLAP

(**Fig. 6-6**) A line is drawn to serve as the anterior border of the gracilis, as mentioned previously. The anterior perimeter of the skin flap can extend 2 or 3 cm beyond the line, and the posterior limitation is 6 to 9 cm beyond. The skin flap should be centered over the gracilis muscle. However, the skin over the distal third of the gracilis is not supplied from the underlying muscle, and it should be excluded from the flap. Maximal reported flap size is 11 × 27 cm. In patients with very lax or redundant skin, this skin paddle is *not* reliable.

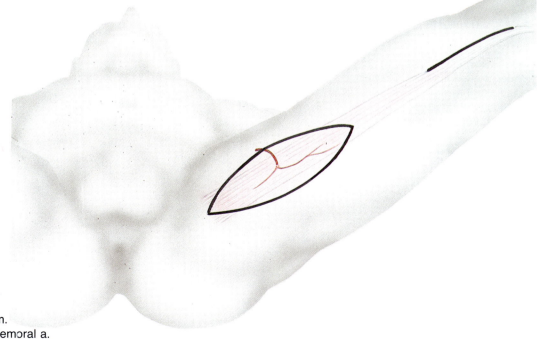

1. Gracilis m.
2. Adductor longus m.
3. Adductor brevis m.
4. Adductor magnus m.
5. Branch from deep femoral a. and v.
6. Anterior branch of obturator n.
7. Semimembranosus m.
8. Sartorius m.

172 ATLAS OF MICROVASCULAR SURGERY

(**Fig. 6-7**) In the procedure to raise the muscle flap, the proximal anterior margin of the skin flap is incised to expose the dominant vessels [5] and nerve. Under traction of the distal muscle portion [1], the skin territory can be accurately outlined.

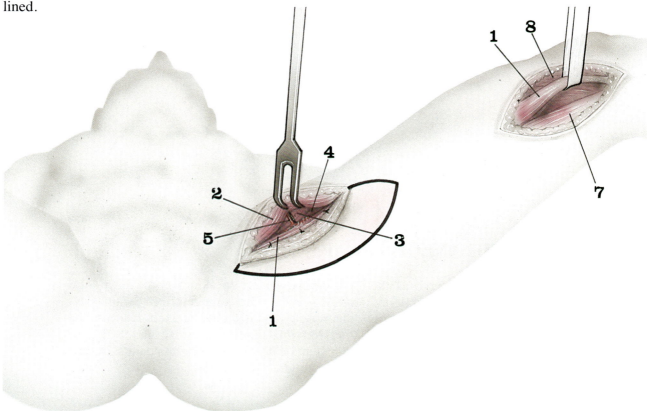

1. Gracilis m.
2. Adductor longus m.
3. Adductor brevis m.
4. Adductor magnus m.
5. Branch from deep femoral a. and v.
7. Semimembranosus m.
8. Sartorius m.

(**Fig. 6-8**) All the skin margins of the flap are incised and the muscle is divided proximally and distally. Several tacking stitches should be used in this procedure.

The musculocutaneous flap is elevated, based on the dominant neurovascular pedicle [5,6].

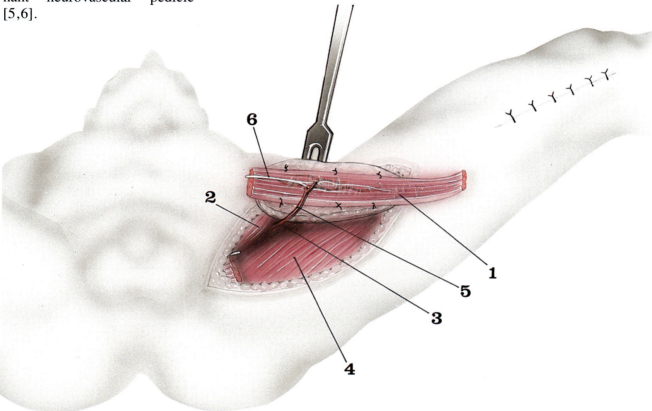

1. Gracilis m.
2. Adductor longus m.
3. Adductor brevis m.
4. Adductor magnus m.
5. Branch from deep femoral a. and v.
6. Anterior branch of obturator n.

Tensor Fascia Lata Flap

Anatomy (Fig. 6-9)

The origin is the anterior 5 cm of the outer lip of the iliac crest and anterior superior iliac spine (ASIS). Insertion is at the iliotibial band at a level a little below the greater trochanter; the iliotibial band is in turn attached below to the lateral condyle of the tibia. The main function of the muscle is as an accessory flexor and medial rotator of the thigh. The muscle is small, broad, flat, and fish-shaped. The average length is 17 cm, width is 5 cm, and thickness is 1.5 cm.

Blood Supply

The lateral circumflex femoral artery [6] commonly arises from the lateral side of the profunda femoris artery [5], passes laterally between the divisions of the femoral nerve behind the sartorius and rectus femoris muscles [3,2], and divides into three major branches.

The ascending branch is the dominant pedicle to the tensor fascia lata (TFL) [7,1]. It passes up between the rectus femoris and vastus lateralis muscles to reach the TFL approximately 8 cm below the ASIS. Immediately before entering the muscle, this branch divides into superior, middle, and inferior twigs. The superior twig feeds the upper muscle and a segment of iliac crest; the middle twig nourishes the main belly of the muscle; and the inferior twig supplies the distal fascia lata and an extensive skin territory of the thigh.

There are five to seven musculocutaneous perforators from the muscle into the overlying skin and iliac crest, and the lower perforator runs longitudinally above the fascia to supply the cutaneous territory over the distal iliotibial band.

	Diameter (mm)		Length of Vascular Pedicle (cm)
	A	V	
Ascending branch (after descending branch)	1.1 0.8–1.5	1.3 0.7–2.0	4–5
Lateral femoral circumflex vessel (at its origin)	1.5–2.5	2.5–4.0	10 (by ligating the descending branch)

There are commonly two venae comitantes.

Innervation

Motor. The inferior branch of the superior gluteal nerve courses between the gluteus medius and minimus, entering the undersurface of the TFL near the vascular pedicle.

Sensory. The branch of T12 pierces the external oblique muscle just above the iliac crest in the anterior axillary line, innervating the upper third of the skin flap.

The lateral cutaneous nerve of the thigh emerges 1 to 2 cm inferomedial to the ASIS and runs over the sartorius, piercing the deep fascia, to supply the distal two thirds of the anterolateral aspect of the thigh.

	Diameter (mm)
Cutaneous branch of T12	0.5–2.0
Lateral cutaneous nerve of thigh	2.0–3.0
Inferior branch of superior gluteal nerve	0.5–2.0

THIGH REGION

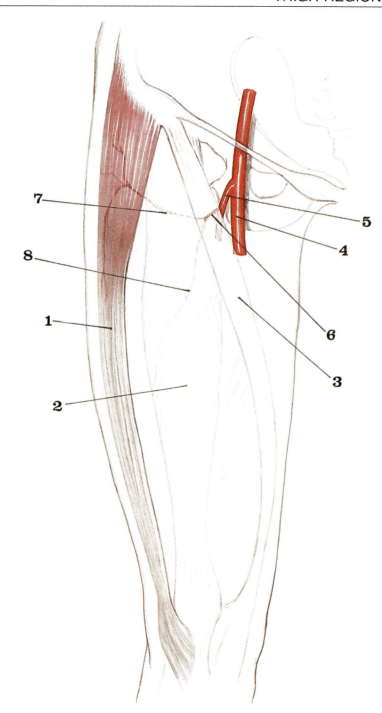

1. Tensor fascia lata
2. Rectus femoris m.
3. Sartorius m.
4. Femoral a.
5. Deep femoral a.
6. Lateral circumflex femoral a.
7. Ascending branch
8. Descending branch

COMMENT AND INSIGHTS

This flap is one of the most reliable and commonly acceptable myocutaneous flaps, because of its constant anatomy and the adequate length and diameter of the vascular pedicle. Even though the tensor fascia lata muscle itself is quite small, its musculocutaneous perforators can nourish almost all the skin of the anterolateral thigh, providing an enormous skin territory. The flap under discussion is a sensory myocutaneous flap and has been widely applied clinically, but it has not been reported as a functional muscular flap.

The widest donor defect that can be closed primarily is about 6 cm, and wider flaps require skin grafting. Any overtight closure may result in a compartment syndrome.

The TFL muscle is expendable and not of primary functional importance. There is minimal donor site morbidity postoperatively. The donor scar may cause some cosmetic problems.

The entrance of the vascular pedicle is located at the center of the undersurface of the muscle; this should be considered during flap design so that the recipient defect and vessels can be adequately matched. Also of some significance is the fact that the proximal part of the flap is thicker, and the distal part somewhat thinner.

Caution needs to be advised, since the distal skin paddle may be unreliable, if extended too far. A safer limit is advised in this chapter.

TENSOR FASCIA LATA MYOCUTANEOUS FLAP

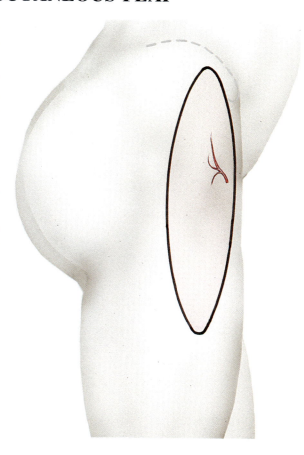

(Fig. 6-10) In the surface anatomy of the muscle, its anterior border corresponds to a line between the ASIS and the lateral edge of the patella. Its posterior border is a line from the iliac crest 5 cm posterior to the ASIS through the anterior edge of the greater trochanter to the lateral condyle of the femur.

Its skin territory can be harvested to a size as large as 20 × 30 cm, three times the size of the muscle. The superior border can exceed the iliac crest for a few centimeters, the inferior border can reach a level 15 cm above the knee, and the anterior and posterior borders can be extended for at least 2 cm on either side of the muscle.

The vascular pedicle is marked on the anterior border of the muscle 8 cm below the ASIS.

1. TFL
2. Rectus femoris m.
3. Vastus lateralis m.
4. Ascending branch
5. Iliotibial band
6. Lateral cutaneous n. of thigh
7. Cutaneous branch of T12 n.
8. Glutei m.
9. Iliac bone

(**Fig. 6-11**) Flap elevation begins from distal to proximal subfascially to raise the fascia lata with the skin flap. Several tacking stitches are applied to protect the musculocutaneous perforator. The vascular pedicle [4] is visualized on the undersurface, about 8 cm below the ASIS.

1. TFL
2. Rectus femoris m.
3. Vastus lateralis m.
4. Ascending branch
5. Iliotibial band

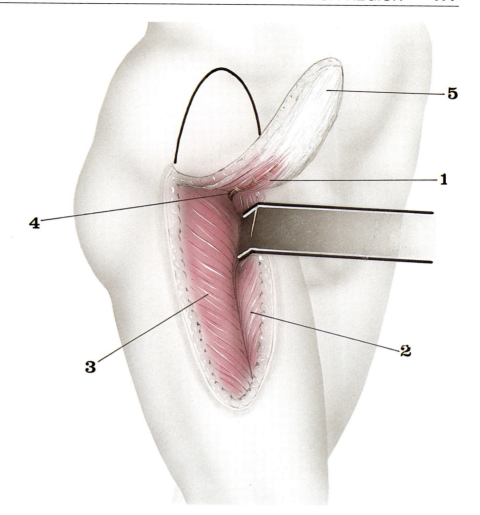

178 ATLAS OF MICROVASCULAR SURGERY

(**Fig. 6-12**) If a sensory flap is required, the cutaneous branch of T12 [7] is identified above the iliac crest in the anterior axillary line, and the lateral cutaneous nerve of the thigh [6] is dissected at a point 1 to 2 cm inferomedial to the ASIS. For a functional musculocutaneous flap, the inferior branch of the superior gluteal nerve should be carefully sought out at the posterior border of the muscle, 4 to 5 cm below the iliac crest.

6. Lateral cutaneous n. of thigh
7. Cutaneous branch of T12 n.

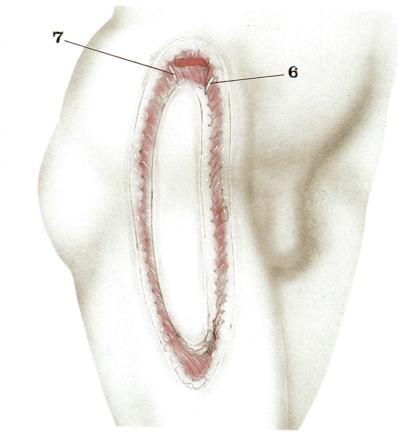

(**Fig. 6-13**) The vascular pedicle [4] is dissected by medial retraction of the rectus femoris [2].

The muscle [1] is detached, dividing all the nerves to the TFL with markers. The musculocutaneous flap is raised based on the ascending branch [4] of the lateral circumflex femoral artery. This can be dissected further to obtain a pedicle as long as 10 cm by ligating all the branches, including the descending branch. During the dissection of the pedicle, care should be taken deep to the rectus femoris [2] where the vessel is intimately related to the muscular branches of the femoral nerve.

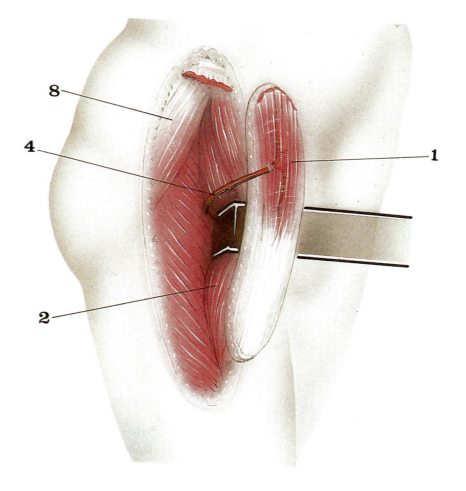

1. TFL
2. Rectus femoris m.
4. Ascending branch
8. Glutei m.

TENSOR FASCIA LATA OSTEOMYOCUTANEOUS FLAP

(Fig. 6-14) An anterior segment of the iliac crest [9], connected with the origin of the TFL and adjacent tissue, can be taken with the flap as a vascularized bone graft.

8. Glutei m.
9. Iliac bone

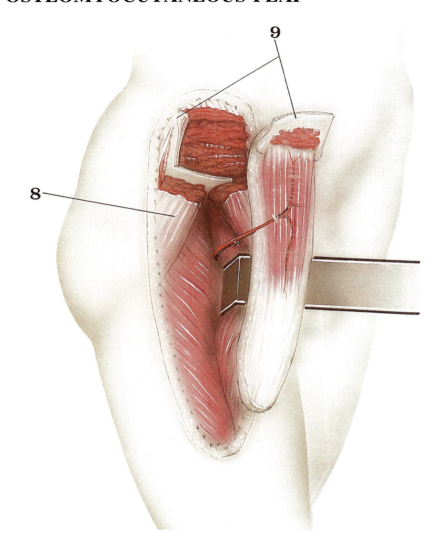

Rectus Femoris Flap

Anatomy (Fig. 6-15)

The origin of the muscle [6] is the anterior inferior iliac spine and the groove above the acetabulum. Insertion is in the upper border of the patella as a central portion of the quadriceps tendon. The muscle is fusiform and bipennate in shape. Its complete length is 36 cm (muscle belly, 30 cm), its thickness is 1.5 cm, and its width is 5.5 cm. The function of the muscle is leg extension and thigh flexion.

Blood Supply

The dominant blood supply usually comes from the descending branch [4] of the lateral circumflex femoral artery [3]. There is a double grouping of the neurovascular bundle, which enters the posterior surface of the muscle 10 and 15 cm below the anterior superior iliac spine, respectively. Each group has two venae comitantes. The length of the pedicle is approximately 4 cm.

Innervation

There are two motor branches from the femoral nerve that enter the muscle, accompanying the vascular pedicle.

			Diameter (mm)	Length of Pedicle (cm)
Group 1	Artery		1.5	
	Veins	1	0.7	3–4
		2	0.7	
	Nerve		1.0	10–12
Group 2	Artery		2.0	
	Veins	1	1.2	3–4
		2	0.5	
	Nerve		1.0	10–12
Descending branch of lateral circumflex femoral a.	Artery		2.5	
	Vein		3.4	

THIGH REGION

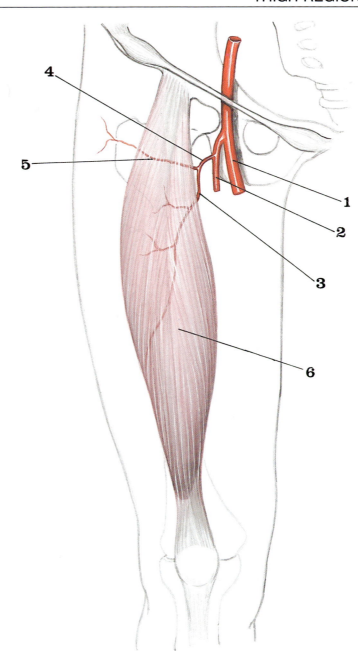

1. Femoral a.
2. Deep femoral a.
3. Lateral circumflex femoral a.
4. Descending branch
5. Ascending branch
6. Rectus femoris m.

COMMENT AND INSIGHTS

The neurovascular anatomy of the rectus femoris is consistent and its vessel diameter adequate for microsurgical transfer in functional reconstruction or wound coverage. Compared with other muscle flaps, the rectus femoris, as a strong portion of the quadriceps, has an important function. Removal of the muscle will decrease the strength of knee extension, especially in the last twenty degrees.

RECTUS FEMORIS MUSCLE FLAP

(**Fig. 6-16**) The incision for harvesting the muscle flap is made in an S-shaped fashion along a line drawn from the anterior superior iliac spine to the midpoint of the upper border of the patella.

1. Rectus femoris m.
2. Sartorius m.
3. TFL
4. Descending branch
5. Lateral circumflex femoral a.
6. Deep femoral a.
7. Femoral n.
8. Vastus intermedialis m.

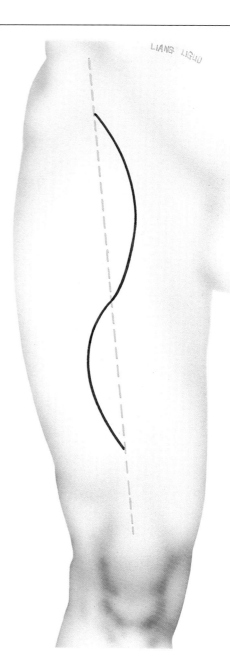

(Fig. 6-17) The medial and lateral borders of the rectus femoris [1] are exposed at the lower part of the muscle. Retracting the sartorius [2] medially, the lateral circumflex femoral vessels [5] and their descending branch [4] are identified about 10 cm below the anterior superior iliac spine.

1. Rectus femoris m.
2. Sartorius m.
3. TFL
4. Descending branch
5. Lateral circumflex femoral a.
6. Deep femoral a.
7. Femoral n.

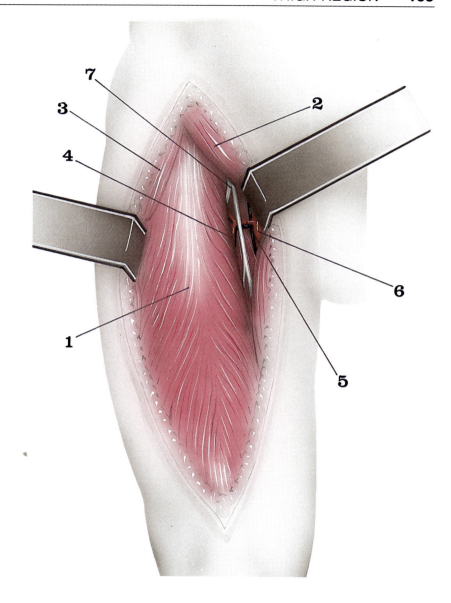

(Fig. 6-18) The muscle [1] is separated from the vastus lateralis intermedialis and medialis, ligating the branches to these muscles. The vascular pedicle [5] and muscular branches of the femoral nerve are further identified and dissected. The muscle is then isolated on its pedicle [5], after detaching its origin and insertion.

1. Rectus femoris m.
5. Lateral circumflex femoral a.
7. Femoral n.
8. Vastus intermedialis m.

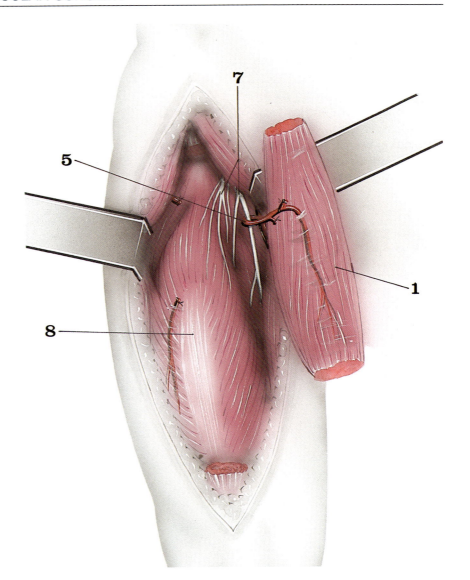

RECTUS FEMORIS MYOCUTANEOUS FLAP

(Fig. 6-19) A line is drawn from the anterior superior iliac spine to the midpoint of the upper border of the patella, as an axis of the musculocutaneous flap. The skin territory is limited to the area between the sartorius and TFL at the upper third. The flap can measure as much as 10 cm in width by 30 cm in length, but the lower third is less reliable.

1. Rectus femoris m.
2. Sartorius m.
3. TFL
4. Descending branch
5. Lateral circumflex femoral a.
6. Deep femoral a.
7. Femoral n.
8. Vastus intermedialis m.

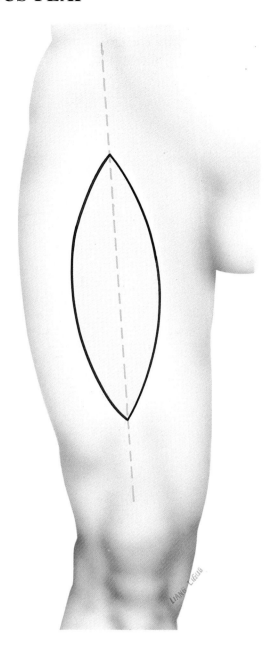

(Fig. 6-20) Keeping the skin territory intact with tacking stitches, the musculocutaneous flap [1] is raised, based on its neurovascular pedicle [5]. The procedure then follows that of the muscle flap described before.

1. Rectus femoris m.
2. Sartorius m.
5. Lateral circumflex femoral a.
7. Femoral n.

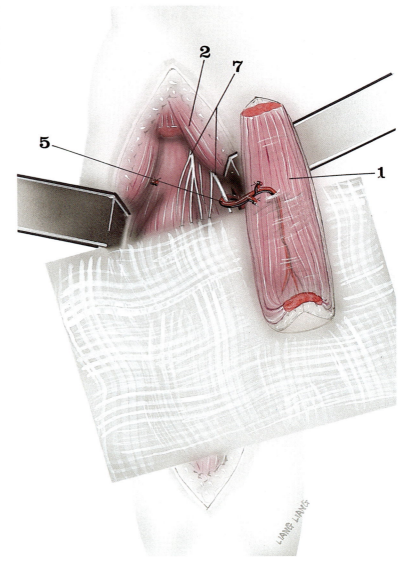

Thigh Skin Flaps

MEDIAL THIGH FLAP

Anatomy (Fig. 6-21)

An unnamed branch [7] arises from the medial aspect of the superficial femoral artery [6], just proximal to the adductor canal [5] at the apex of the femoral triangle that is formed by the medial borders of the sartorius [1] and adductor longus [2], and inguinal ligament. The branch continues as a cutaneous artery, emerging near the apex of the femoral triangle to supply the skin of the medial thigh. The diameter at its origin is 2.0 to 4.0 mm, and its venae comitantes provide venous drainage.

Innervation

The medial femoral cutaneous nerve runs from the femoral nerve, crossing superficially to the femoral vessels at the apex of the femoral triangle.

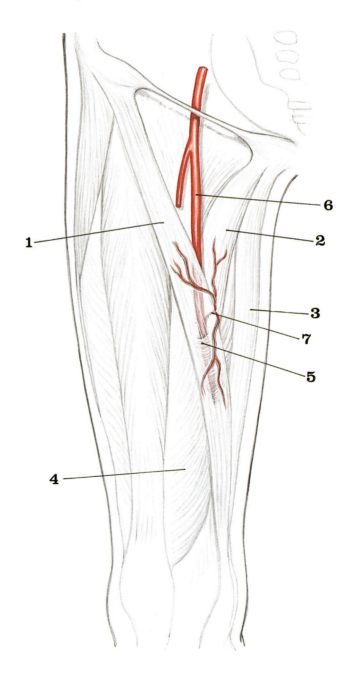

COMMENT AND INSIGHTS

Experience with this flap is limited, and cadaver dissection of these vessels is recommended prior to clinical application.

The skin of the medial thigh is generally uniformly thin and hairless, and it could be provided with sensibility through the medial femoral cutaneous nerve. Therefore this flap can be considered for use in the reconstruction of the head, neck, and hand.

The common size of this flap is reported as about 6 × 12 cm, and the donor defect could be closed primarily. Donor site morbidity is minimal, but a resulting linear scar or skin graft may create some cosmetic problems in females.

Harvesting Technique

(Fig. 6-22) The course of the superficial femoral artery is traced from the midpoint of the inguinal ligament to the adductor tubercle. The vascular pedicle is marked on the apex of the femoral triangle approximately at the midpoint of the line, and the upper border of the flap is placed at the level of this apex. Flap outline is in the medial aspect of the thigh, and its area has been reported as 6 × 12 cm.

1. Sartorius m.
2. Adductor longus m.
3. Adductor magnus m.
4. Adductor canal
5. Femoral a. and v.
6. Medial femoral cutaneous n.
7. Unnamed a. and v.
8. Vastus medialis m.
9. Gracilis m.

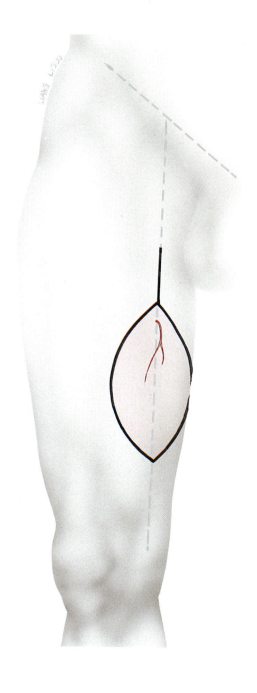

(**Fig. 6-23**) A straight incision is made at the proximal course of the femoral artery, and the femoral vessel [5] is identified, dissected, and traced toward the adductor canal [4]. Retracting the sartorius [1] laterally, the unnamed vascular pedicle [7] is located just proximal to the adductor canal. The branch to the sartorius is ligated. The medial femoral cutaneous nerve [6] appears superficial to the femoral vessels, if a sensory flap is desired.

1. Sartorius m.
2. Adductor longus m.
3. Adductor magnus m.
4. Adductor canal
5. Femoral a. and v.
6. Medial femoral cutaneous n.
7. Unnamed a. and v.

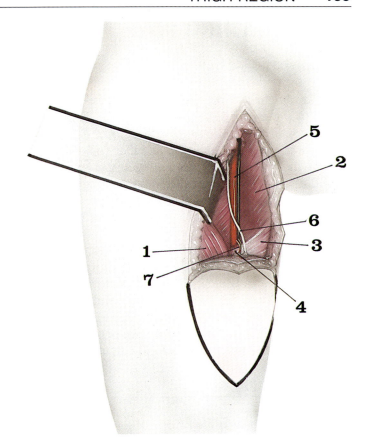

(**Fig. 6-24**) The medial thigh flap, based on the unnamed vascular pedicle [7], is raised from the deep fascia, leaving the saphenous vein intact. The average length of the vascular pedicle of medial thigh flaps is 5 cm.

5. Femoral a. and v.
6. Medial femoral cutaneous n.
7. Unnamed a. and v.
8. Vastus medialis m.
9. Gracilis m.

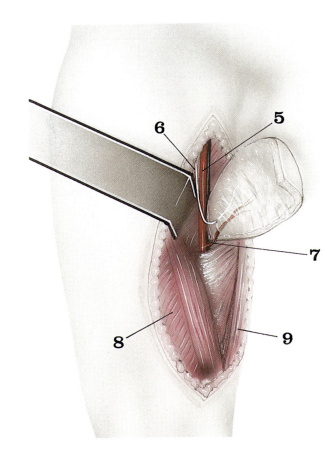

LATERAL THIGH FLAP

Anatomy (Fig. 6-25)

This flap is based on the third perforating branch of the profunda femoris artery [1]. The vessel arises from the femoral artery about 3.5 cm below the inguinal ligament and then runs in front of the pectineus [9] and adductor brevis [7] and magnus [8] behind the adductor longus [6], near the linea aspera of the femur. It terminates as the fourth perforating artery [5].

The third perforating artery [4] begins below the adductor brevis [7] and pierces the insertion of the adductor magnus [8]. After giving off branches to the muscles, the third perforator traverses between the biceps femoris and the vastus lateralis and then pierces the deep fascia. It then emerges at about the midpoint between the greater trochanter and the lateral epicondyle of the femur.

Vessel Landmarks	Arterial Diameter (mm)
At the piercing of the adductor magnus	3–5
Between the biceps femoris and vastus lateralis	2
At its emergence as a cutaneous branch	1.0–1.5

The venae comitantes terminate in the profunda femoris vein. Occasionally, the cutaneous branch may originate from the superficial femoral branch.

Innervation

Sensibility is provided by the lateral cutaneous nerve of the thigh.

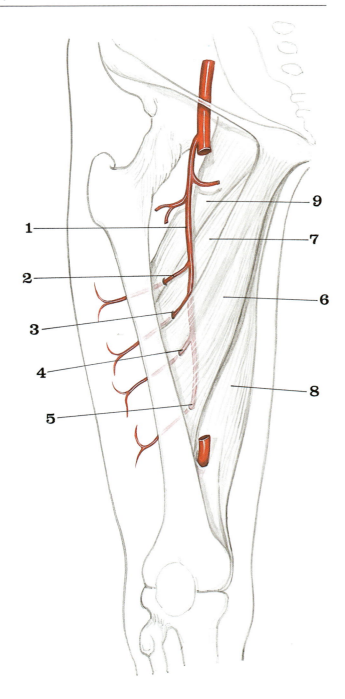

1. Deep femoral a.
2. First perforator
3. Second perforator
4. Third perforator
5. Fourth perforator
6. Adductor longus m.
7. Adductor brevis m.
8. Adductor magnus m.
9. Pectineus m.

COMMENT AND INSIGHTS

There have been several cases of free lateral thigh flaps reported. This flap is a typical septofasciocutaneous flap based on the perforating branches of the deep femoral artery in the lateral septum of the thigh.

The vascular anatomy of the flap is quite constant, and the diameter and length of pedicle vessels are quite enough for anastomosis at the recipient site. If the patient is properly positioned, the harvesting procedure should not be difficult.

Thigh skin is generally uniformly thin, but the skin of the lateral side of the thigh is hairy in males. The flap may be somewhat bulky and stiff because of the thick dermis and fascia lata, if the fascia layer is included in the flap, even though there is less subcutaneous tissue there.

The skin territory of this flap should be quite large, especially when the deep fascia is included. A flap size of 8 × 25 cm has been reported.

Flap sensibility can be provided through the lateral cutaneous nerve of the thigh.

If the width of the flap is less than 8 cm, the donor defect can be closed primarily. Donor site morbidity is minimal, but a resulting linear scar or skin graft may create some cosmetic problems in females.

Harvesting Technique

(Fig. 6-26) The patient is placed in a prone position. As the axis of the flap, a line is drawn from the greater trochanter to the lateral condyle of the femur. This corresponds to the lateral intermuscular septum and the posterior edge of the iliotibial tract. The vascular pedicle of the third perforator is marked at the midpoint of this line. The flap can be adjusted along its axis to suit the siting requirements of the vascular pedicle.

1. Second perforator
2. Third perforator
3. Fourth perforator
4. Iliotibial tract
5. Vastus lateralis m.
6. Short head of biceps femoris m.
7. Long head of biceps femoris m.
8. Deep femoral a.
9. Adductor magnus m.

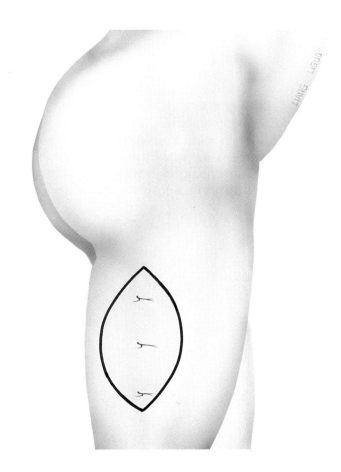

(Fig. 6-27) The anterior part of the flap is elevated toward the lateral intermuscular septum (the axis of the flap). The fascia lata is included or excluded, as desired. The septofasciocutaneous branch of the third perforator [2] is identified, with the second and fourth perforating branches [1,3] appearing about 2 inches cephalic and caudal to it.

1. Second perforator
2. Third perforator
3. Fourth perforator
4. Iliotibial tract
5. Vastus lateralis m.

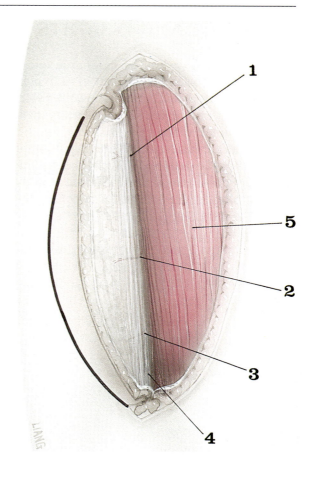

(Fig. 6-28) Retracting the vastus lateralis [5] anteriorly and ligating the muscular branches to the vastus lateralis and biceps femoris [6], the vascular pedicle is dissected toward the linea aspera. The fasciocutaneous branches from the second and fourth perforating branches are then ligated.

2. Third perforator
5. Vastus lateralis m.
6. Short head of biceps femoris m.

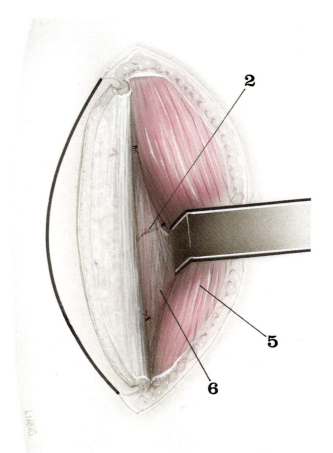

(**Fig. 6-29**) Once the vascular pedicle is isolated, the posterior part of the flap is raised, and the entire flap is isolated on its vascular pedicle. The origin of the short head of the biceps [6] is detached from the femur.

2. Third perforator
5. Vastus lateralis m.
6. Short head of biceps femoris m.
7. Long head of biceps femoris m.

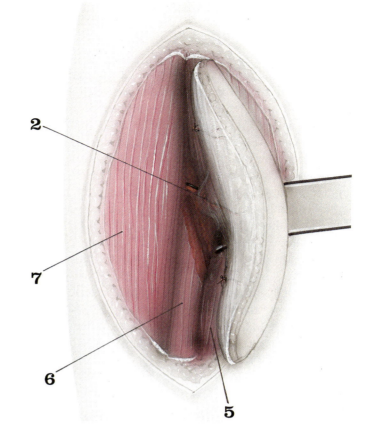

(**Fig. 6-30**) After detaching a part of the origin of the short head of the biceps [6] from the femur around the vascular pedicle and retracting the biceps femoris [7] from the other hamstring muscles, the vascular pedicle of the third perforator [2] can be traced up to the deep femoral vessels [8] by windowing the adductor magnus muscle [9]. The pedicle length can reach 10 cm.

If a sensory flap is required, the lateral cutaneous nerve of the thigh is preserved at the superoanterior edge of the flap.

2. Third perforator
5. Vastus lateralis m.
6. Short head of biceps femoris m.
7. Long head of biceps femoris m.
8. Deep femoral a.
9. Adductor magnus m.

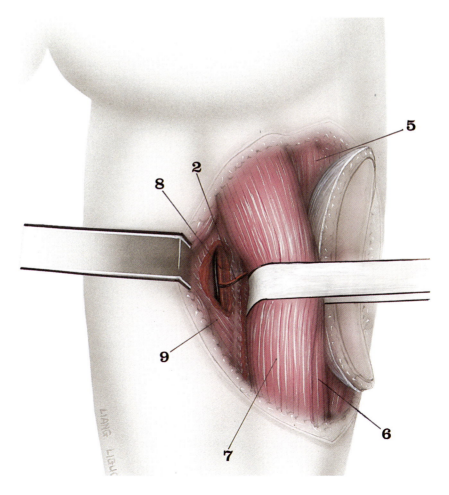

ANTEROLATERAL THIGH FLAP

Anatomy (Fig. 6-31)

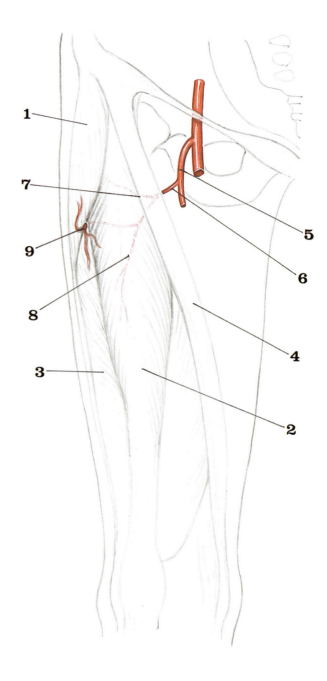

The fasciocutaneous branch [9] that supplies this area of the skin originates from the descending branch [8] of the lateral femoral circumflex artery [6]. The descending branch [8] runs downward between the rectus femoris [2] and vastus lateralis [3], giving off some muscular branches to these two muscles and a fasciocutaneous branch to the skin. The latter branch emerges through the intermuscular space formed by the muscles of the rectus femoris [2], vastus lateralis [3], and TFL [1], at the level of the junction of the upper and middle thirds of the thigh.

There may be accessory cutaneous arteries found above and below the fasciocutaneous branch along the intermuscular space. When a large flap is required, all the branches should be included in the flap.

The descending branch has a diameter of more than 2 mm, and the length of the pedicle can reach 8 cm.

Innervation

Sensibility is provided by the anterior femoral cutaneous and lateral femoral cutaneous nerves.

1. TFL
2. Rectus femoris m.
3. Vastus lateralis m.
4. Sartorius m.
5. Deep femoral a.
6. Lateral femoral circumflex a.
7. Ascending branch
8. Descending branch
9. Fasciocutaneous perforator

COMMENT AND INSIGHTS

The skin on the anterolateral side of the thigh is usually thin, but somewhat hairy in males. Flap sensibility can be provided through the anterior femoral cutaneous nerve and lateral femoral cutaneous nerve.

A flap size of 20 × 15 cm has been reported. Donor site morbidity is minimal, but a resulting linear scar or skin graft may create some cosmetic problems in females.

The anterolateral thigh flap could be combined with the TFL, vastus lateralis, and rectus femoris muscles on the common pedicle of the lateral femoral circumflex vessels, to provide a large amount of soft tissue. A case of a large chest wall defect covered with this kind of composite flap has been reported.

Harvesting Technique

(Fig. 6-32) A line is drawn from the anterior superior iliac spine to the lateral edge of the patella. The cutaneous perforator is marked at the junction of the upper and middle thirds of this line. In the design, the pedicle can be at the center or on one side of the flap.

1. Rectus femoris m.
2. Fasciocutaneous perforator
3. Vastus lateralis m.
4. Descending branch
5. TFL

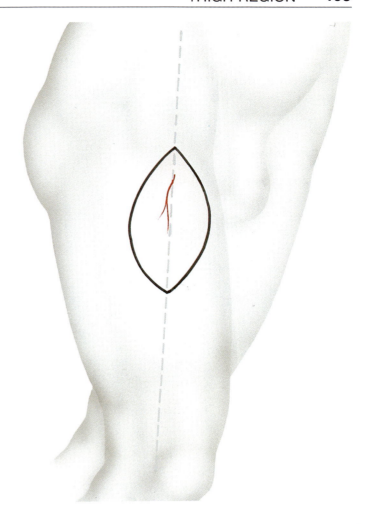

(Fig. 6-33) The anterior part of the flap, with or without deep fascia, is raised from the rectus femoris [1] toward the intermuscular septum, to expose the emergence of the cutaneous branch [2].

1. Rectus femoris m.
2. Fasciocutaneous perforator

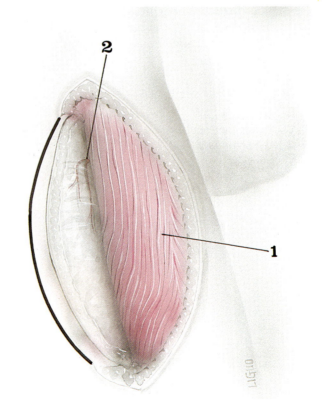

(Fig. 6-34) Retracting the rectus femoris [1] medially and ligating the branches to the muscle, the descending branch [4] of the lateral femoral circumflex artery is dissected toward its origin.

1. Rectus femoris m.
3. Vastus lateralis m.
4. Descending branch

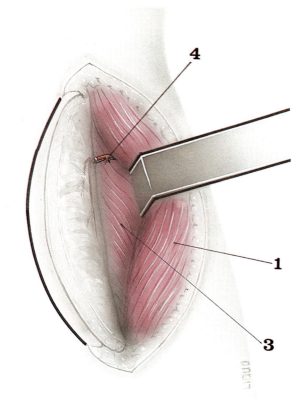

(Fig. 6-35) The posterior part of the flap is elevated from the vastus lateralis [3] and TFL [5], and the entire flap is isolated on its vascular pedicle. The pedicle can be dissected proximally under the rectus femoris to reach the lateral femoral circumflex artery, and the pedicle length can be about 8 cm.

1. Rectus femoris m.
3. Vastus lateralis m.
4. Descending branch
5. TFL

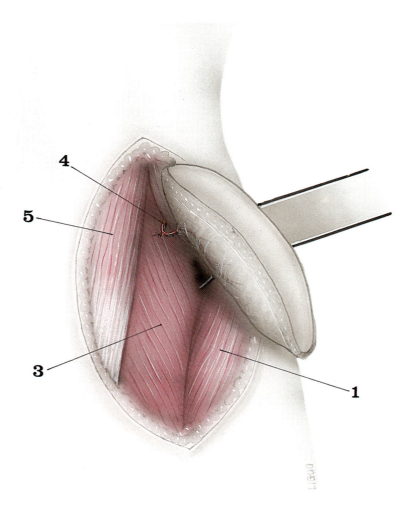

ANTEROMEDIAL THIGH FLAP

Anatomy (Fig. 6-36)

An unnamed branch [8] arises directly from the lateral circumflex femoral artery [5] and runs inferomedially along the medial aspect of the rectus femoris [1] and between the sartorius [2] and vastus medialis [3], emerging from the intermuscular space formed by the sartorius [2], rectus femoris [1], and vastus medialis [3] at the level of the midpoint of the thigh.

The diameter of the branch at its origin is approximately 2 mm, and the length of the pedicle can reach 12 cm.

Venous drainage is provided by the venae comitantes and by the superficial tributary of the anterior femoral vein that drains into the greater saphenous vein.

Innervation

Sensibility is provided by the medial cutaneous femoral nerve.

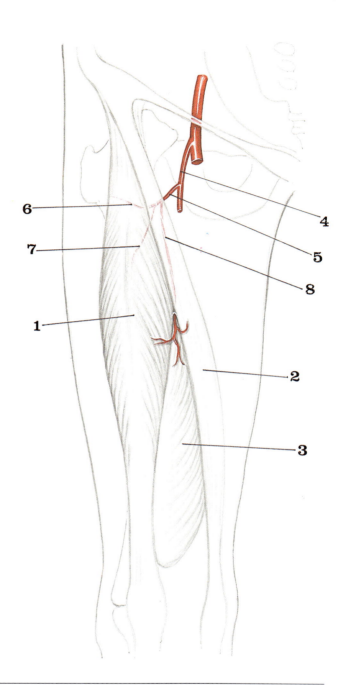

1. Rectus femoris m.
2. Sartorius m.
3. Vastus medialis m.
4. Deep femoral a.
5. Lateral circumflex femoral a.
6. Ascending branch
7. Descending branch
8. Unnamed branch

COMMENT AND INSIGHTS

Experience with this flap is limited, and cadaver dissection of these vessels is recommended prior to clinical application.

The skin of the anteromedial aspect of the thigh is generally uniformly thin and hairless, and it might be provided with sensibility through the medial femoral cutaneous nerve.

As a septocutaneous flap, the anteromedial thigh flap may include the deep fascia. When the fasciae are used, increased blood supply may be obtained by employing the vascular plexus of the deep fascia, so that the skin territory of this flap should be quite large. The maximal flap size reported is 10 × 25 cm.

This flap has also been reported for repair of herniation of the abdominal wall and for reconstruction of a defect of the cerebral dura, incorporating the strong fascia lata in the flap.

Donor site morbidity is minimal, but a resulting linear scar or skin graft may create some cosmetic problems in females.

Harvesting Technique

(Fig. 6-37) A line is drawn from the anterior superior iliac spine to the adductor tubercle of the femur. The midpoint of the line corresponds approximately to the emergence of the unnamed branch of the lateral circumflex femoral artery. The flap is designed using the line as an axis.

1. Rectus femoris m.
2. Unnamed branch
3. Sartorius m.
4. Vastus medialis m.

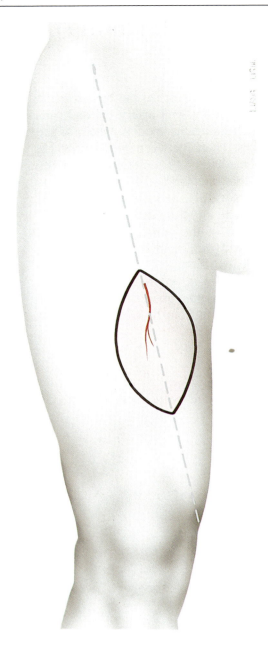

(Fig. 6-38) The anterior part of the flap, with or without deep fascia, is raised from the rectus femoris [1]. Lower medial border of the rectus femoris [1] and upper lateral border of the sartorius [3] are identified and traced, to find the narrow triangular intermuscular space formed by the sartorius, rectus femoris, and vastus medialis. Careful dissection should be undertaken to reveal the emergence of the fasciocutaneous perforator [2].

1. Rectus femoris m.
2. Unnamed branch
3. Sartorius m.

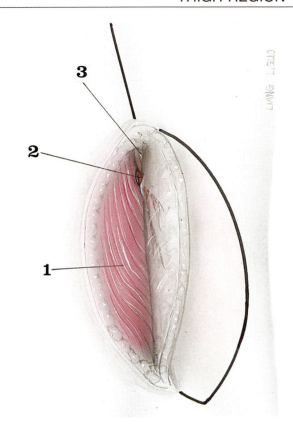

(Fig. 6-39) After assessing its position, the fasciocutaneous perforator [2] is dissected as a vascular pedicle toward its origin at the lateral circumflex femoral artery. Then, the rectus femoris [1] is retracted laterally and the sartorius [3] medially, and the muscular branches ligated.

1. Rectus femoris m.
2. Unnamed branch
3. Sartorius m.
4. Vastus medialis m.

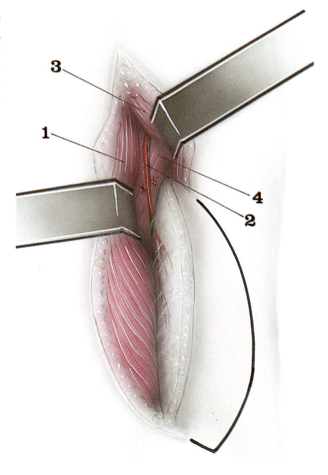

(Fig. 6-40) The medial portion of the flap is elevated from the sartorius [3] and vastus medialis [4], preserving the superficial vein on the upper border of the flap. The entire flap is isolated on its vascular pedicle.

1. Rectus femoris m.
2. Unnamed branch
3. Sartorius m.
4. Vastus medialis m.

If a sensory flap is required, the medial cutaneous femoral nerve is dissected on the upper medial flap border.

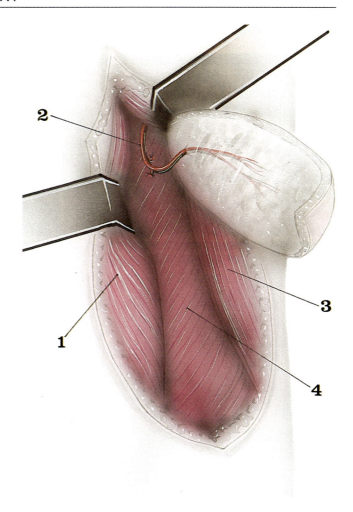

RECIPIENT SITE EXPOSURES

Anterior Approach to the Common and Superficial Femoral Arteries

(**Fig. 6-41**) A line is drawn from the midpoint of the inguinal ligament to the adductor tubercle of the femur. An incision is made on the proximal part of this line for a length of about 10 cm.

1. Saphenous v.
2. Superficial circumflex iliac v.
3. Lymph node
4. Cribriform fascia
5. Common femoral a. and v.
6. Superficial femoral a. and v.
7. Deep femoral a. and v.
8. Femoral n.
9. Sartorius m.

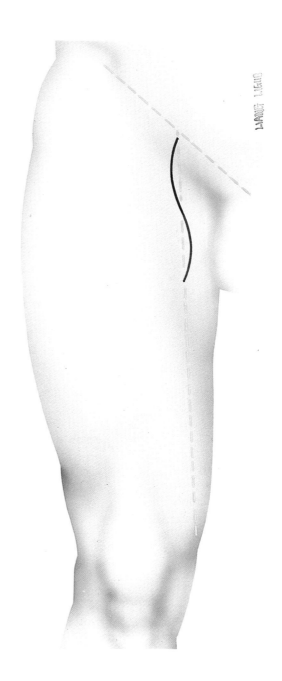

(Fig. 6-42) The greater saphenous vein [1] is identified beneath the superficial fascia. At the saphenous opening, it pierces the cribriform fascia [4] to join the femoral vein about 3 cm below the inguinal ligament. The superficial circumflex iliac vein [2] that branches from the greater saphenous vein and runs transversely should be ligated.

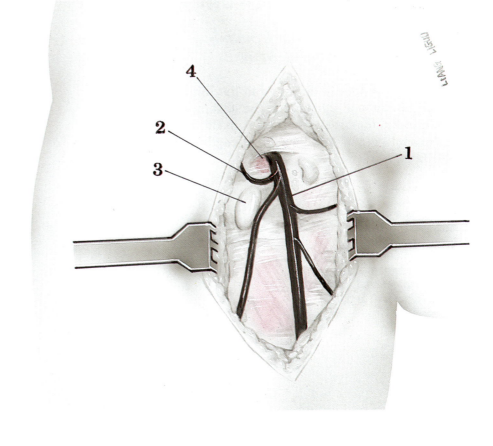

1. Saphenous v.
2. Superficial circumflex iliac v.
3. Lymph node
4. Cribriform fascia

(Fig. 6-43) Dividing the deep fascia, the sartorius muscle [9] is mobilized and retracted laterally. The femoral sheath is identified and opened to expose the common femoral artery [5], which is located lateral to the femoral vein [5]. Further dissection proceeds to expose the proximal portion of the superficial femoral artery [6] as its continuation. On its posterolateral aspect, the deep femoral artery [7] originates from the femoral artery about 3 to 4 cm below the inguinal ligament.

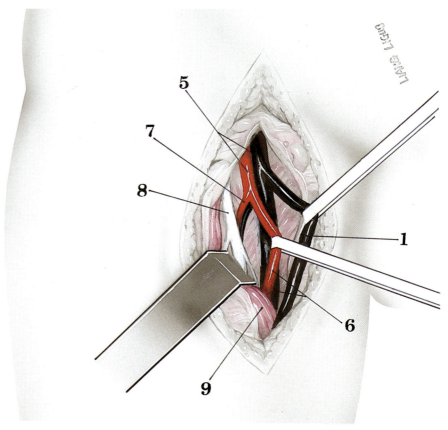

1. Saphenous v.
5. Common femoral a. and v.
6. Superficial femoral a. and v.
7. Deep femoral a. and v.
8. Femoral n.
9. Sartorius m.

Anterior Approach to the Superficial Femoral Artery in Hunter's Canal

(**Fig. 6-44**) An incision is made on the middle third of the line described above in the exposure of the common femoral artery.

1. Superficial femoral a. and v.
2. Saphenous a.,v., and n.
3. Roof of adductor canal
4. Sartorius m.
5. Vastus medialis m.
6. Gracilis m.
7. Adductor magnus m.
8. Adductor longus m.

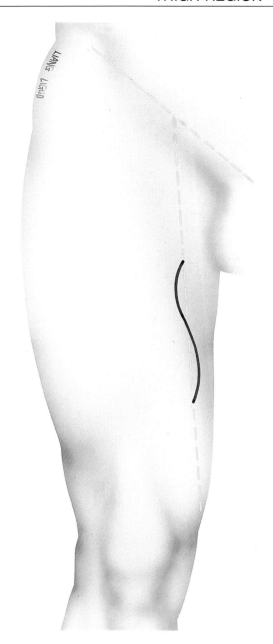

(Fig. 6-45) The deep fascia is incised, and the sartorius [4] and gracilis [6] are identified, mobilized, and retracted anteriorly and posteriorly, respectively. The fibrous roof of Hunter's canal [3], which extends from the adductor longus and magnus [8,7] to the vastus medialis [5], is exposed in the wound.

1. Superficial femoral a. and v.
2. Saphenous a., v., and n.
3. Roof of adductor canal
4. Sartorius m.
5. Vastus medialis m.
6. Gracilis m.
7. Adductor magnus m.
8. Adductor longus m.

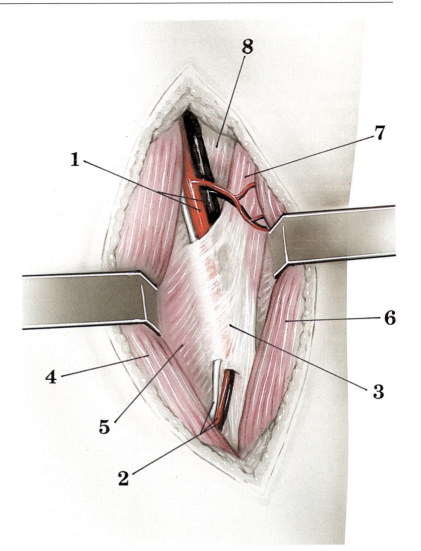

(Fig. 6-46) The fibrous roof is divided longitudinally. The saphenous nerve [2] can be seen in front of the artery running from lateral to medial; it should be carefully protected. Then, the superficial femoral artery [1] is dissected out from the femoral vein [1], which lies posterior to the artery.

1. Superficial femoral a. and v.
2. Saphenous a., v., and n.
4. Sartorius m.
5. Vastus medialis m.
6. Gracilis m.
7. Adductor magnus m.
8. Adductor longus m.

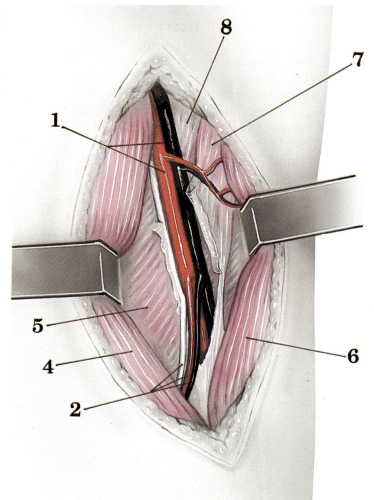

Posterior Approach to the Superficial Femoral Artery

(Fig. 6-47) The incision begins on the posterior midline of the thigh at the top of the popliteal fossa (at the level of the junction of the middle and distal thirds of the thigh). The incision runs proximally along the semitendinosus tendon to the medial aspect of the tuberosity of the ischium.

1. Popliteal a. and v.
2. Adductor magnus m.
3. Gracilis m.
4. Gluteus maximus m.
5. Semitendinosus m.
6. Semimembranosus m.
7. Sartorius m.
8. Superficial femoral a. and v.
9. Adductor longus m.
10. Roof of adductor canal divided

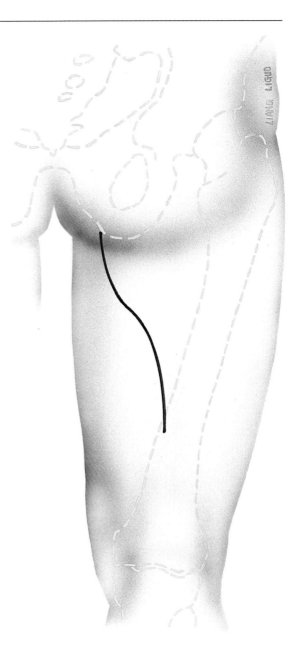

(**Fig. 6-48**) The deep fascia is incised, and the semitendinosus [5], semimembranosus [6], and gracilis [3] are identified, to determine the intermuscular septum between the gracilis [3] and semimembranosus [6].

A dissection is carried out to separate the semimembranosus [6] from the gracilis [3], which is retracted with the semitendinosus [5] laterally. Then, the medial edges and posterior surface of the adductor magnus [2] are exposed.

1. Popliteal a. and v.
2. Adductor magnus m.
3. Gracilis m.
4. Gluteus maximus m.
5. Semitendinosus m.
6. Semimembranosus m.

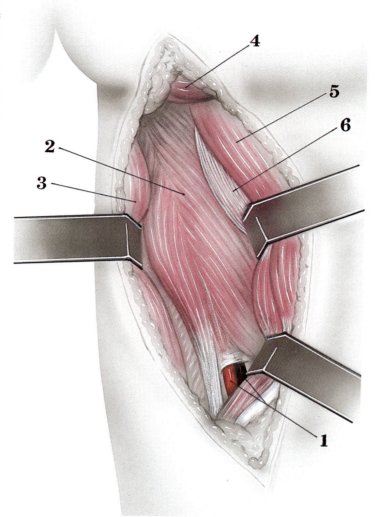

208 ATLAS OF MICROVASCULAR SURGERY

(**Fig. 6-49**) The adductor magnus [2] and the adductor longus [9] are separated from the deep surfaces of the gracilis [3] and sartorius [7] muscles, and then retracted with the semimembranosus [6] and semitendinosus [5] laterally toward the femoral shaft.

At this stage, tracing the adductor tendon [2], the adductor canal is identified along the posteromedial aspect of the femur in the lower half of the wound. The aponeurosis roof of the canal [10] is incised along the medial edge of the adductor magnus, to expose the femoral vessels [8]. The proximal portion of the superficial femoral vessels [8] can be dissected out from underneath the adductor longus [9].

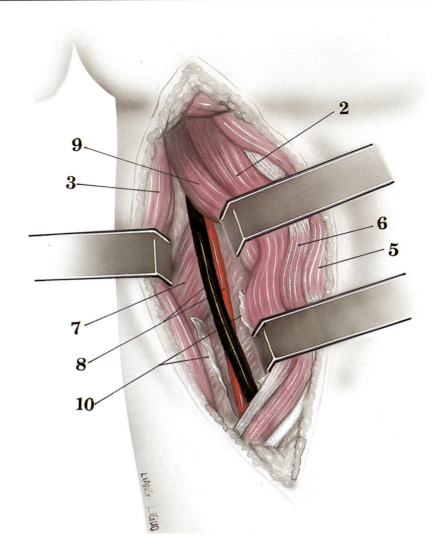

2. Adductor magnus m.
3. Gracilis m.
5. Semitendinosus m.
6. Semimembranosus m.
7. Sartorius m.
8. Superficial femoral a. and v.
9. Adductor longus m.
10. Roof of adductor canal divided

(Fig. 6-50) The posterior approach to the superficial femoral artery is shown in a cross-sectional diagram.

2. Adductor magnus m.
3. Gracilis m.
5. Semitendinosus m.
6. Semimembranosus m.
7. Sartorius m.
8. Superficial femoral a. and v.
9. Adductor longus m.

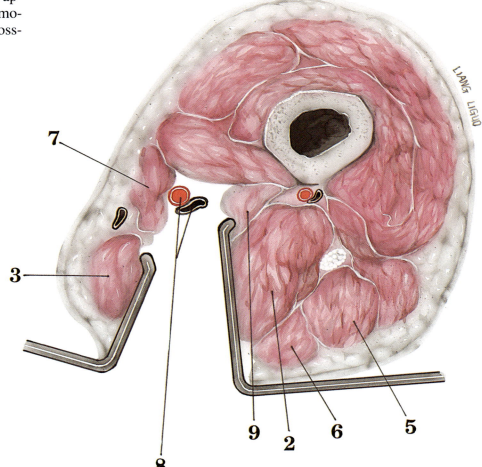

Anterior Approach to the Deep Femoral Artery

After takeoff from the main femoral trunk, the deep femoral artery lies deeply behind the thick cluster of the thigh muscles, the branches of the femoral nerve, and the main trunk of the superficial femoral vessels.

(Fig. 6-51) A line is drawn from a point 4 cm medial to the anterior superior iliac spine, to the medial edge of the patella. The incision is made on the proximal and middle thirds of the line.

1. Inguinal ligament
2. Greater saphenous v.
3. Femoral n.
4. Femoral a. and v.
5. Deep femoral a.
6. Lateral circumflex femoral a.
7. Sartorius m.
8. Rectus femoris m.
9. Vastus medialis m.
10. Adductor longus m.
11. Adductor brevis m.
12. First and second perforators
13. Adductor magnus m.
14. Pectineus m.

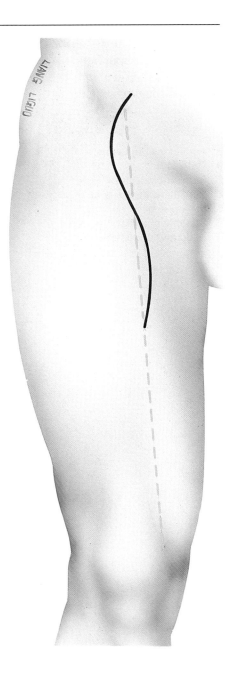

(Fig. 6-52) While dividing the deep fascia along the medial edge of the sartorius [7], the anterior cutaneous branches of the femoral nerve are preserved as much as possible. The sartorius [7] and rectus femoris [8] muscles are mobilized from their medial edge and retracted laterally. At this stage, the many branches of the femoral nerve [3] and the sheath of the femoral vessels [4] are exposed.

1. Inguinal ligament
2. Greater saphenous v.
3. Femoral n.
4. Femoral a. and v.
5. Deep femoral a.
6. Lateral circumflex femoral a.
7. Sartorius m.
8. Rectus femoris m.
9. Vastus medialis m.

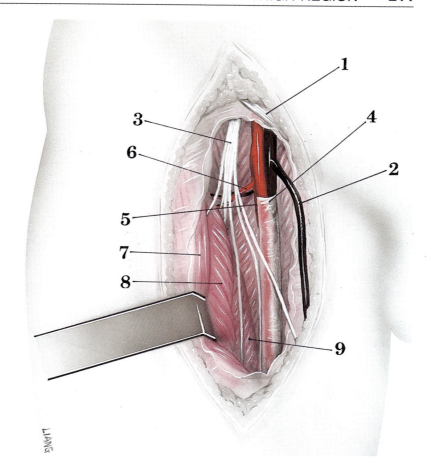

(Fig. 6-53) The branches of the femoral nerve [3] are carefully dissected from the anterior and lateral aspects of the main femoral vessels [4], and retracted laterally. The saphenous nerve or fine branches that enter the sheath of the artery can be divided, if required, for greater exposure.

Retracting the nerve branches [3] and vastus medialis muscle [9] laterally and the main femoral vessels [4] medially, the deep femoral artery [5] is identified running in front of the pectineus [14] toward the medial slope of the femur. It then disappears between the adductor longus and brevis muscles [10,11]. If needed, the adductor longus [10] can be detached from the femur, to obtain 3 to 4 cm more of distal exposure of the deep femoral artery [5].

In the course of this segment, the deep femoral artery gives off the lateral circumflex femoral artery [6], about 6 cm below the inguinal ligament, the three perforating arteries [12], and terminates as a fourth perforating artery.

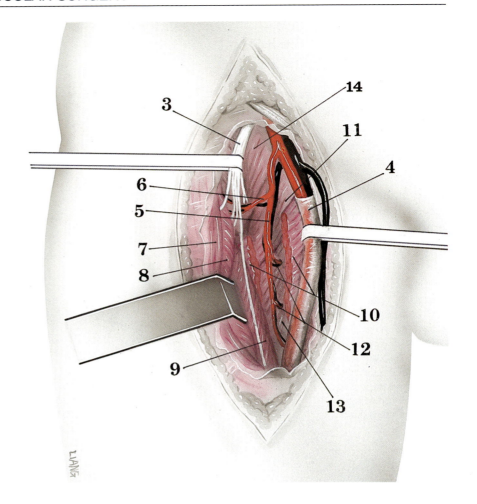

3. Femoral n.
4. Femoral a. and v.
5. Deep femoral a.
6. Lateral circumflex femoral a.
7. Sartorius m.
8. Rectus femoris m.
9. Vastus medialis m.
10. Adductor longus m.
11. Adductor brevis m.
12. First and second perforators
13. Adductor magnus m.
14. Pectineus m.

Posterior Approach to the Deep Femoral Artery

(**Fig. 6-54**) An incision is made from the top of the popliteal fossa (on the posterior midline and at the level of the junction of the middle and distal thirds of the thigh) to the tuberosity of the ischium.

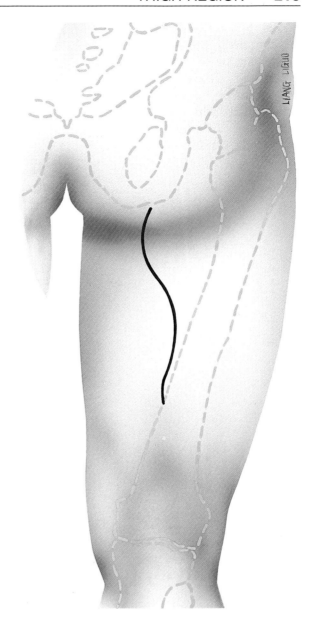

1. Gluteus maximus m.
2. Semimembranosus m.
3. Semitendinosus m.
4. Long head of biceps femoris
5. Short head of biceps femoris
6. Adductor magnus m.
7. Linea aspera
8. Sciatic n.
9. Second perforating a.
10. Third perforating a.
11. Deep femoral a. and v.

(Fig. 6-55) After dividing the deep fascia, the intermuscular septum between the medial [2,3] and lateral [4] hamstrings is identified and entered with blunt dissection to expose the sciatic nerve [8].

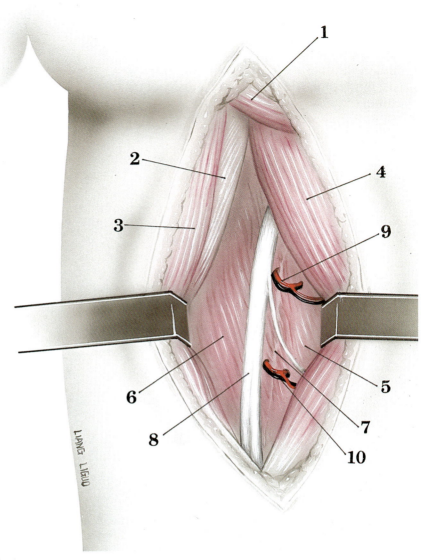

1. Gluteus maximus m.
2. Semimembranosus m.
3. Semitendinosus m.
4. Long head of biceps femoris
5. Short head of biceps femoris
6. Adductor magnus m.
7. Linea aspera
8. Sciatic n.
9. Second perforating a.
10. Third perforating a.

THIGH REGION

(**Fig. 6-56**) The sciatic nerve [8] is mobilized and displaced medially or laterally. Retracting the long head of the biceps femoris [4] laterally and the semitendinosus [3] and semimembranosus [2] medially, the linea aspera [7] is defined. The adductor magnus muscle [6] is detached from the medial edge of the linea aspera, between the levels of 10 to 15 cm distal to the greater trochanter, and the deep femoral artery [11] then appears before the asperal aponeurosis of the adductor longus or vastus medialis.

The second [9] and third [10] perforating arteries arise from the deep femoral artery and pierce the insertion of the adductors to the posterior and lateral aspects of the thigh.

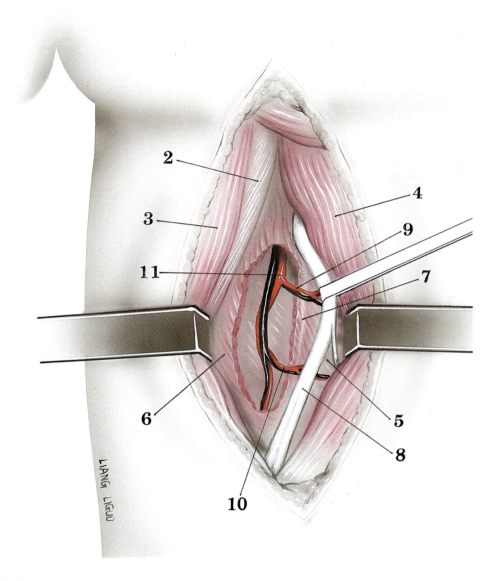

2. Semimembranosus m.
3. Semitendinosus m.
4. Long head of biceps femoris
5. Short head of biceps femoris
6. Adductor magnus m.
7. Linea aspera
8. Sciatic n.
9. Second perforating a.
10. Third perforating a.
11. Deep femoral a. and v.

216 ATLAS OF MICROVASCULAR SURGERY

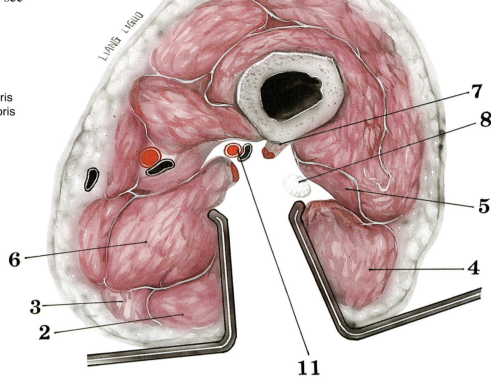

(Fig. 6-57) The posterior approach to the deep femoral artery is shown in a cross-sectional diagram.

2. Semimembranosus m.
3. Semitendinosus m.
4. Long head of biceps femoris
5. Short head of biceps femoris
6. Adductor magnus m.
7. Linea aspera
8. Sciatic n.
11. Deep femoral a. and v.

BIBLIOGRAPHY

Gracilis Flap

Harii K: Microneurovascular free transfer of a gracilis muscle flap to the face. In: Strauch B, Vasconez LO, Hall-Findlay E (eds): *Grabb's Encyclopedia of Flaps,* vol 3. Boston: Little, Brown, 1990, pp. 604–607.

Harii K, Ohmori K, Sekiguchi J: The free musculocutaneous flap. Plast Reconstr Surg 57:294, 1976.

Manktelow RT, McKee NH: Free muscle transplantation to provide active finger flexion. J Hand Surg 3:416, 1978.

Manktelow RT, Zuker RM: Microvascular free gracilis muscle and musculocutaneous flap to the forearm. In: Strauch B, Vasconez LO, Hall-Findlay E (eds): *Grabb's Encyclopedia of Flaps,* vol 2. Boston: Little, Brown, 1990, pp. 1207–1211.

Manktelow RT, Zuker RM: Microvascular free gracilis muscle and musculocutaneous flap. In: Strauch B, Vasconez LO, Hall-Findlay E (eds): *Grabb's Encyclopedia of Flaps,* vol 3. Boston: Little, Brown, pp. 1783–1784.

Manktelow RT, Zuker RM: Muscle transplantation by fascicular territory. Plast Reconstr Surg 73:751, 1984.

Mathes SJ, Nahai F, Vasconez LO: Myocutaneous free-flap transfer: Anatomical and experimental considerations. Plast Reconstr Surg 62:162, 1978.

McCraw JB, Massey FM, Shanklin KD, Horton CE: Vaginal reconstruction with gracilis myocutaneous flaps. Plast Reconstr Surg 58:176, 1976.

Wellisz T, Rechnic M, Dougherty W, Sherman R: Coverage of bilateral lower extremity calcaneal fractures with osteomyelitis using a single split free gracilis muscle transfer. Plast Reconstr Surg 85:457, 1990.

Wingate GB, Friedland JA: Repair of ischial pressure ulcers with gracilis myocutaneous island flaps. Plast Reconstr Surg 62:245, 1978.

Zhu SX, Lu SB, Zhang BX, et al: Free transfer of the gracilis musculocutaneous flap: A report of seven cases. Chin J Surg 19:143, 1981.

Tensor Fascia Lata Flap

Armenta E, Fisher J: Vascular pedicle of the tensor fascia lata myocutaneous flap. Ann Plast Surg 6:112, 1981.

Caffee HH, Asokan R: Tensor fascia lata myocutaneous free flaps. Plast Reconstr Surg 68:195, 1981.

Elliott LF, Beegle PH, Hartrampf CR Jr: The lateral transverse thigh free flap: An alternative for autogenous-tissue breast reconstruction. Plast Reconstr Surg 85:169, 1990.

Hill HL, Nahai F, Vasconez LO: The tensor fascia lata myocutaneous free flap. Plast Reconstr Surg 61:517, 1978.

Katsaros J: Use of the island tensor fasciae latae flap to cover a chest-wall defect. Plast Reconstr Surg 69:1007, 1982.

Little JW, Lyons JR: The gluteus medius-tensor fasciae latae flap. Plast Reconstr Surg 71:366, 1983.

Mathes SJ, Buchanan RT: Tensor fascia lata: Neurosensory musculo-cutaneous free flap. Br J Plast Surg 32:184, 1979.

Nahai F, Hill L, Hester TR: Experiences with the tensor fascia lata flap. Plast Reconstr Surg 63:788, 1979.

O'Hare PM, Leonard AG, Brennen MD: Experience with the tensor fasciae latae free flap. Br J Plast Surg 36:98, 1983.

Rectus Femoris Flap

Bhagwat BM, Pearl RM, Laub DR: Uses of the rectus femoris myocutaneous flap. Plast Reconstr Surg 62:698, 1978.

Dibbell DG Jr, Mixter RC, Dibbell DG Sr: Abdominal wall reconstruction (the "mutton chop" flap. Plast Reconstr Surg 87:60, 1991.

Schenck RR: Microneurovascular transfer of rectus femoris muscle and musculocutaneous flaps. In: Strauch B, Vasconez LO, Hall-Findlay E (eds): *Grabb's Encyclopedia of Flaps,* vol 2. Boston: Little, Brown, 1990, pp 1201–1204.

Schenck RR: Rectus femoris muscle and composite skin transplantation by microneurovascular anastomoses for avulsion of forearm muscles: A case report. J Hand Surg 3:60, 1978.

Thigh Flap

Baek SM: Two new cutaneous free flaps: The medial and lateral thigh flaps. Plast Reconstr Surg 71:354, 1983.

Cormack GC, Lamberty BGH: The blood supply of thigh skin. Plast Reconstr Surg 75:342, 1985.

Koshima I, Soeda S, Yamasaki M, Kyou J: The free or pedicled anteromedial thigh flap. Ann Plast Surg 21:480, 1988.

Kuo ET, Ji ZL, Zhao YC, et al: Microvascular free flap based on the medial femoral main cutaneous artery. J Reconstr Microsurg 1:305, 1985.

Maruyama Y, Ohnishi K, Takeuchi S: The lateral thigh fascio-cutaneous flap in the repair of ischial and trochanteric defects. Br J Plast Surg 37:103, 1984.

Press BHJ, Colen SR, Boyd A, Golomb F: Reconstruction of a large chest wall defect with a musculocutaneous free flap using anterolateral thigh musculature. Ann Plast Surg 20:238, 1988.

Song YG, Chen GZ, Song YL: The free thigh flap: A new free flap concept based on the septocutaneous artery. Br J Plast Surg 37:149, 1984.

7 LOWER LEG AND KNEE

Fibula and Adjacent Tissue Transfer

Anatomy of the Peroneal Artery
(Fig. 7-1)

The peroneal artery [3] arises from the posterior tibial artery [2] about 3 cm below the lower border of the popliteal muscle [8], at a level 7 cm below the head of the fibula, passing inferolaterally toward the fibula between the soleus and the tibialis posterior. It then enters a fibrous canal between the tibialis posterior and the flexor hallucis longus [7] or in the substance of the latter muscle, descending along the medial crest of the fibula toward the tibiofibular syndesmosis. Finally, it divides into the calcaneus branches.

In its course, the peroneal artery gives off the following significant branches:

1. A nutrient artery [5] that originates 6.8 cm after the origin of the peroneal artery [3] at a level 13.8 cm below the head of the fibula. The nutrient artery is directed downward into the fibula, with an average length of 1.8 cm and a diameter of 1.2 mm.

2. Four to six circular or arcade arteries [6] run around the posterior aspect of the fibula, segmentally nourish it, the periosteum, and surrounding muscles, at intervals of 3 to 5 cm, and then pass through the posterior crural intermuscular septum as septocutaneous branches to supply the lateral skin of the leg. The first circular artery [6] arises mostly from the popliteal artery, anterior or posterior tibial arteries, whereas the second, third, and fourth circular arteries almost constantly originate from the peroneal artery. These vessels have diameters of 0.6 to 0.8 mm; they emerge through the posterior crural septum at points about 9, 15, and 20 cm, respectively, below the head of the fibula.

3. Among a number of the muscular branches (excepting those from the circular artery), there usually are two large branches with a diameter of 1.8 mm to the lateral part of the soleus muscle directly from the peroneal artery, reaching the muscle at about its middle part.

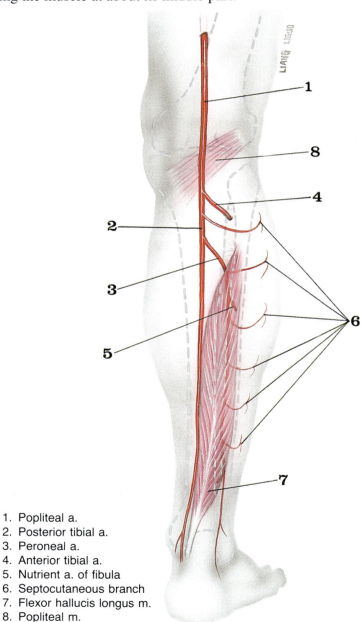

1. Popliteal a.
2. Posterior tibial a.
3. Peroneal a.
4. Anterior tibial a.
5. Nutrient a. of fibula
6. Septocutaneous branch
7. Flexor hallucis longus m.
8. Popliteal m.

Variations of the Peroneal Artery (Fig. 7-2)

Type A. The peroneal artery arises from the posterior tibial artery in 90% of cases.

Type B. It arises from the anterior tibial artery in 1% of cases.

Type C. It arises from the popliteal artery in 1% of cases.

Type D. It takes the place of the posterior tibial artery in 8% of cases.

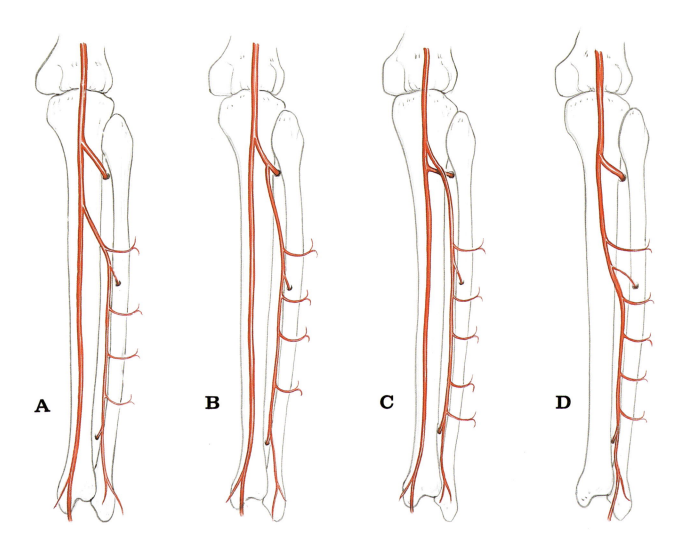

Anatomy of the Fibula (Fig. 7-3)

As a compact, straight, tubed bone, the fibula is relatively strong mechanically. The cross-sectional area of the upper part of the fibula is quadrilateral in shape and the lower part, triangular. The fibula plays a minor role in weight-bearing and in the stability of the lower extremity. Its diameter is 1.5 to 2.0 cm, and it is somewhat comparable to the femur, tibia, and humerus. In adults, the average total length is 33 cm, and a straight segment of up to 25 cm is available for grafting. This does not include the lower portion, which forms an integral part of the ankle joint.

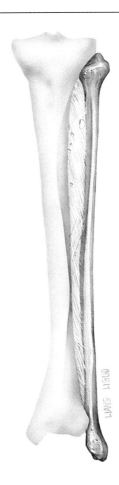

COMMENT AND INSIGHTS

The donor site is one of the most useful for harvesting a vascularized bone graft. The fibula is a straight, long, tubed bone, much stronger than any other available bone that can be currently used for a vascularized graft. It has a reliable peroneal vascular pedicle with large diameters and moderate length. There is a definite nutrient artery that enters the medullary cavity, as well as multiple arcade vessels that add to the supply of the bone through periosteal circulation.

The vascularized fibula graft is used mainly for long segment defects of the long tubed bone of the upper and lower extremities. It can provide a long, straight length of up to 25 cm in an adult. The fibula can be easily osteotomized and can be used to reconstruct the curved mandible.

As the anatomy has been more precisely investigated and the approach improved, harvesting techniques have become easier and faster. The bone can be combined with skin and muscle as a composite flap graft.

Osteocutaneous and osteomuscular fibular flaps are applicable in reconstruction of both bone and skin defects of the extremity, which are frequently encountered clinically.

Compared with some other types of skin flaps, the peroneal flap is not a primary choice, because the dissection of the septocutaneous branches, the circular vessels, and the peroneal vascular pedicle is more time-consuming and complicated under the intact fibular bone. However, a reversed peroneal flap is a useful method for reconstructing a badly injured foot.

Removal of the fibula usually does not result in morbidity, but the lower 8 cm length of the bone should be retained for stability of the ankle joint.

The peroneal flap or osteocutaneous flap usually requires split-thickness skin grafts on the donor defect, sometimes causing a problem with cosmesis.

VASCULARIZED FIBULA BONE GRAFT

(Fig. 7-4) The patient is placed in a supine position with the knee bent. A straight incision is made along the posterior edge of the fibula.

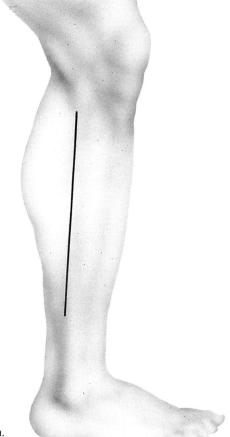

1. Soleus and gastrocnemius m.
2. Peroneus longus and brevis m.
3. Extensor digitorum and hallucis longus m.
4. Flexor hallucis longus m.
5. Fibula bone
6. Common peroneal n.
7. Interosseous membrane
8. Posterior tibialis m.
9. Peroneal a. and v.
10. Posterior tibial a., v., and n.

(**Fig. 7-5**) After cutting through the deep fascia and ligating the septocutaneous branches, the space between the peroneus longus [2] and soleus muscles [1] is entered.

1. Soleus and gastrocnemius m.
2. Peroneus longus and brevis m.

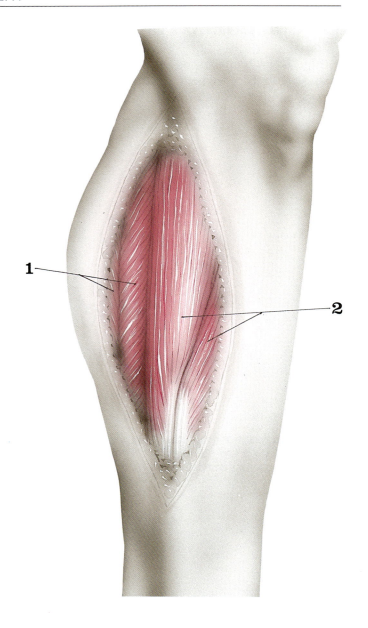

(Fig. 7-6) The sharp and extraperiosteal dissection is carried on anteriorly to detach the peroneus longus and brevis [2] and the extensor digitalis and hallucis longus muscles [3] from the anterolateral aspect of the fibula, leaving a minimal muscle cuff to the bone up to the interosseous membrane [7]. Posteriorly, the soleus muscle [1] is separated from the fibula [5] in the same way to expose the flexor hallucis longus [4].

If a longer segment of the fibula is required, reaching toward its neck, the common peroneal nerve [6] should be identified and meticulously preserved.

1. Soleus and gastrocnemius m.
2. Peroneus longus and brevis m.
3. Extensor digitorum and hallucis longus m.
4. Flexor hallucis longus m.
5. Fibula bone
6. Common peroneal n.
7. Interosseous membrane

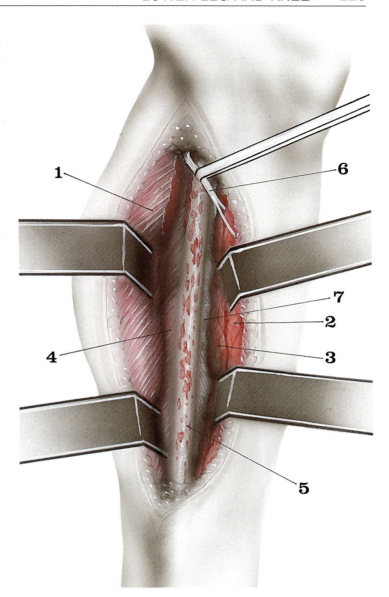

(Fig. 7-7) Although the peroneal artery has not been visible up to this point, to facilitate further exposure, the fibula [5] should then be cut at its proximal and distal ends with a Gigli saw and measurements made according to the length needed. This segment must include the middle third of the fibula, so that the nutrient artery is kept intact to nourish the bone.

4. Flexor hallucis longus m.
5. Fibula bone
7. Interosseous membrane
8. Posterior tibialis m.

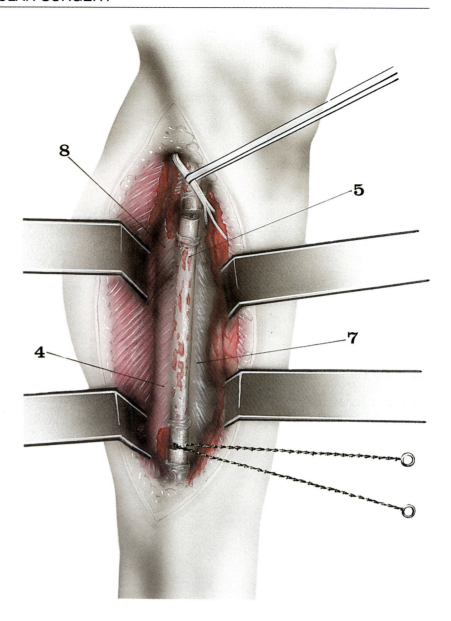

(Fig. 7-8) Using small bone hooks, the graft is gently retracted anteriorly and the soleus muscle retracted posteriorly. The peroneal vessel [9] can be seen at the upper inner border of the origin of the flexor hallucis longus [4], passing into its deeper substance.

4. Flexor hallucis longus m.
8. Posterior tibialis m.
9. Peroneal a. and v.
10. Posterior tibial a., v., and n.

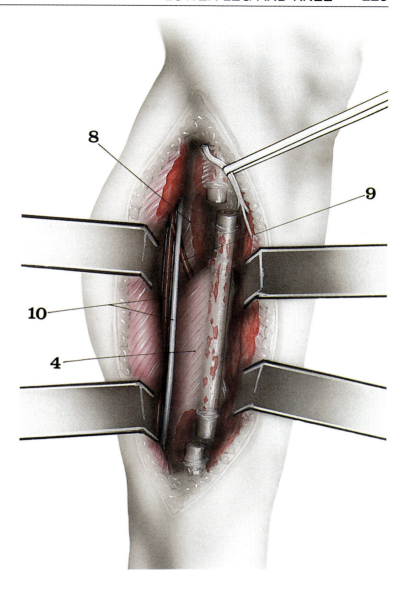

(Fig. 7-9) Separating the flexor hallucis longus [4], the peroneal bundle [9] is seen passing along the posterior aspect of the fibula. It is then ligated and sectioned at the severed distal level of the fibula.

After the interosseous membrane [7] is divided, the posterior tibialis [8] is severed from below upward, between the peroneal vascular bundle [9] and the lateral side of the posterior tibial nerve [10], leaving a 0.5- to 1.0-cm muscle fringe to the fibula.

At this point, the whole graft is freed from the donor site, except for the peroneal vascular pedicle [9] which can be dissected further toward the bifurcation of the posterior tibial artery [10], to obtain a pedicle length of less than 3 cm.

4. Flexor hallucis longus m.
5. Fibula bone
7. Interosseous membrane
8. Posterior tibialis m.
9. Peroneal a. and v.
10. Posterior tibial a., v., and n.

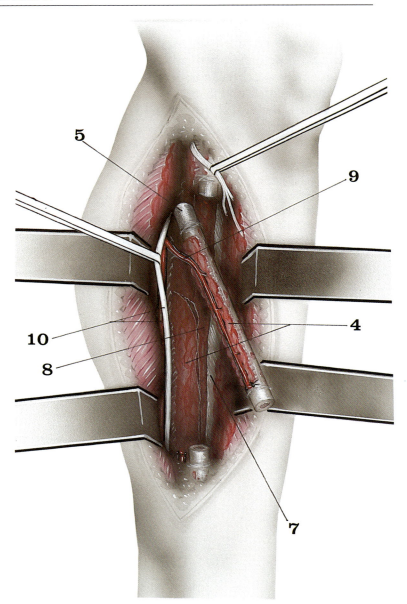

(**Fig. 7-10**) This is a diagram of a cross section of vascularized fibular bone graft.

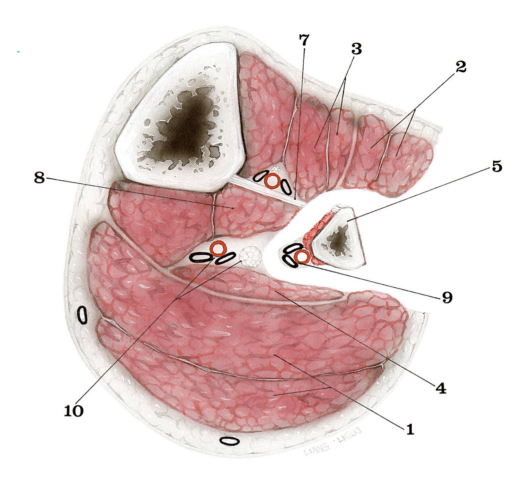

1. Soleus and gastrocnemius m.
2. Peroneus longus and brevis m.
3. Extensor digitorum and hallucis longus m.
4. Flexor hallucis longus m.
5. Fibula bone
7. Interosseous membrane
8. Posterior tibialis m.
9. Peroneal a. and v.
10. Posterior tibial a., v., and n.

PERONEAL FLAP (Lateral Leg Skin Flap)

(**Fig. 7-11**) A line is drawn as the axis of the flap, from the head of the fibula along its posterior edge to the malleolus. A point 2 cm above the midpoint of this line is marked as the center of the flap. The largest flap size reported is 32 × 10 cm.

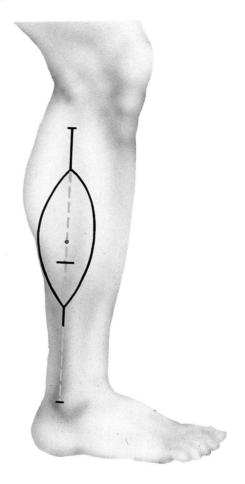

1. Soleus and gastrocnemius m.
2. Septocutaneous branches
3. Flexor hallucis longus m.
4. Fibula bone
5. Peroneal a. and v.
6. Posterior tibial a., v., and n.
7. Extensor m.
8. Peroneus longus and brevis m.

(**Fig. 7-12**) The posterior part of the flap, along with the deep fascia, is elevated toward the posterior crural septum, corresponding to the axial line of the flap. The lesser saphenous vein and the lateral sural nerve are preserved, while the proximal edge of the flap is being dissected.

The septocutaneous or musculocutaneous branches [2] can be found near the septum, usually at levels 9, 15, or 20 cm below the head of the fibula.

1. Soleus and gastrocnemius m.
2. Septocutaneous branches

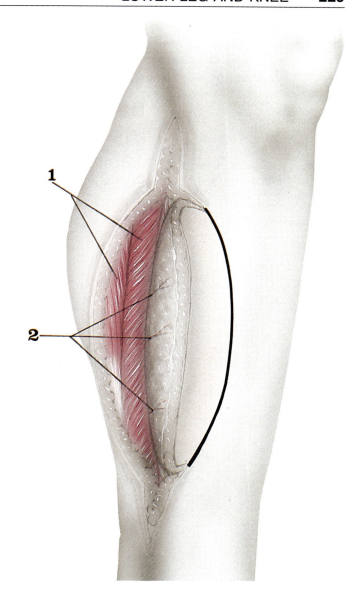

(Fig. 7-13) A meticulous dissection is carried out on the cutaneous branches, separating the soleus [1] and the flexor hallucis longus muscles [3] from the branches and the fibula [4], to expose their origins from the peroneal vessels [5].

1. Soleus and gastrocnemius m.
3. Flexor hallucis longus m.
4. Fibula bone
5. Peroneal a. and v.
6. Posterior tibial a., v., and n.

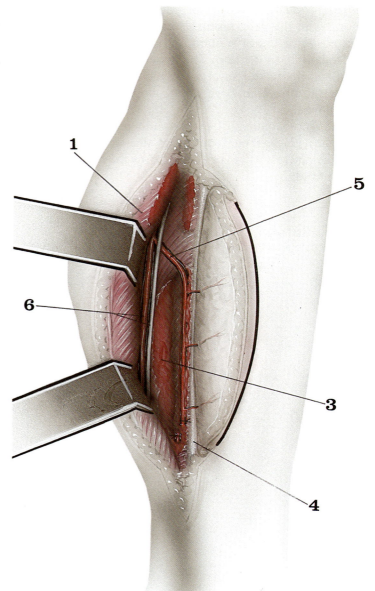

(Fig. 7-14) Then, the anterior part of the flap is raised from the extensor [7] and peroneus muscles [8] toward the septum. The septocutaneous or musculocutaneous branches are dissected from the peroneus muscles and the fibula, ligating the peroneal vessels [5] just distal to the origin of the lowest cutaneous branches of the flap. The peroneal flap is isolated on the proximal peroneal pedicle.

5. Peroneal a. and v.
6. Posterior tibial a., v., and n.
7. Extensor m.
8. Peroneus longus and brevis m.

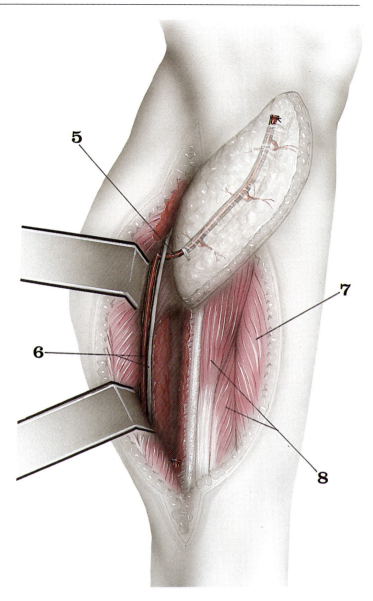

(Fig. 7-15) If a reversed skin flap is required, the peroneal vessels [5] are severed proximal to the origin of the upper cutaneous branch of the flap. The distal pedicle can be dissected up to the ankle region. However, the proximal ends of the peroneal vein should be anastomosed to the veins in the recipient site. If the lesser saphenous vein has been taken with the flap, this can serve as additional venous drainage.

5. Peroneal a. and v.
6. Posterior tibial a., v., and n.

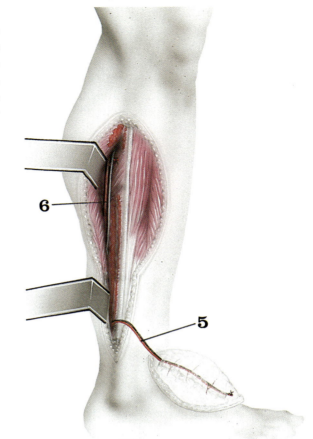

(Fig. 7-16) This is a diagram of the cross-section of the peroneal flap.

1. Soleus and gastrocnemius m.
2. Septocutaneous branches
3. Flexor hallucis longus m.
4. Fibula bone
5. Peroneal a. and v.
6. Posterior tibial a., v., and n.
7. Extensor m.
8. Peroneus longus and brevis m.

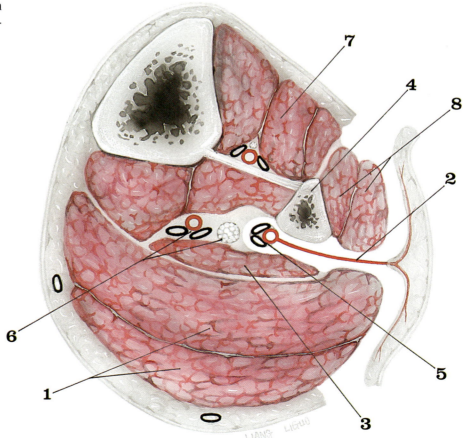

FIBULAR OSTEOCUTANEOUS FLAP

(**Fig. 7-17**) The skin flap is designed and the fibula marked, as in the peroneal flap and vascularized fibula bone graft procedures. The size and shape of the skin markings, the length of the fibula, and the relationship of the skin and bone should follow requirements at the recipient site. Usually, the skin flap should be about one fifth larger than the size of the defect, and the fibular graft should be 4 cm longer than the defect, for proper fixation of both ends.

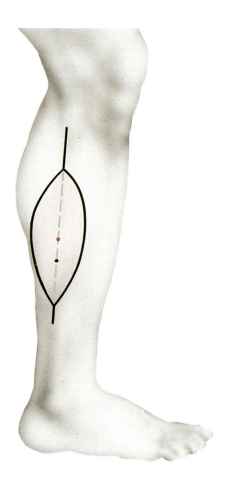

1. Soleus and gastrocnemius m.
2. Septocutaneous branches
3. Flexor hallucis longus m.
4. Fibula bone
5. Peroneal a. and v.
6. Posterior tibial a., v., and n.
7. Extensor m.
8. Peroneus longus and brevis m.
9. Interosseous membrane

(**Fig. 7-18**) The posterior and anterior parts of the flap, along with the deep fascia, are elevated toward the posterior crural septum, near to where the septocutaneous or musculocutaneous branches [2] can be seen emerging from the septum or muscles into the subcutaneous layer.

1. Soleus and gastrocnemius m.
2. Septocutaneous branches
7. Extensor m.
8. Peroneus longus and brevis m.

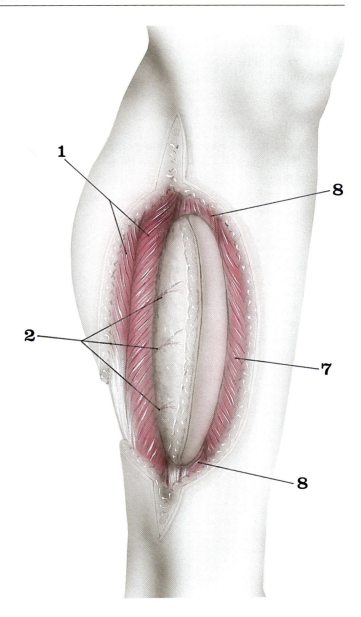

(**Fig. 7-19**) The fibula [4] is divided at each end with a Gigli saw, according to the length needed. The severed fibula can then be rotated on its long axis to facilitate further dissection.

The septocutaneous branches are traced and dissected toward their origins from the peroneal vessels [5], while the soleus muscle is being detached from the fibula (leaving a 0.5 cm muscle fringe to the fibula), and the flexor hallucis longus muscle [3] is separated.

The peroneal vessels [5] are ligated distally and cut, with the proximal side vessels kept intact as a pedicle.

3. Flexor hallucis longus m.
4. Fibula bone
5. Peroneal a. and v.
6. Posterior tibial a., v., and n.

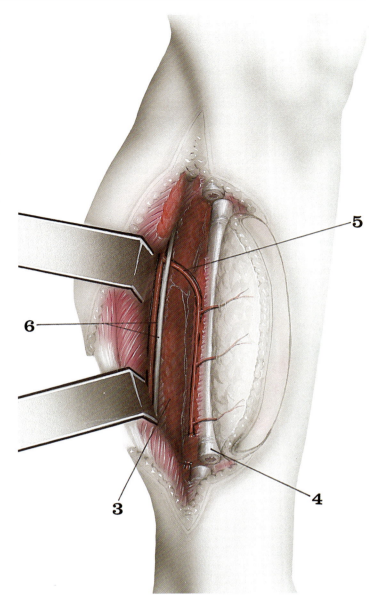

(Fig. 7-20) Subsequent procedures on the anterior and medial aspect of the fibula are similar to a free fibula transfer. However, special attention should be paid to keep the bone and skin flap intact, with the peroneal vessels [5] and their circular arteries and the posterior crural septum; the cutaneous branches should not be injured.

The entire fibular osteocutaneous flap is then isolated, connected to the lower leg only by its vascular pedicle [5].

5. Peroneal a. and v.
6. Posterior tibial a., v., and n.
8. Peroneus longus and brevis m.
9. Interosseous membrane

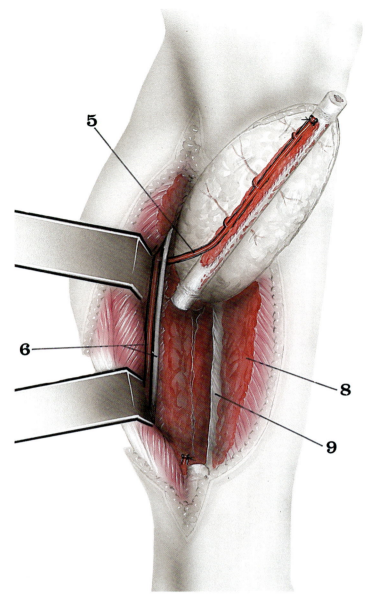

(Fig. 7-21) This is a diagram of the cross-section of a fibular osteocutaneous flap.

1. Soleus and gastrocnemius m.
2. Septocutaneous branches
3. Flexor hallucis longus m.
4. Fibula bone
5. Peroneal a. and v.
6. Posterior tibial a., v., and n.
7. Extensor m.
8. Peroneus longus and brevis m.
9. Interosseous membrane

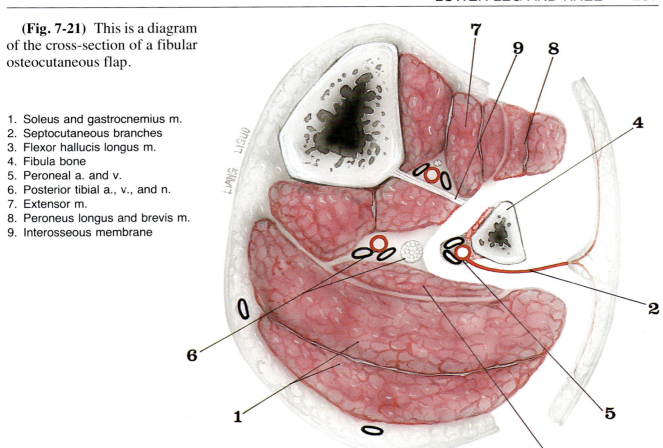

FIBULAR OSTEOMUSCULAR TRANSFER (with the Soleus Muscle)

(Fig. 7-22) The patient is placed in a prone position.

The incision begins from the popliteal fossa, running inferolaterally to the back of the head of the fibula, then proceeding downward along the posterior edge of the fibula.

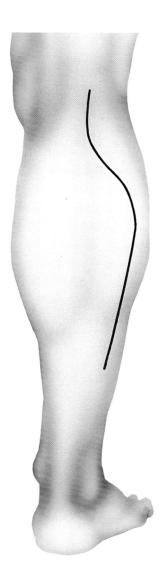

1. Lateral head of gastrocnemius m.
2. Soleus m.
3. Popliteal m.
4. Popliteal a. and v. and tibial n.
5. Flexor hallucis longus m.
6. Peroneal a. and v.
7. Tibialis posterior m.
8. Fibula bone
9. Interosseous membrane
10. Peroneotibial a. and v.

(Fig. 7-23) The skin and deep fascia are incised, and the superior attachment of the lateral gastrocnemius [1] then detached from the femur. The gastrocnemius, with its overlying skin as a flap, is turned medially to expose the soleus muscle [2].

1. Lateral head of gastrocnemius m.
2. Soleus m.
3. Popliteal m.
4. Popliteal a. and v. and tibial n.

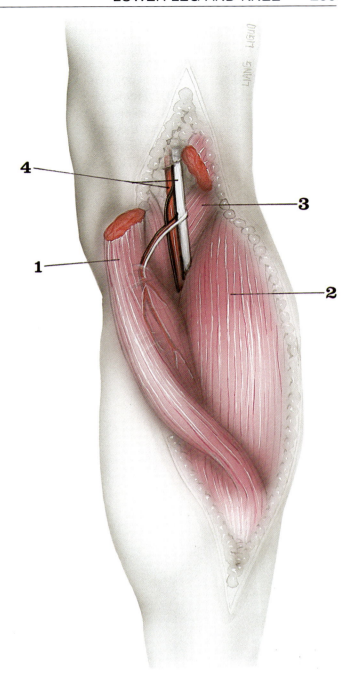

(**Fig. 7-24**) The muscle [2] is split longitudinally on its midline, and the muscle belly (its lateral portion) is retracted laterally to expose the peroneotibial vessels [10], accompanied by the posterior tibial nerve [4]. Tracing the vessels downward, the peroneal vessels [6] can be seen running obliquely toward the fibula and giving off one or two muscular branches to the soleus with a diameter of more than 1 mm, usually about 4 cm after the origin of the peroneal artery.

2. Soleus m.
4. Popliteal a. and v. and tibial n.
5. Flexor hallucis longus m.
6. Peroneal a. and v.
7. Tibialis posterior m.
10. Peroneotibial a. and v.

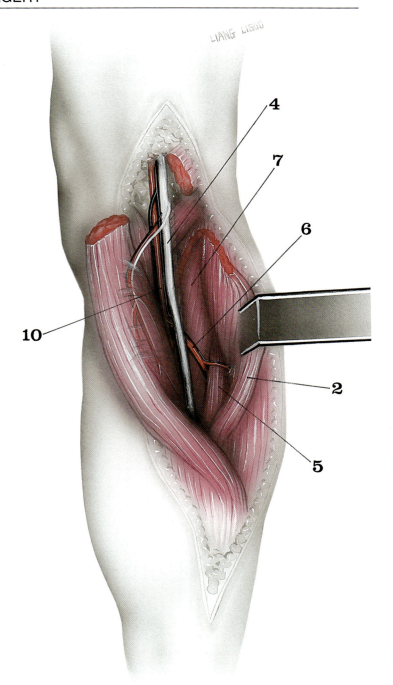

(Fig. 7-25) The required length of fibula [8] is divided by a Gigli saw, and the lateral part of the soleus muscle [2] is severed at the same levels as the divided upper and lower ends of the fibula. The peroneal vessels [6] are ligated and divided distally. It is not necessary to separate the soleus from the fibular segment, if it is to be used only for coverage of the fibular graft.

2. Soleus m.
5. Flexor hallucis longus m.
6. Peroneal a. and v.
7. Tibialis posterior m.
8. Fibula bone

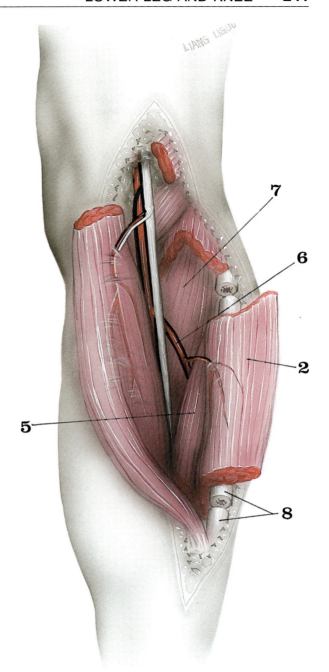

(Fig. 7-26) Subsequent steps, such as detaching the peroneus, extensor, and tibialis posterior muscles, are similar to those for a free fibular transfer. Care should be taken not to damage the muscular branches to the soleus muscle [2].

2. Soleus m.
5. Flexor hallucis longus m.
6. Peroneal a. and v.
7. Tibialis posterior m.
8. Fibula bone
9. Interosseous membrane

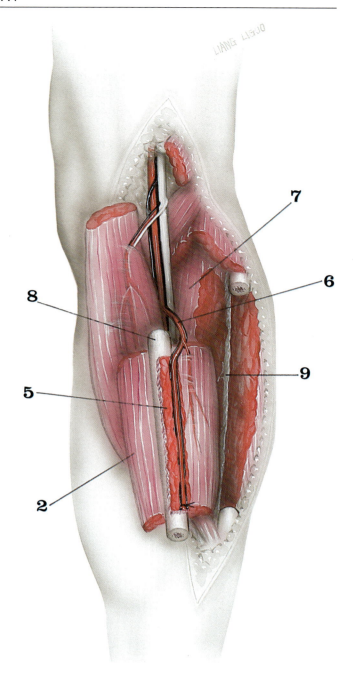

LOWER LEG AND KNEE 243

(Fig. 7-27) This is a diagram of the cross-section of a fibular osteomuscular transfer.

1. Lateral head of gastrocnemius m.
2. Soleus m.
5. Flexor hallucis longus m.
6. Peroneal a. and v.
7. Tibialis posterior m.
8. Fibula bone
9. Interosseous membrane

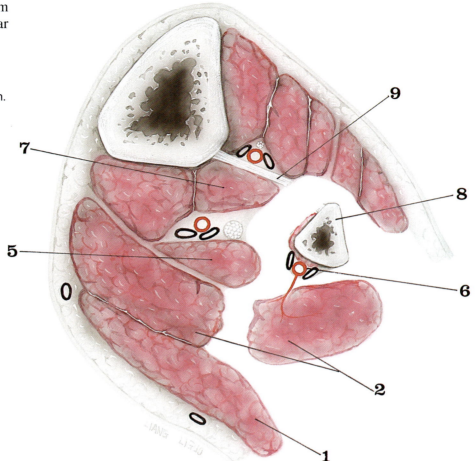

Gastrocnemius Flap

Anatomy (Fig. 7-28)

The origin of the muscle involves two heads [6,5] arising from the lateral and medial condyles of the femur, the adjacent capsule of the knee, and the insertion is the calcaneal tendon [3]. The gastrocnemius functions for plantar flexion of the foot and flexion of the knee joint. The two muscle heads, medial [1] and lateral [2], unite at about the level of the head of the fibula; they join the tendon of the soleus at the middle level of the leg to form the Achilles tendon [3].

Muscle Belly	Length (cm)	Width (cm)	Thickness (cm)
Medial head	23	7.0	1.7
Lateral head	23	8.1	1.7

The broadest parts of both heads are located 6 cm below the head of the fibula.

Blood Supply

Each head has an independent vascular unit. The medial and lateral sural arteries [5,6] arise from the popliteal artery [4], 3 to 4 cm above the head of the fibula and, respectively, enter the medial [1] and lateral [2] heads of the gastrocnemius at about the level of the fibular head.

	Medial Sural Vessels		Lateral Sural Vessels	
	Artery	Vein	Artery	Vein
Diameter	1.4 mm	1.4 mm	1.5 mm	1.4 mm
Pedicle length	2.6 cm		2.2 cm	

Innervation

The paired motor nerves come from the tibial nerve and enter each head of the muscle adjacent to the vascular pedicle.

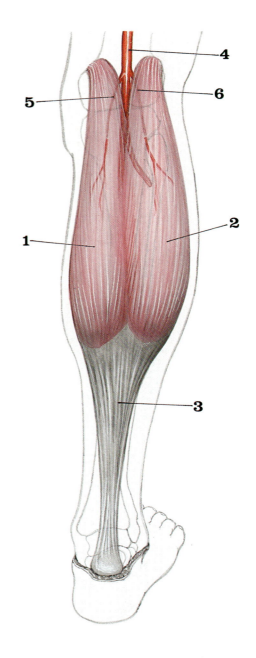

1. Medial head of gastrocnemius
2. Lateral head of gastrocnemius
3. Achilles tendon
4. Popliteal a.
5. Medial sural a.
6. Lateral sural a.

COMMENT AND INSIGHTS

Microvascular transfer of the gastrocnemius muscle or myocutaneous flap is not widely applied clinically. The vascular anatomy is, however, quite constant and the calibers of the pedicle are adequate, but pedicle length is somewhat short. Removal of the muscle does not result in obvious disability or morbidity, although loss of part of the plantar flexor may lessen jumping and running ability to a certain extent. Local transfer of the muscle or musculocutaneous flap as an island flap, applied to cover the upper half of the tibia or the knee joint, is more commonly utilized.

For coverage of the lower half of the tibia using microvascular technique, a free medial gastrocnemius flap can be transferred by lengthening the medial sural artery with a segment graft of the lesser saphenous vein. (The sural vein can be directly anastomosed to the lesser or greater saphenous.)

Myocutaneous flap transfer causes substantial contour deformity, either from depression and scar in the donor calf or from bulk in the recipient area. For these reasons, the muscle flap with split-thickness skin graft might be preferred.

MEDIAL GASTROCNEMIUS MUSCLE FLAP

(**Fig. 7-29**) With the patient in a prone or semilateral position, a midposterior S-shaped incision is made, starting 5 cm above the popliteal crease and extending down to the distal end of the muscle belly.

1. Medial head of gastrocnemius
2. Lateral head of gastrocnemius
3. Lesser saphenous v. and medial sural n.
4. Popliteal a. and v. and tibial n.
5. Soleus m.
6. Medial sural a. and v. and muscular branch of tibial n.
7. Plantaris m.

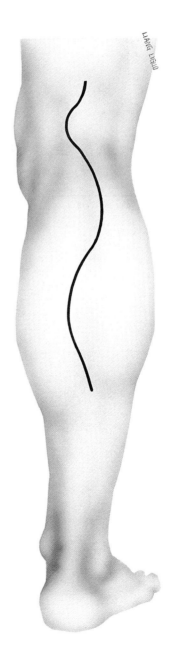

(**Fig. 7-30**) The lesser saphenous vein and medial sural nerve [3] are identified and retracted laterally. The medial and lateral heads of the muscle [1,2] are then separated to expose the tibial nerve [4] and the popliteal vessel [4].

1. Medial head of gastrocnemius
2. Lateral head of gastrocnemius
3. Lesser saphenous v. and medial sural n.
4. Popliteal a. and v. and tibial n.

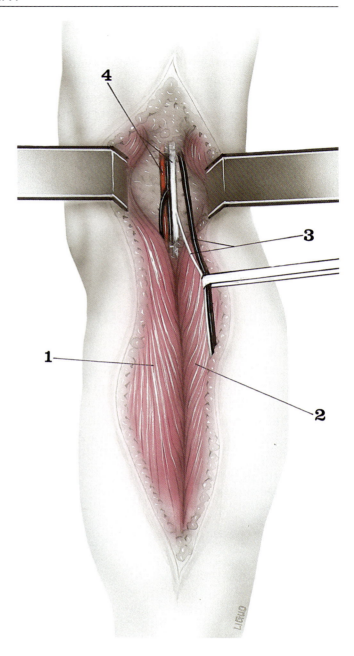

(**Fig. 7-31**) Tracing along the medial and anterior surface of the medial head of the muscle [1], the medial sural vessels [6] and accompanying nerve [6] are identified and dissected from the entrance of the muscle [1] to the origins of the popliteal vessels [4] and tibial nerve [4].

1. Medial head of gastrocnemius
4. Popliteal a. and v. and tibial n.
5. Soleus m.
6. Medial sural a. and v. and muscular branch of tibial n.
7. Plantaris m.

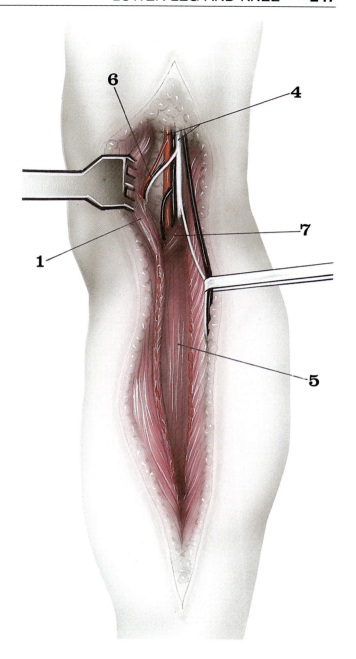

(**Fig. 7-32**) The superficial surface of the medial head [1] is exposed, and the plane between the gastrocnemius [1] and soleus [5] is developed by blunt dissection, with care being taken to protect the neurovascular bundle [6].

1. Medial head of gastrocnemius
5. Soleus m.
6. Medial sural a. and v. and muscular branch of tibial n.
7. Plantaris m.

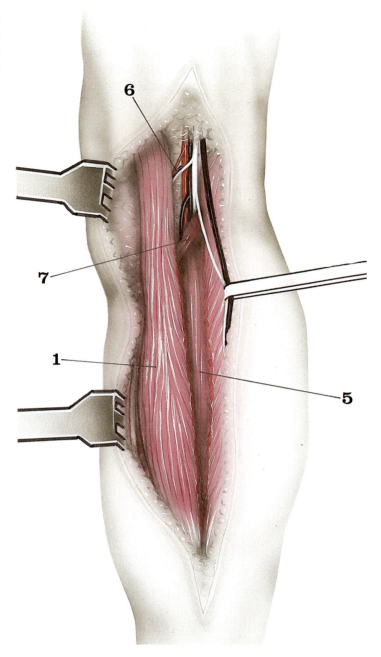

(**Fig. 7-33**) Detaching its origin on the medial condyle of the femur and separating its lower muscle fibers from the Achilles tendon, the medial gastrocnemius muscle flap [1] is isolated on the medial sural neurovascular pedicle [6] with a length of about 3 cm.

1. Medial head of gastrocnemius
5. Soleus m.
6. Medial sural a. and v. and muscular branch of tibial n.
7. Plantaris m.

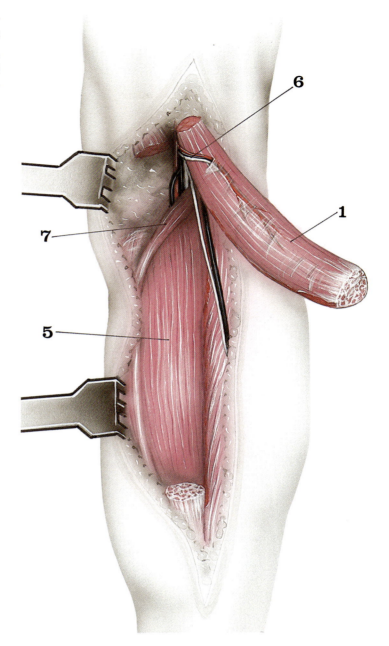

LATERAL GASTROCNEMIUS MUSCLE FLAP

(**Fig. 7-34**) The lateral gastrocnemius muscle flap can be raised with a maneuver similar to the medial flap, but the incision is Z-shaped.

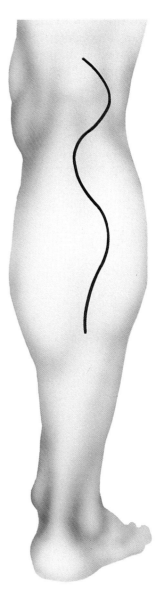

1. Medial head of gastrocnemius
2. Lateral head of gastrocnemius
3. Lesser saphenous v. and medial sural n.
4. Popliteal a. and v. and tibial n.
5. Soleus m.
6. Lateral sural a. and v. and muscular branch of tibial n.
7. Plantaris m.
8. Common peroneal n.
9. Biceps femoris tendon

(**Fig. 7-35**) Since the common peroneal nerve [8] passes between the lateral head of the gastrocnemius [2] and the tendon of the biceps femoris [9], particular attention should be paid to preserve the nerve during isolation of the origin of the lateral head.

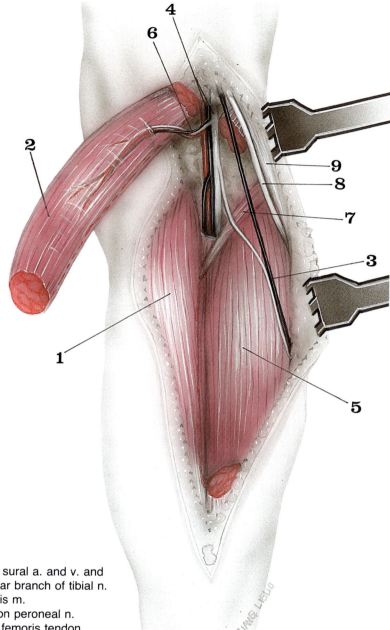

1. Medial head of gastrocnemius
2. Lateral head of gastrocnemius
3. Lesser saphenous v. and medial sural n.
4. Popliteal a. and v. and tibial n.
5. Soleus m.
6. Lateral sural a. and v. and muscular branch of tibial n.
7. Plantaris m.
8. Common peroneal n.
9. Biceps femoris tendon

Saphenous Flap

Anatomy (Fig. 7-36)

The territory of the skin flap is nourished by the saphenous artery [6], a branch of the *descending genicular artery* [5], which arises from the femoral artery [4] about 15 cm above the knee. This is just proximal to the opening in the adductor magnus in the lower part of the adductor canal [3]. The descending genicular artery [5] immediately divides into two equal branches, the musculoarticular branch [7] and the saphenous artery [6]. The diameter of the latter ranges from 1.2 to 1.8 mm.

The *saphenous artery* [6] pierces the aponeurosis roof of the adductor canal [3] within 2 cm of its origin, and then runs downward between the sartorius [1] and vastus medialis [2] muscles and the adductor tendon for a distance of 12 to 15 cm. It then gives off one to four important cutaneous branches, to supply a large area of skin medially above the knee. Some branches pass anterior to the sartorius, and others posterior to it.

The terminal (distal) saphenous artery passes between the sartorius [1] and gracilis [8] tendons and is distributed to the skin of the upper and medial portions of the leg below the knee.

There are two systems for venous drainage: the paired venae comitantes and the greater saphenous vein that lies about 1.5 cm posterior to the course of the saphenous artery.

Variations

In 5% of cases, the artery is absent and in 6.7% of cases, there is an additional unnamed cutaneous artery from the popliteal artery or musculoarticular branch of the descending genicular artery.

Innervation

The *medial femoral cutaneous nerve* supplies the skin territory above the knee. It runs near the anterior border of the sartorius close to the deep fascia.

The *saphenous nerve* supplies the anteromedial aspect of the leg below the knee. It courses sequentially in close proximity to the femoral artery, the descending genicular artery, the saphenous artery, and the greater saphenous vein.

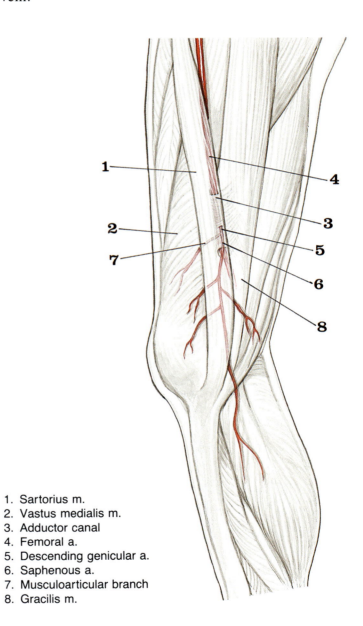

1. Sartorius m.
2. Vastus medialis m.
3. Adductor canal
4. Femoral a.
5. Descending genicular a.
6. Saphenous a.
7. Musculoarticular branch
8. Gracilis m.

COMMENT AND INSIGHTS

The donor site provides a sensory skin flap innervated by two nerves that can be easily identified during flap dissection. The skin of the flap is quite thin, less than 1 cm in thickness. Anatomically, the length and caliber of the vascular pedicle are generally adequate, but there can be anatomic variation of the saphenous vessels and their cutaneous branches. It is sometimes necessary that final flap design must follow a tedious vascular dissection and exploration.

A split-thickness skin graft should be used whenever the width of the donor defect is more than 7 cm. Postoperatively, there is no resultant morbidity, but the scar left after skin graft is not cosmetically acceptable.

Harvesting Technique

(Fig. 7-37) The anatomy of the saphenous artery and its cutaneous branches is intimately involved with the sartorius muscle. Therefore a line is drawn from the anterior superior iliac spine to the medial supracondyle of the tibia, to follow the course of the sartorius. The flap can be designed primarily along the distal part of this line as an axis, with its proximal edge 12 cm above the knee joint. The largest flaps reported are 29 × 8 cm and 15 × 11 cm.

1. Vastus medialis m.
2. Gracilis m.
3. Greater saphenous v.
4. Medial femoral cutaneous n.
5. Sartorius m.
6. Saphenous a., v., and n.
7. Anterior cutaneous branch
8. Roof of adductor canal

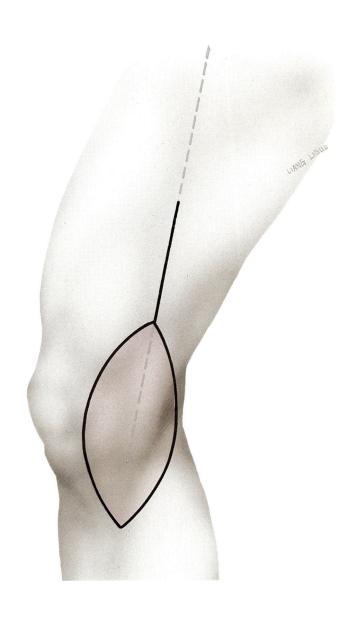

254 ATLAS OF MICROVASCULAR SURGERY

(Fig. 7-38) A 10 cm incision is made along the course of the sartorius above the designed flap. The medial femoral cutaneous nerve [4] and greater saphenous vein [3] are first isolated near the anterior and posterior borders of the sartorius [5].

1. Vastus medialis m.
2. Gracilis m.
3. Greater saphenous v.
4. Medial femoral cutaneous n.
5. Sartorius m.

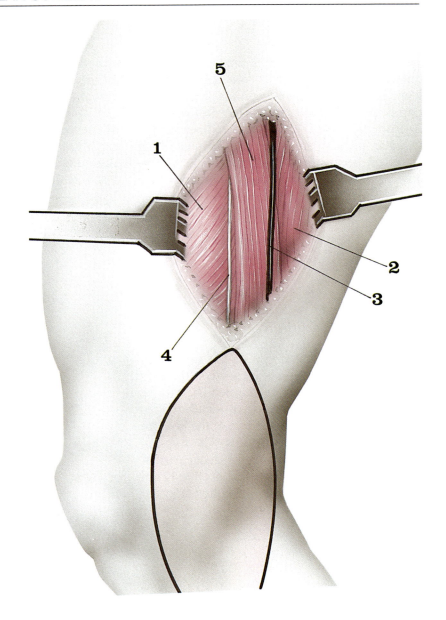

(**Fig. 7-39**) The deep fascia is incised and the sartorius [5] is bluntly dissected in the upper part of the incision and separated from the vastus medialis [1] to expose the saphenous neurovascular bundle [6].

Tracing the saphenous vessel [6] distally, the cutaneous branches [7] can be found passing over the anterior or posterior border of the sartorius [5] to supply the overlying skin. If it is necessary to expose and dissect the cutaneous branches [7] more easily and safely, the sartorius [5] can be divided or even a segment of the muscle can be included in the flap.

1. Vastus medialis m.
3. Greater saphenous v.
4. Medial femoral cutaneous n.
5. Sartorius m.
6. Saphenous a., v., and n.
7. Anterior cutaneous branch
8. Roof of adductor canal

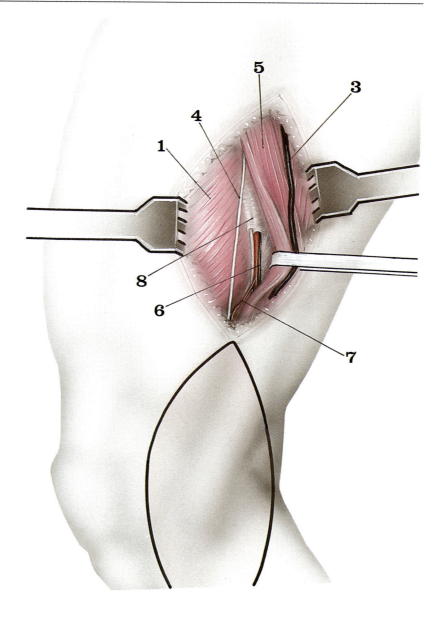

(Fig. 7-40) The designed flap is adjusted anteriorly or posteriorly, according to the major cutaneous branches uncovered.

The greater saphenous vein [3] is ligated at the distal flap margin and the saphenous flap, including deep fascia, is raised based on the saphenous neurovascular pedicle [6], the greater saphenous vein [3], and the medial femoral cutaneous nerve [4]. The saphenous neurovascular bundle can be further dissected to achieve a length varying from 4 to 16 cm.

1. Vastus medialis m.
3. Greater saphenous v.
4. Medial femoral cutaneous n.
5. Sartorius m.
6. Saphenous a., v., and n.
7. Anterior cutaneous branch
8. Roof of adductor canal

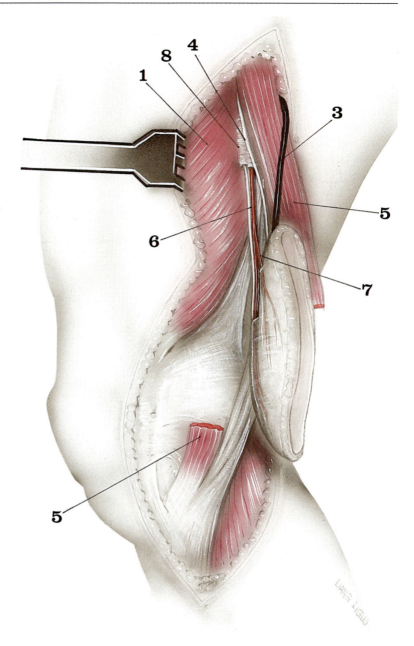

Leg Skin Flaps

ANTERIOR TIBIAL FLAP

Anatomy (Fig. 7-41)

The anterior tibial artery [2] arises from the popliteal artery [1] at the lower border of the popliteus muscle. It passes through the tibialis posterior muscle and the interosseous membrane to the anterior compartment medial to the neck of the fibula, then descends in front of the interosseous membrane and the tibia in the lower part of the leg, accompanied by the deep peroneal nerve [7]. In front of the ankle, it appears midway between the malleoli.

In its course, the artery gives off two septocutaneous branches into the anterior crural intermuscular septum between the anterior and peroneal compartments.

The *superior lateral peroneal artery* [3] originates about 8 cm below the head of the fibula. Accompanying the superficial peroneal nerve, it runs downward and superficially in the septum in the upper third of the leg, under the fascia in the middle third, and above the fascia in the lower third, giving off a cutaneous branch in the middle third. The artery, with an average diameter of 1.6 mm, is present in 100% of cases.

The *inferior lateral peroneal artery* [4] originates about 17 cm below the head of the fibula, that is, at the level of the fibular midpoint. Accompanying the superficial peroneal nerve [6], it communicates with the superior lateral peroneal artery [3]. The artery, with an average diameter of 1.4 mm, is present in 70% of cases.

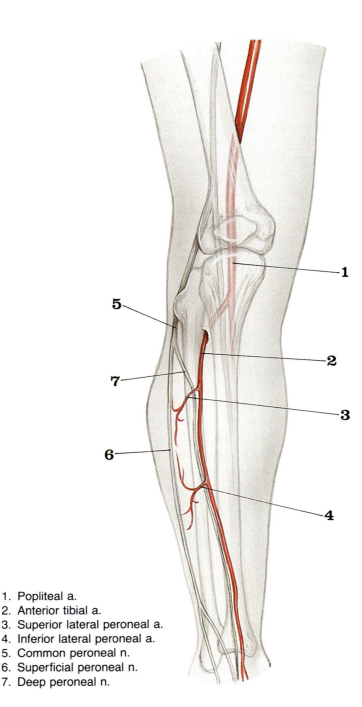

1. Popliteal a.
2. Anterior tibial a.
3. Superior lateral peroneal a.
4. Inferior lateral peroneal a.
5. Common peroneal n.
6. Superficial peroneal n.
7. Deep peroneal n.

COMMENT AND INSIGHTS

The anterior tibial flap is a septocutaneous flap, and its septocutaneous branches come from the anterior tibial artery through the anterior crural intermuscular septum between the anterior and peroneal compartments.

There have been relatively few cases of revascularized anterior tibial flaps reported, because use of the flap demands sacrifice of the anterior tibial artery, even though the arterial anatomy is quite constant. For this reason, arteriography should routinely be done to confirm the existence of both the posterior and anterior tibial arteries, if the flap is to be used.

There are several case reports indicating that the superior or inferior lateral peroneal artery can provide an independent vascular pedicle for this flap in a local transfer, to cover soft-tissue defects of the knee or ankle joint. Since there may be no communication between the superior and inferior lateral peroneal arteries in about 40% of cases, these kinds of pedicle flaps are not introduced here.

The skin in the anterior aspect of the lower leg has moderate thickness and is quite hairy in males. The donor site generally needs a split-thickness skin graft after removal of a skin flap more than 3 cm wide.

Compared with other donor sites, the anterior tibial flap is not a primary choice for revascularized transfer; local transfers as island flaps are acceptable.

Harvesting Technique

(Fig. 7-42) A line is drawn from the anterior edge of the head of the fibula to the anterior edge of the lateral malleolus. The flap is designed on the middle and lower thirds of the leg, with this line as an axis. Maximum size may be as large as 10 cm wide and 20 cm long.

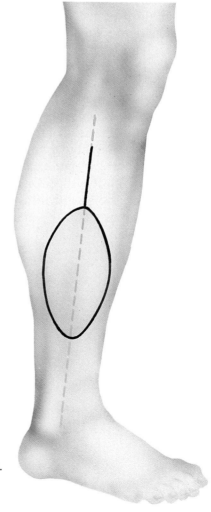

1. Anterior tibial artery and deep peroneal n.
2. Inferior lateral peroneal a.
3. Superior lateral peroneal a.
4. Extensor digitorum longus m.
5. Tibialis anterior m.
6. Interosseous membrane
7. Peroneus longus and brevis m.
8. Soleus m.
9. Superficial peroneal n.

(**Fig. 7-43**) The anterior part of the flap with deep fascia is raised from the extensor muscles [4,5] toward the anterior crural intermuscular septum between the anterior and peroneal compartments. Usually, the neurovascular bundle is first found at the distal margin of the flap. The superficial peroneal nerve [9] is large, but the septocutaneous artery is small. The nerves are traced to identify the inferior lateral peroneal [2] and the anterior tibial arteries [1], and the latter is ligated distal to the origin of the artery.

1. Anterior tibial a. and deep peroneal n.
2. Inferior lateral peroneal a.
4. Extensor digitorum longus m.
5. Tibialis anterior m.
9. Superficial peroneal n.

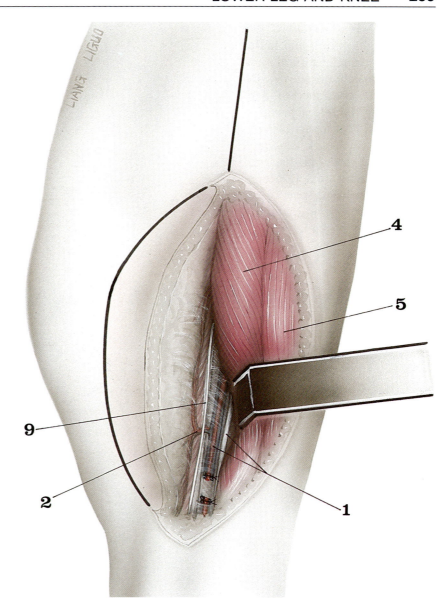

(Fig. 7-44) Detaching the extensors digitorum and hallucis longus from the fibula and interosseous membrane [6], the dissection is continued to identify the superior lateral peroneal artery [3]. The superficial peroneal nerve [9] is separated from the septocutaneous vessels, leaving it intact. Meanwhile, the posterior part of the flap is developed gradually, from distal to proximal.

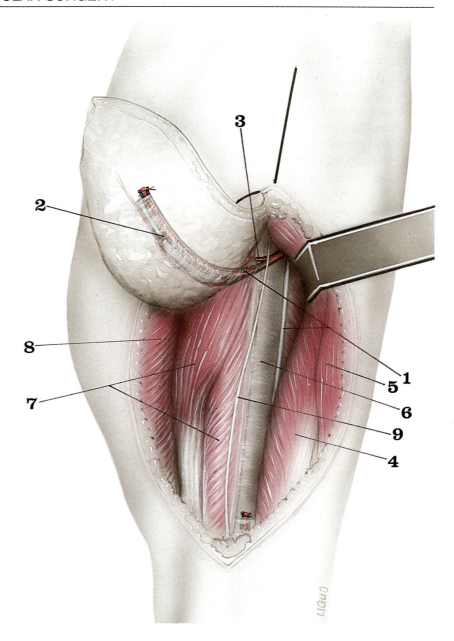

1. Anterior tibial a. and deep peroneal n.
2. Inferior lateral peroneal a.
3. Superior lateral peroneal a.
4. Extensor digitorum longus m.
5. Tibialis anterior m.
6. Interosseous membrane
7. Peroneus longus and brevis m.
8. Soleus m.
9. Superficial peroneal n.

(**Fig. 7-45**) The superior lateral peroneal artery [3] is dissected to its origin on the anterior tibial artery [1].

The entire flap is raised, based on the superior and inferior lateral peroneal vessels and the anterior tibial vessels, with a pedicle length ranging from 6 to 9 cm, depending on the location of the designed flap.

1. Anterior tibial a. and deep peroneal n.
2. Inferior lateral peroneal a.
3. Superior lateral peroneal a.

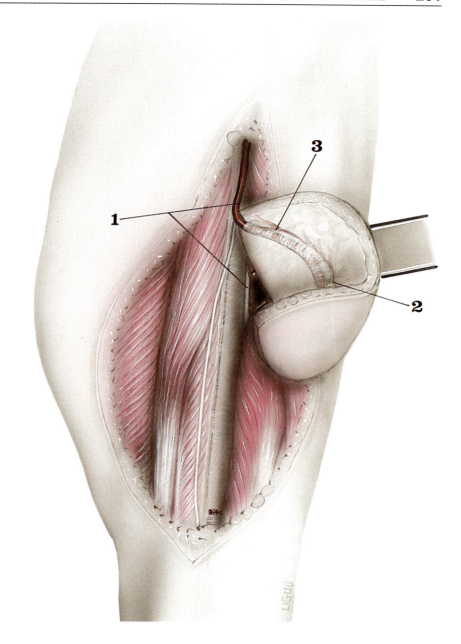

REVERSE ANTERIOR TIBIAL ISLAND FLAP

(Fig. 7-46) This flap is designed on the upper and middle thirds of the leg. After raising the flap with the superior and inferior lateral peroneal vessels and the septum isolated, the anterior tibial vessels are ligated above the origin of these septocutaneous vessels. They are then freed downward from the deep peroneal nerve, to reach a sufficient pedicle length for a distal transfer. It is suggested that the proximal end of the anterior tibial vein be anastomosed to a vein in the recipient site.

1. Anterior tibial a. and deep peroneal n.
4. Extensor digitorum longus m.
5. Tibialis anterior m.
6. Interosseous membrane
7. Peroneus longus and brevis m.
8. Soleus m.

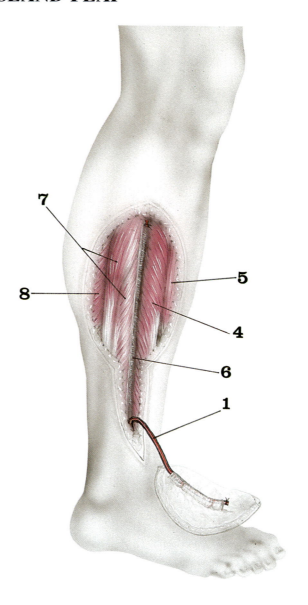

LOWER LEG AND KNEE 263

(Fig. 7-47) This is a diagram of the cross-section of the anterior tibial flap.

1. Anterior tibial a. and deep peroneal n.
2. Inferior lateral peroneal a.
3. Superior lateral peroneal a.
4. Extensor digitorum longus m.
5. Tibialis anterior m.
7. Peroneus longus and brevis m.
8. Soleus m.

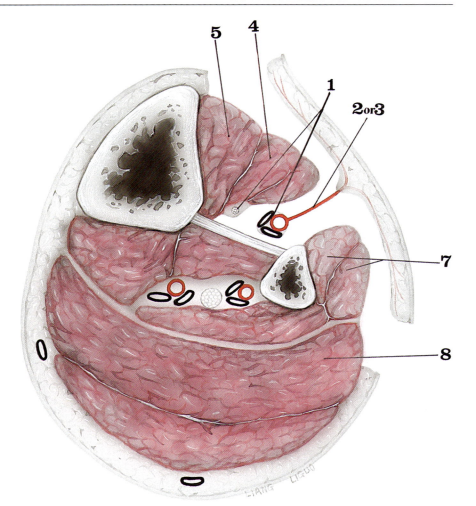

MEDIAL LEG FLAP

Anatomy of the Posterior Tibial Artery (Fig. 7-48)

After bifurcating from the anterior tibial artery [2], the vessel [1] runs between the soleus and flexor digitorum longus or tibialis posterior, accompanied by two veins and the tibial nerve.

In its course, it gives off about four or more septocutaneous branches [4] along the medial border of the tibia, passing through the deep transverse fascial septum. These septocutaneous branches emerge to the subcutaneous layer, just behind the medial border of the tibia. The diameter of these arteries varies from 0.5 to 1.5 cm.

1. Posterior tibial a.
2. Anterior tibial a.
3. Peroneal a.
4. Septocutaneous branches

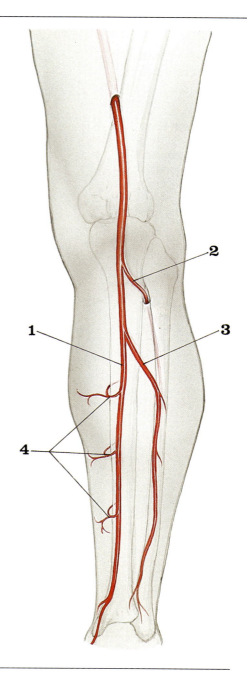

COMMENT AND INSIGHTS

The medial tibial flap is a septocutaneous flap, and its septocutaneous branches come from the posterior tibial artery through the deep transverse fascial septum, emerging along the medial border of the tibia.

There have been relatively few cases of revascularized medial leg flaps reported, since the flap requires the sacrifice of the posterior tibial artery, even though the arterial anatomy is quite reliable. For this reason, arteriography should be routinely done to confirm the existence of both the posterior and anterior tibial arteries before harvesting this flap.

The skin in the medial aspect of the lower leg has moderate thickness, but the donor site generally needs a split-thickness skin graft after removal of a skin flap more than 3 cm wide. Even so, a cosmetic problem remains.

Compared with other donor sites, the medial leg flap is not a primary choice for transfer; local transfers as island flaps may be acceptable.

The medial leg flap also can be combined with the medial plantar flap on the same pedicle of the posterior tibial artery and its continuation, as "twin" flaps. (For the harvesting technique of the medial plantar flap, see Chapter 8.)

Harvesting Technique

(**Fig. 7-49**) The posterior edge of the tibia corresponds to the vascular axis, but the anterior border is drawn only a little over this line to avoid exposing the tibia and its periosteum; the posterior border is limited to the posterior midline. The flap should be sited on the midportion of the leg, and a successful flap size of 22 × 9 cm has been reported.

1. Soleus m.
2. Tibia
3. Septocutaneous branches
4. Posterior tibial a., v., and tibial n.
5. Flexor digitorum longus m.
6. Gastrocnemius m.

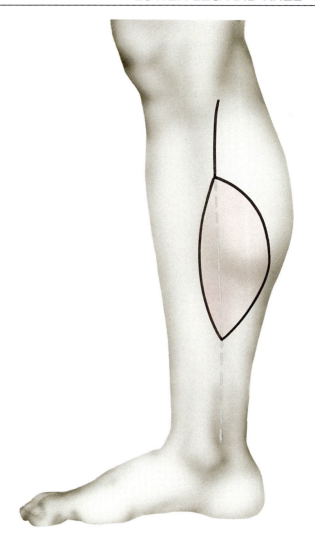

(Fig. 7-50) The anterior border of the flap is incised, and the dominant septocutaneous branches [3] are identified within the midportion of the leg. Detaching the soleus muscle [1] from the tibia [2], the septocutaneous branches are carefully dissected.

1. Soleus m.
2. Tibia
3. Septocutaneous branches
5. Flexor digitorum longus m.

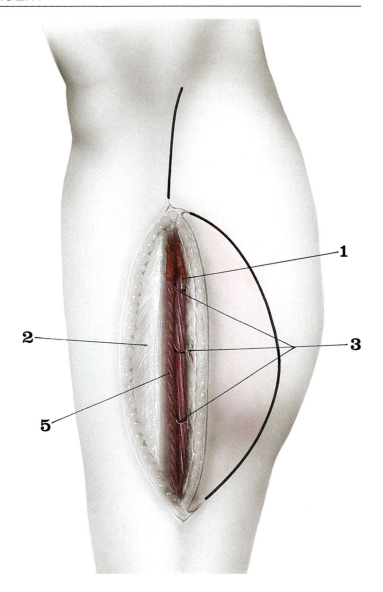

(Fig. 7-51) The posterior part of the flap with deep fascia is raised toward the septum behind the tibia [2]. Tracing these branches, the posterior tibial vessels [4] are widely exposed. Ligating the several muscular branches, a segment of the posterior tibial vessels can be provided, in case it should be required for graft at the recipient site.

1. Soleus m.
4. Posterior tibial a. and v., and tibial n.
5. Flexor digitorum longus m.
6. Gastrocnemius m.

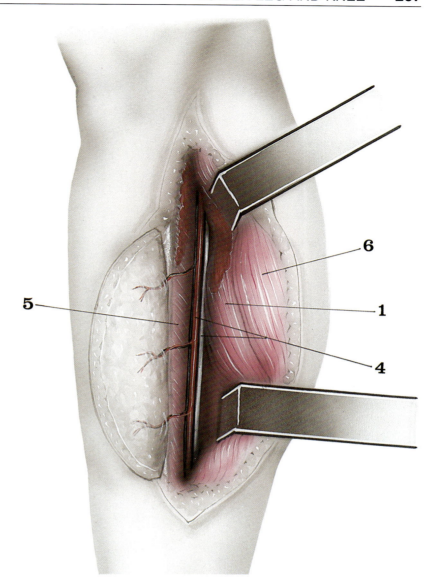

(Fig. 7-52) Ligating and dividing the distal end of the vascular segment, the entire flap is raised on the proximal pedicle of the posterior tibial vessels [4].

If a sensory flap is needed, the saphenous nerve should be included with the flap.

4. Posterior tibial a. and v., and tibial n.
5. Flexor digitorum longus m.
6. Gastrocnemius m.

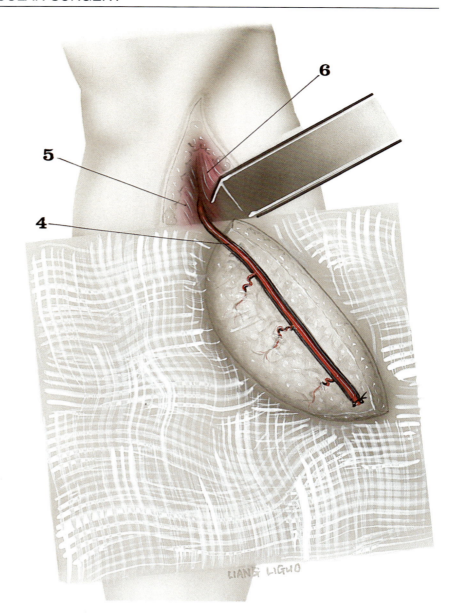

(Fig. 7-53) A diagram of the cross-section of the medial leg flap.

1. Soleus m.
2. Tibia
3. Septocutaneous branches
4. Posterior tibial a. and v., and tibial n.
5. Flexor digitorum longus m.
6. Gastrocnemius m.

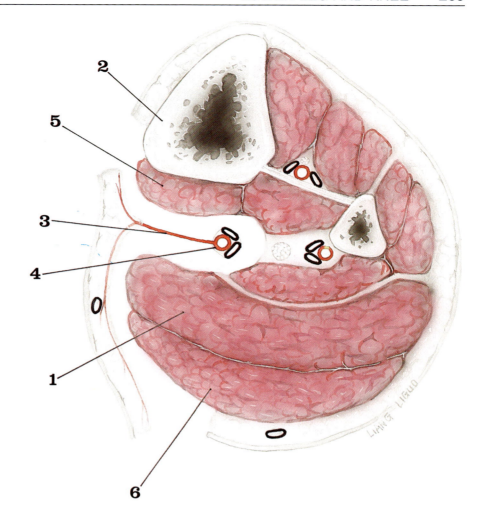

POSTERIOR LEG FLAP

Anatomy (Fig. 7-54)

There are two to three axial fasciocutaneous branches from the popliteal artery [1] or medial and lateral sural arteries to supply the posterior skin of the leg. One of them, the superficial sural artery [3], accompanies the lesser saphenous vein and the medial sural nerve [3]. However the dominant axial artery, the *lateral popliteal cutaneous artery* [2], arises at the level of the tibial condyle in the cleft between the heads of the gastrocnemius. It then runs inferolaterally to accompany the lateral sural nerve [5] under the deep fascia. Usually, it can be identified at the midpoint between the posterior midline and the fibular head.

The artery pierces the deep fascia about 4 cm below the tibial condyle and continues downward, terminating at the medial side of the Achilles tendon. The vessel has an average diameter of 1.2 mm, with a range from 1.0 to 1.7 mm. It is accompanied by two venae comitantes with diameters of 2.0 mm.

Innervation

The upper part of the flap is innervated by the posterior cutaneous nerve of the thigh. That of the lower part of the flap is from the lateral sural nerve.

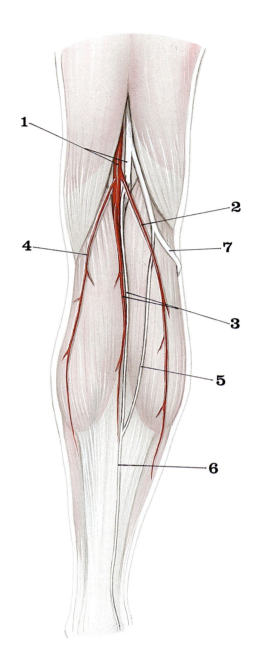

1. Popliteal a. and tibial n.
2. Lateral popliteal cutaneous a.
3. Superficial sural a. and medial sural n.
4. Medial popliteal cutaneous a.
5. Lateral sural n.
6. Sural n.
7. Common peroneal n.
8. Medial sural a.
9. Lateral sural a.

(Fig. 7-55) Variations in origin of the lateral popliteal cutaneous artery are:

Type A. directly from the popliteal artery (65%)

Type B. from the lateral sural artery (10%)

Type C. from the medial sural artery (15%)

Type D. from another cutaneous artery (20%)

1. Popliteal a. and tibial n.
2. Lateral popliteal cutaneous a.
8. Medial sural a.
9. Lateral sural a.

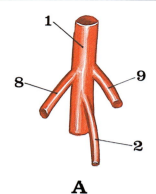
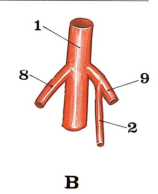
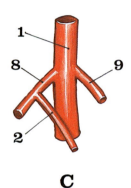
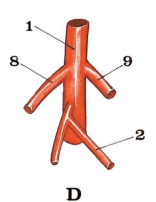

COMMENT AND INSIGHTS

The posterior leg flap is an axial fasciocutaneous flap; its axial fasciocutaneous branches come from the popliteal artery.

Because of the variable anatomy and relatively small size of the axial fasciocutaneous branches from the popliteal artery, the posterior leg flap may be somewhat difficult to harvest and therefore less reliable.

The skin on the posterior aspect of the lower leg has moderate thickness, but the donor site generally needs a split-thickness skin graft after removal of a skin flap more than 3 cm wide. Even so, a cosmetic problem remains.

Compared with other donor sites, the posterior leg flap is not a primary choice for transfer; local transfers as island flaps are acceptable. The island fasciocutaneous flap is based on the proximal fascial layer below the popliteal fossa as the pedicle of the flap; the vascular structure is included in the fascia and need not be dissected out.

272 ATLAS OF MICROVASCULAR SURGERY

Harvesting Technique

(Fig. 7-56) The patient is placed in a prone or lateral decubitus position. The posterior midline is marked and the flap is designed within the following boundaries: medially and laterally, up to each midline of the leg; superiorly, up to the superior flexion crease of the calf; inferiorly, up to the junction of the middle and lower thirds of the leg. The largest flap size reported is 11 × 19 cm.

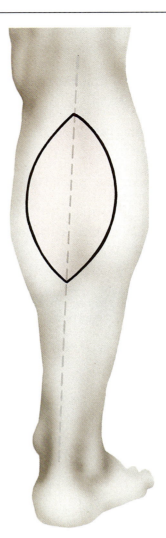

1. Gastrocnemius m.
2. Lateral popliteal cutaneous a.
3. Lateral sural n.
4. Sural n.
5. Lesser saphenous v., superficial sural a., and medial sural n.
6. Popliteal a. and tibial n.
7. Posterior cutaneous n. of thigh

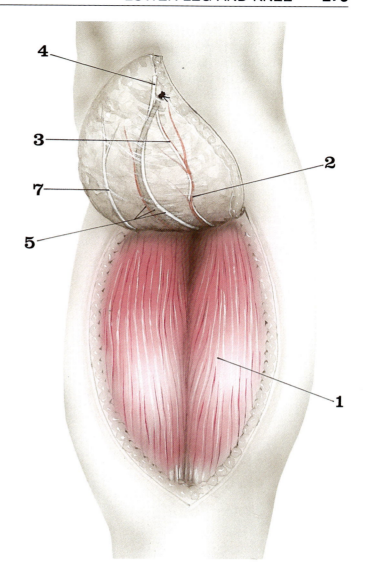

(Fig. 7-57) The flap with deep fascia is elevated from distal to proximal. The sural nerve [4] and lesser saphenous vein [5] are divided at the lower border of the flap and included with it.

Special attention should be paid to the dissection on the superior lateral flap edge to identify the lateral sural nerve [3] and the dominant vessel [2] that is located between the posterior midline and the head of the fibula under deep fascia.

1. Gastrocnemius m.
2. Lateral popliteal cutaneous a.
3. Lateral sural n.
4. Sural n.
5. Lesser saphenous v., superficial sural a., and medial sural n.
7. Posterior cutaneous n. of thigh

(Fig. 7-58) The posterior cutaneous nerve of the thigh [7], the medial sural nerve [5], and the lesser saphenous vein [5] are isolated and divided on the superior border of the flap under deep fascia. The posterior leg flap is isolated on the lateral popliteal cutaneous vessels [2]; these can be dissected further to the vessel origin to achieve a pedicle length of 8 to 12 cm.

1. Gastrocnemius m.
2. Lateral popliteal cutaneous a.
5. Lesser saphenous v., superficial sural a., and medial sural n.
6. Popliteal a. and tibial n.
7. Posterior cutaneous n. of thigh

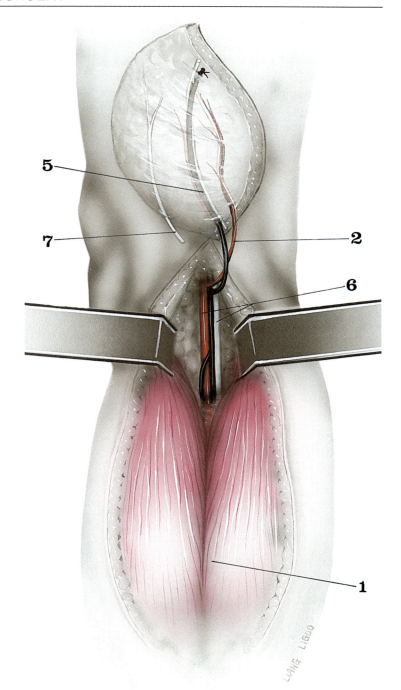

RECIPIENT SITE EXPOSURES

Popliteal Artery

The popliteal artery commences at the opening of the adductor magnus, at the junction of the middle and distal thirds of the thigh. The vessel extends downward and slightly laterally, to the intercondylar fossa of the femur. Thence, it continues obliquely to the lower border of the popliteus.

The artery may be considered as having three portions. The proximal portion begins at the opening of the adductor; the middle portion lies between the heads of the gastrocnemius, at about the level of the knee joint; and the distal portion lies behind the upper part of the tibia and fibula.

There are three approaches to the artery. Compared to a posterior and lateral approach, the medial approach has the following advantages: (1) The popliteal artery is more accessible and can be easily drawn forward toward the skin, when the knee is flexed; (2) the tibial nerve and popliteal veins are more easily avoided; and (3) the patient is in the supine position, so that surgeons may work simultaneously on the donor site in this position.

Medial Approach to the Proximal Portion of the Popliteal Artery

(**Fig. 7-59**) The patient is placed in the supine position. The affected foot is placed on the contralateral shin, with the knee flexed and the thigh externally rotated. An incision 15 cm in length is made from the adductor tubercle of the femur [4], running proximally toward the midpoint of the inguinal ligament, and ending at the junction of the middle and distal thirds of the thigh.

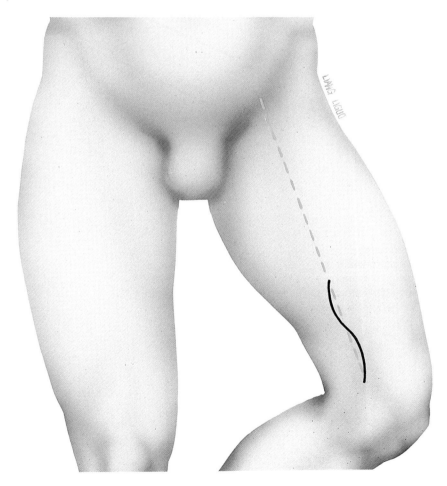

1. Sartorius m.
2. Vastus medialis m.
3. Adductor tendon
4. Adductor tubercle
5. Saphenous a. and n.
6. Popliteal a. and v.
7. Posterior edge of femur

(**Fig. 7-60**) While undermining, the greater saphenous vein can be seen posterior to the incisions. The deep fascia is divided anterior to the sartorius muscle [1], which is then retracted posteriorly. The saphenous vessels and nerve [5] are beneath the muscle, piercing the aponeurosis roof of the adductor canal and running over the adductor tendon [3]. The saphenous nerve should be preserved.

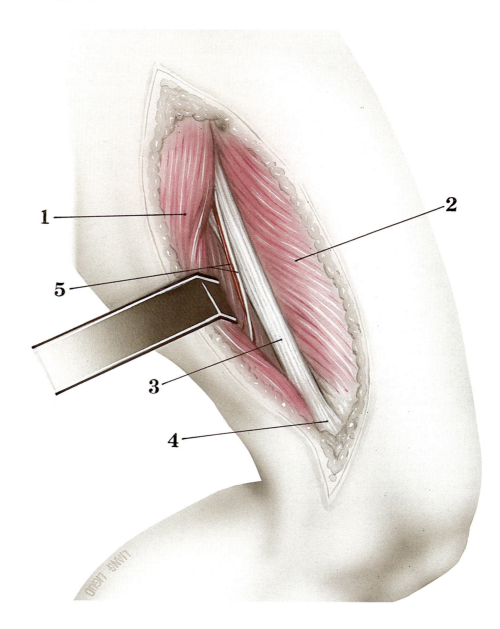

1. Sartorius m.
2. Vastus medialis m.
3. Adductor tendon
4. Adductor tubercle
5. Saphenous a. and n.

LOWER LEG AND KNEE

(Fig. 7-61) The vastus medialis muscle [2] is retracted anteriorly and the adductor tendon [3] is divided. The popliteal artery [6] is identified posterior to the femur [7]; it is the most superficial (medial) vessel in the neurovascular structure in the fossa. The medial superior genicular artery and medial sural artery may arise from the medial aspect of the popliteal artery.

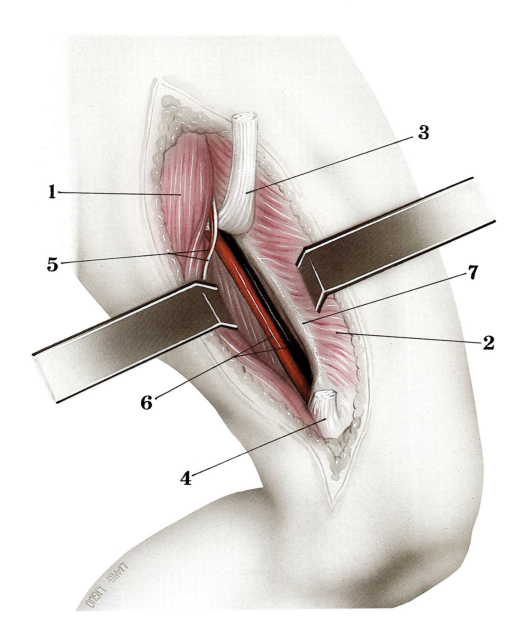

1. Sartorius m.
2. Vastus medialis m.
3. Adductor tendon
4. Adductor tubercle
5. Saphenous a. and n.
6. Popliteal a. and v.
7. Posterior edge of femur

Medial Approach to the Middle Portion of the Popliteal Artery

(**Fig. 7-62**) The patient is placed in the supine position and the affected foot is placed on the contralateral shin, with the knee flexed. The skin incision used for the proximal portion of the artery is extended distally to the medial condyle of the tibia.

1. Sartorius m.
2. Vastus medialis m.
3. Medial head of gastrocnemius m.
4. Common tendon of gracilis, semimembranosus, and semitendinosus
5. Saphenous a. and n.
6. Greater saphenous v.
7. Popliteal a. and v.
8. Tibial n.

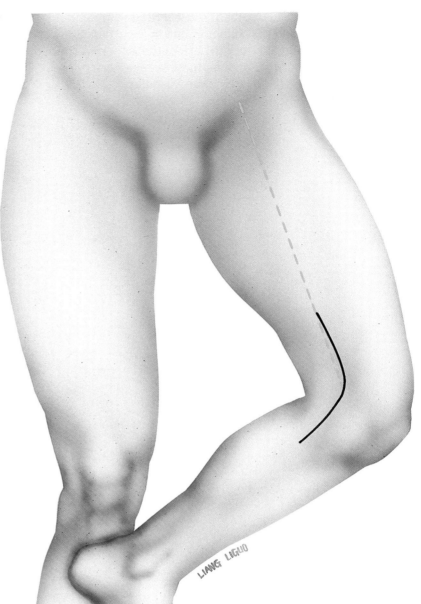

(**Fig. 7-63**) After the greater saphenous vein [6] and sartorius muscle [1] are identified, the deep fascia is divided between the sartorius and medial hamstring tendons [4]. The gracilis [4], semimembranosus [4], and semitendinosus [4] tendons are usually combined to form a common tendon [4]. While dissecting between them, the saphenous vessels and nerve [5] are seen emerging between the sartorius and gracilis at the knee joint at a subcutaneous level and running distally with the greater saphenous vein.

1. Sartorius m.
2. Vastus medialis m.
3. Medial head of gastrocnemius m.
4. Common tendon of gracilis, semimembranosus, and semitendinosus
5. Saphenous a. and n.
6. Greater saphenous v.

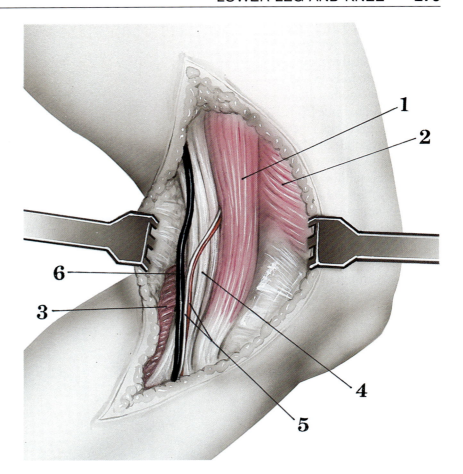

(Fig. 7-64) After the sartorius [1] is retracted anteriorly and the medial hamstring tendons [4] are divided, the medial head of the gastrocnemius [3] is identified and detached from the medial condyle of the femur. One centimeter of the tendinous attachment is left, to facilitate later suturing and to avoid injuring the synovial membrane of the knee joint.

While turning the medial head of the muscle downward to expose the popliteal fossa, care should be taken not to injure the neurovascular bundle to the muscle.

The sheath of the popliteal artery [7] is incised. It may be necessary to divide venous tributaries that cross the artery. The tibial nerve [8] is deep to the popliteal vein and well out of the way.

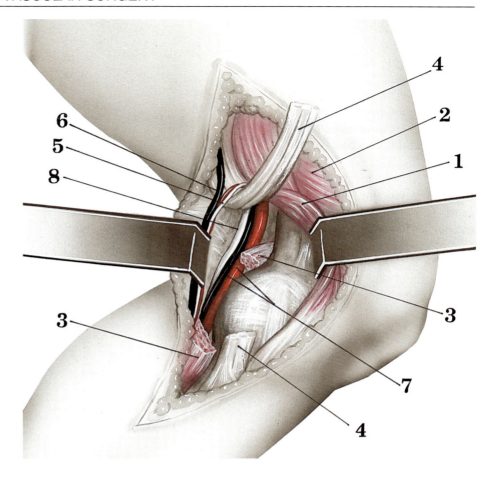

1. Sartorius m.
2. Vastus medialis m.
3. Medial head of gastrocnemius m.
4. Common tendon of gracilis, semimembranosus, and semitendinosus
5. Saphenous a. and n.
6. Greater saphenous v.
7. Popliteal a. and v.
8. Tibial n.

LOWER LEG AND KNEE

Medial Approach to the Distal Portion of the Popliteal Artery

(**Fig. 7-65**) The patient is placed in the supine position; the affected foot is placed on the contralateral shin, with the knee flexed. An incision is made from the adductor tubercle of the femur via the medial condyle of the tibia, and extending distally along the posteromedial border of the tibia.

1. Capsule of the knee joint
2. Tendon of sartorius
3. Common tendon of medial hamstring
4. Medial head of gastrocnemius m.
5. Soleus m.
6. Popliteal a. and v.
7. Anterior tibial a. and v.
8. Tibial n.

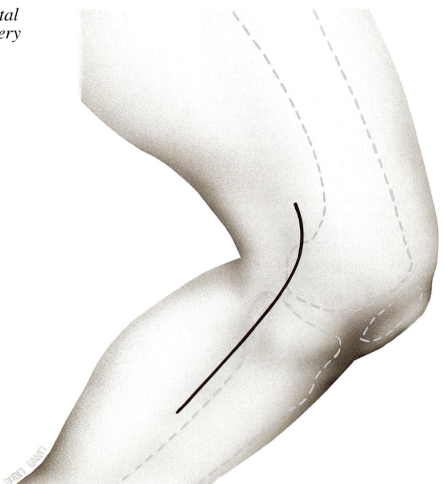

(**Fig. 7-66**) The deep fascia is incised along the posterior edge of the tibia. The tendons of insertion of the sartorius [2] and other medial hamstring [3] muscles are divided to expose the medial head of the gastrocnemius [4].

1. Capsule of the knee joint
2. Tendon of sartorius
3. Common tendon of medial hamstring
4. Medial head of gastrocnemius m.

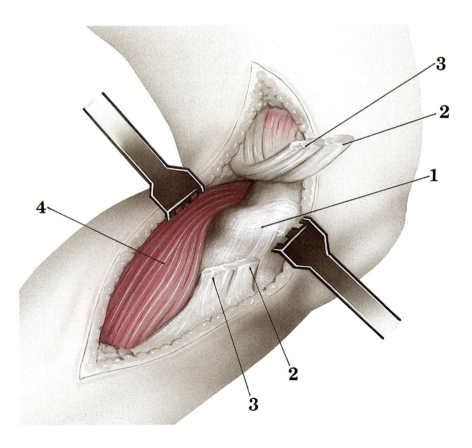

(**Fig. 7-67**) The medial head of the gastrocnemius [4] is retracted posteriorly away from the tibia; the origin of the soleus [5] on the posterior aspect of the tibia is exposed. Along the superomedial edge of the soleus, the popliteal vein [6] is first identified, then dissected and retracted to expose the popliteal artery [6].

Dissecting the medial origin of the soleus muscle and tracing the popliteal vessel distally, the origin of the anterior tibial artery [7] is found on the opposite side of the popliteal artery at the lower border of the popliteus muscle.

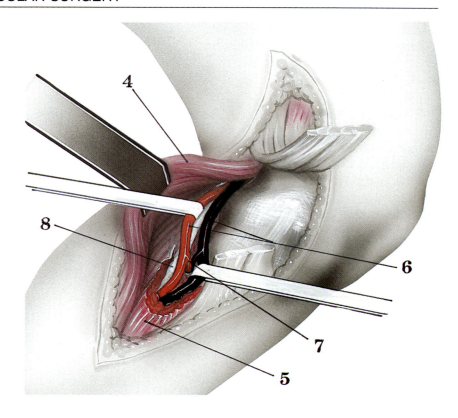

4. Medial head of gastrocnemius m.
5. Soleus m.
6. Popliteal a. and v.
7. Anterior tibial a. and v.
8. Tibial n.

Posterior Approach to the Popliteal Artery

(**Fig. 7-68**) The patient is placed in a prone position. An S-shaped incision is made along the tendons of the medial hamstring vertically and the skin crease of the popliteal fossa transversely, turning toward the lateral head of the gastrocnemius.

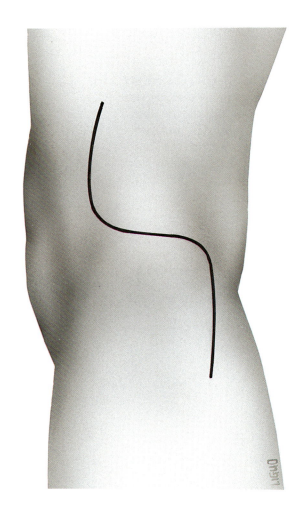

1. Medial hamstring
2. Biceps femoris
3. Medial head of gastrocnemius
4. Lateral head of gastrocnemius
5. Lesser saphenous v. and medial sural n.
6. Popliteal a. and v.
7. Peroneal n.
8. Tibial n.
9. Soleus m.
10. Popliteal m.

(Fig. 7-69) After undermining, the skin flaps are retracted and the deep fascia is incised in the midline. The lesser saphenous vein and medial sural nerve [5] should be preserved, especially if the vein is to be used as a recipient.

1. Medial hamstring
2. Biceps femoris
3. Medial head of gastrocnemius
4. Lateral head of gastrocnemius
5. Lesser saphenous v. and medial sural n.

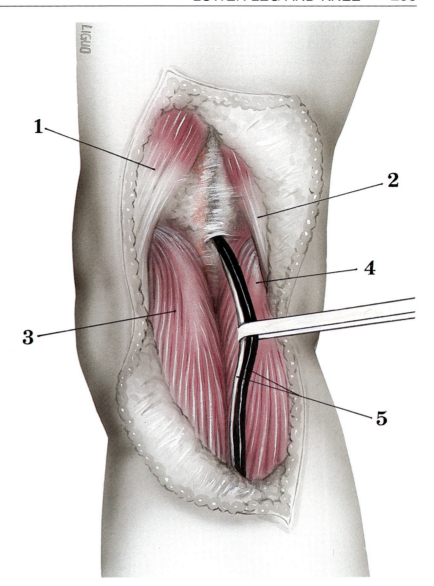

(Fig. 7-70) For exposure of the proximal portion of the artery, the biceps femoris [2] is retracted laterally and the hamstring [1] medially. The tibial nerve [8] and common peroneal nerve [7] are identified and protected in the lateral wall of the fossa. The popliteal vein [6] is exposed, following the lesser saphenous vein [5], and retracted laterally. The popliteal artery [6] is located behind and medial to the vein.

1. Medial hamstring
2. Biceps femoris
5. Lesser saphenous v. and medial sural n.
6. Popliteal a. and v.
7. Peroneal n.
8. Tibial n.

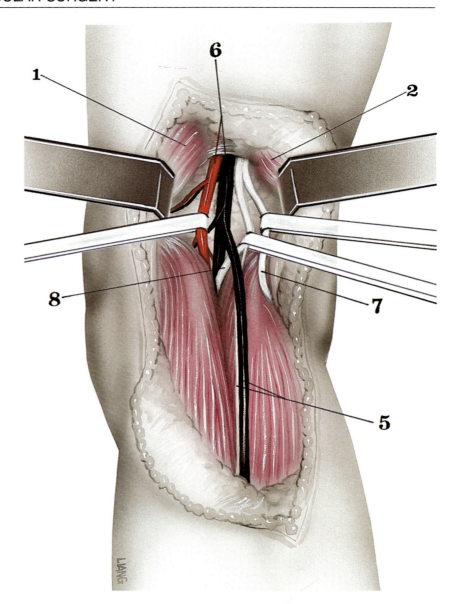

(**Fig. 7-71**) For exposure of the distal portion, the heads of the gastrocnemius [3,4] are retracted. The tibial nerve [8] and the medial sural nerve [5] are encountered first, then isolated and retracted laterally with nerve tape. There may be two popliteal veins [6] behind them, and the artery [6] may be located at the deepest level and between the two veins.

3. Medial head of gastrocnemius
4. Lateral head of gastrocnemius
5. Lesser saphenous v. and medial sural n.
6. Popliteal a. and v.
8. Tibial n.
9. Soleus m.
10. Popliteal m.

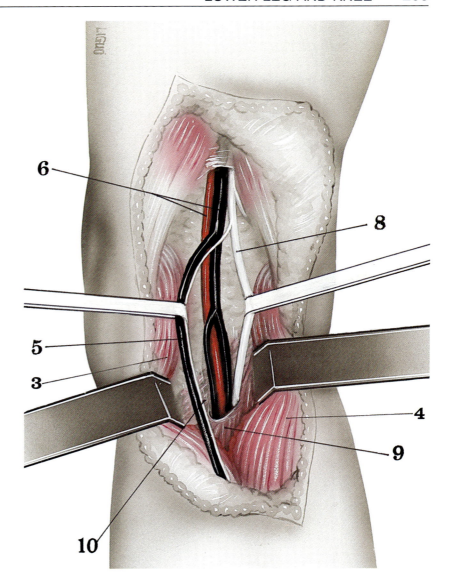

Lateral Approach to the Popliteal Artery (Proximal Portion)

(Fig. 7-72) The patient is placed on the normal side, with the normal limb straight. The affected knee joint is flexed 30° to 60°. A longitudinal incision is made along the posterior edge of the iliotibial tract for about 15 cm to the head of the fibula.

1. Iliotibial tract
2. Vastus lateralis m.
3. Fibular collateral ligament
4. Tendon of biceps femoris
5. Short head of biceps femoris
6. Popliteal a. and v.
7. Peroneal n.
8. Tibial n.
9. Femur

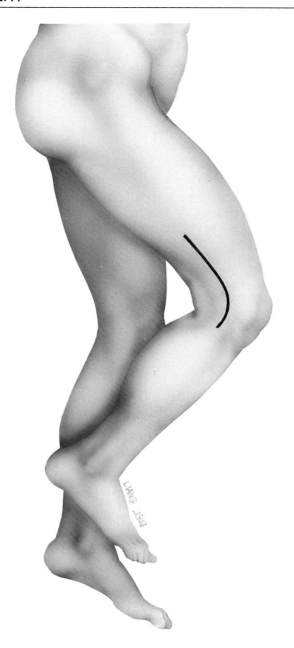

(Fig. 7-73) The deep fascia is divided along the posterior edge of the iliotibial tract [1]. Then, the lateral intermuscular septum between the biceps femoris tendon [4] and the vastus lateralis muscle [2] is identified.

1. Iliotibial tract
2. Vastus lateralis m.
3. Fibular collateral ligament
4. Tendon of biceps femoris
5. Short head of biceps femoris

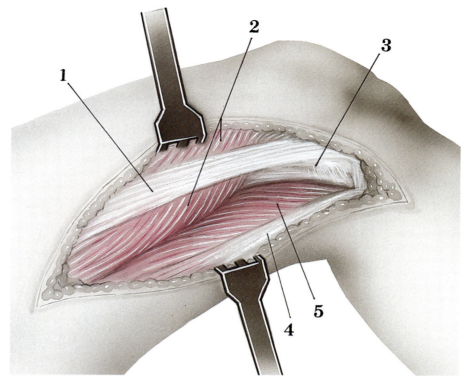

(Fig. 7-74) Ligating the perforating branches to both muscles, the iliotibial tract [1] and vastus lateralis [2] are retracted anteriorly and the biceps [5] posteriorly.

A gap between the short head of the biceps [5] and the posterolateral edge of the femur [9] is reached above the lateral condyle. The gap is enlarged by detaching the attachment of the short head on the femur proximally, and the popliteal fossa is approached by blunt finger dissection. At first, the common peroneal and tibial nerves [7,8] are encountered in the front of the fossa; they should be carefully protected. The popliteal artery [6] is located behind the popliteal vein [6]. There are some branches arising from the lateral aspect of the artery: the lateral superior genicular artery and the lateral sural artery.

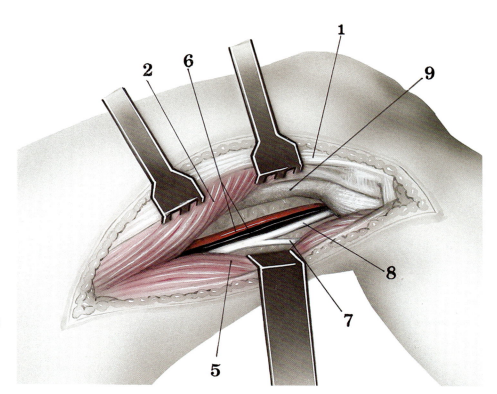

1. Iliotibial tract
2. Vastus lateralis m.
5. Short head of biceps femoris
6. Popliteal a. and v.
7. Peroneal n.
8. Tibial n.
9. Femur

Tibioperoneal Trunk

Medial Approach to the Tibioperoneal Trunk

(**Fig. 7-75**) The patient is placed in the supine position, with the thigh abducted and externally rotated and the knee flexed and supported. The skin incision begins from the medial condyle of the tibia, running distally parallel to and 3 cm posterior to the posteromedial edge of the tibia for about 10 cm.

1. Tibia
2. Medial head of gastrocnemius m.
3. Soleus m.
4. Popliteus m.
5. Popliteal a. and v.
6. Tibial n.
7. Tibioperoneal trunk
8. Posterior tibial a. and v.
9. Anterior tibial a. and v.
10. Peroneal a. and v.
11. Tibialis posterior m.
12. Flexor digitorum longus m.

(Fig. 7-76) The deep fascia is divided, and the medial head of the gastrocnemius [2] is retracted posteriorly; then, the soleus muscle [3] is identified.

1. Tibia
2. Medial head of gastrocnemius m.
3. Soleus m.
4. Popliteus m.
5. Popliteal a. and v.
6. Tibial n.

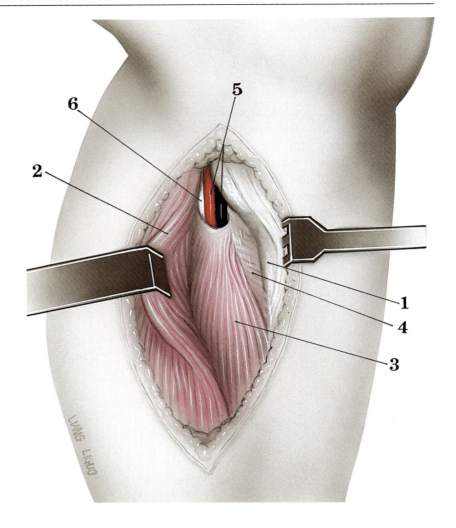

(**Fig. 7-77**) The longitudinal attachment of the soleus [3] is detached from the medial edge of the tibia [1], and the tibioperoneal trunk [7] appears between the soleus [3] and the tibialis posterior [11].

Detachment continues proximally, until the medial pier of the soleus arch is divided. At this stage, this segment of the artery is sufficiently exposed. Dissection proceeds deeply, to isolate the tibial nerve [6] and to identify the takeoffs of the anterior tibial and peroneal arteries [9,10], which are usually located about 2.5 and 5 cm, respectively, below the medial condyle of the tibia.

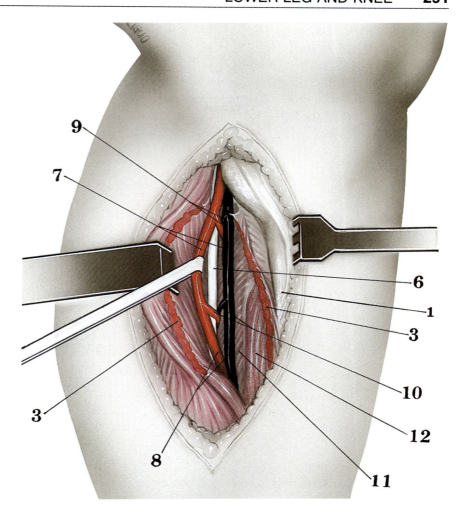

1. Tibia
3. Soleus m.
6. Tibial n.
7. Tibioperoneal trunk
8. Posterior tibial a. and v.
9. Anterior tibial a. and v.
10. Peroneal a. and v.
11. Tibialis posterior m.
12. Flexor digitorum longus m.

292 ATLAS OF MICROVASCULAR SURGERY

Posterior Approach to the Tibioperoneal Trunk

(Fig. 7-78) The incision begins at the level of the knee joint, for about 10 cm along the posterior midline of the calf.

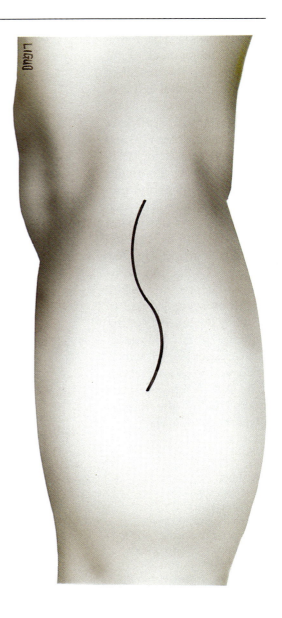

1. Medial head of gastrocnemius m.
2. Lateral head of gastrocnemius m.
3. Popliteal a. and v.
4. Tibial n.
5. Lesser saphenous v. and medial sural n.
6. Soleus m.
7. Popliteus m.
8. Tibioperoneal trunk
9. Anterior tibial a. and v.
10. Posterior tibial a. and v.
11. Peroneal a. and v.
12. Tibialis posterior m.

(**Fig. 7-79**) Isolating the lesser saphenous vein [5] and medial sural nerve [5], the lateral and medial heads of the gastrocnemius [1,2] are split apart along the groove between them. The superior edge of the soleus [6] and neurovascular bundle of the popliteal vessel [3], as well as the tibial nerve [4] about it, are exposed.

1. Medial head of gastrocnemius m.
2. Lateral head of gastrocnemius m.
3. Popliteal a. and v.
4. Tibial n.
5. Lesser saphenous v. and medial sural n.
6. Soleus m.
7. Popliteus m.

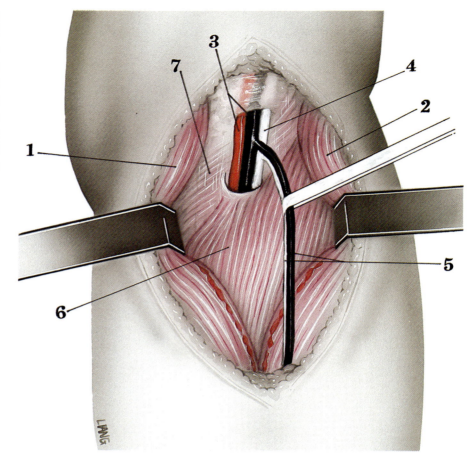

(**Fig. 7-80**) The fibrous band between the tibia and fibula that arches over the popliteal vessels [3] and the tibial nerve [4], is identified and divided. From this point, the soleus muscle [6] is split longitudinally, and the underlying neurovascular bundle [8] is then revealed. Below the lower border of the popliteus muscle [7], the takeoffs of the anterior tibial and peroneal arteries [9,11] are dissected out on the lateral aspect of the tibioperoneal trunk.

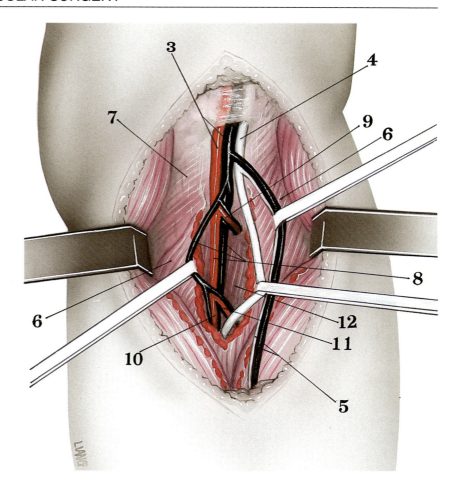

3. Popliteal a. and v.
4. Tibial n.
5. Lesser saphenous v. and medial sural n.
6. Soleus m.
7. Popliteus m.
8. Tibioperoneal trunk
9. Anterior tibial a. and v.
10. Posterior tibial a. and v.
11. Peroneal a. and v.
12. Tibialis posterior m.

Lateral Approach to the Tibioperoneal Trunk

(Fig. 7-81) The incision begins at the popliteal fossa, curving via the posterior aspect of the head of the fibula, and running distally along the posterior edge of the fibula for about 10 cm.

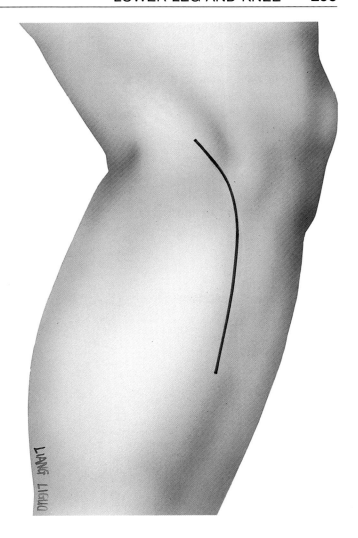

1. Head of fibula
2. Lateral head of gastrocnemius m.
3. Peroneus longus m.
4. Soleus m.
5. Popliteus m.
6. Popliteal a. and v.
7. Tibial n.
8. Peroneal n.
9. Tibioperoneal trunk
10. Anterior tibial a. and v.
11. Peroneal a. and v.
12. Flexor hallucis longus m.
13. Tibialis posterior m.

296 ATLAS OF MICROVASCULAR SURGERY

(Fig. 7-82) The common peroneal nerve [8] is identified between the lateral head of the gastrocnemius [2] and the biceps femoris tendon and should be carefully protected. Retracting the lateral head of the gastrocnemius [2] posteriorly, the lateral proximal portion of the soleus [4] appears in the wound.

1. Head of fibula
2. Lateral head of gastrocnemius m.
3. Peroneus longus m.
4. Soleus m.
5. Popliteus m.
6. Popliteal a. and v.
7. Tibial n.
8. Peroneal n.

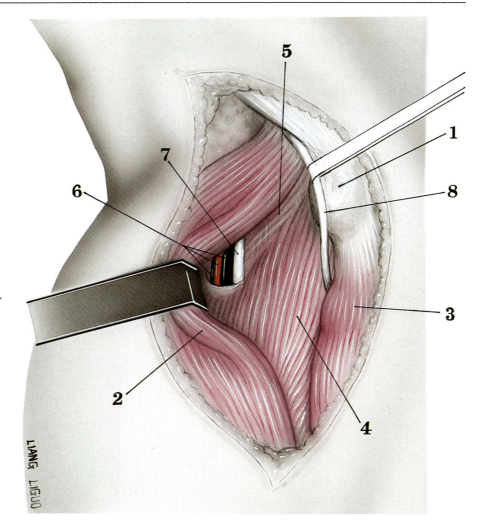

(Fig. 7-83) The soleus [4] is detached from the posterior aspect of the head and the proximal third of the fibula and retracted posteriorly with the gastrocnemius. The anterior tibial and peroneal arteries [10,11] are identified. The tibioperoneal trunk [9] lies deeply behind the tibial nerve [7]. For better exposure, the lateral head of the gastrocnemius can be detached from the lateral condyle of the femur.

3. Peroneus longus m.
4. Soleus m.
7. Tibial n.
8. Peroneal n.
9. Tibioperoneal trunk
10. Anterior tibial a. and v.
11. Peroneal a. and v.
12. Flexor hallucis longus m.
13. Tibialis posterior m.

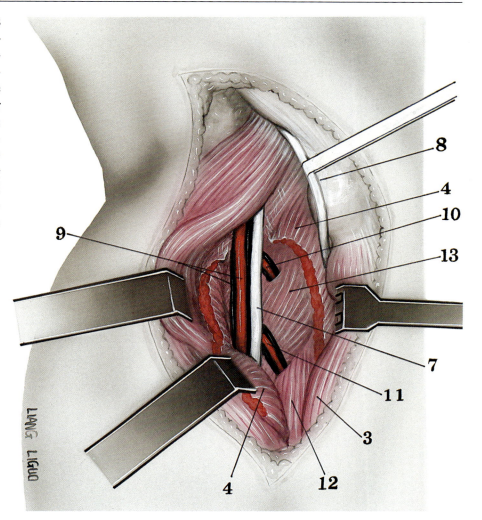

Exposure of the Arched Segment of the Anterior Tibial Artery by Resection of the Fibula

(Fig. 7-84) An incision is made from the lateral wall of the popliteal fossa, along the medial border of the biceps femoris tendon, to the head of the fibula. It then runs distally along the shaft of the fibula for about 8 cm.

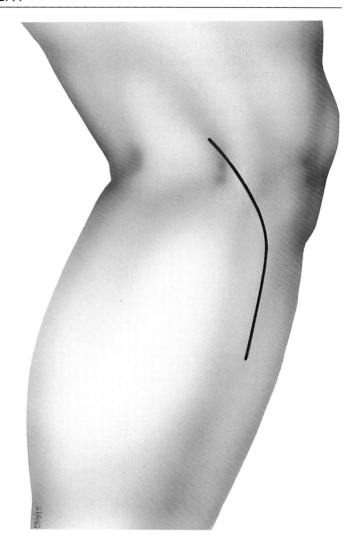

1. Lateral head of gastrocnemius m.
2. Soleus m.
3. Fibula
4. Peroneus longus m.
5. Biceps femoris tendon
6. Tibialis anterior m.
7. Extensor digitorum longus m.
8. Common peroneal n.
9. Tibialis posterior m.
10. Popliteal a. and v.
11. Tibioperoneal trunk
12. Tibial n.
13. Articular facet on tibia
14. Anterior tibial a. and v.
15. Deep peroneal n.

LOWER LEG AND KNEE

(Fig. 7-85) The common peroneal nerve [8] is first identified behind the biceps femoris tendon [5]. The peroneus longus [4] is detached from the head of the fibula; then the nerve can be mobilized from the neck of the fibula. The soleus [2] and peronei [4] are stripped from the fibula, and the interosseous membrane is exposed from the posterior and anterior aspects.

1. Lateral head of gastrocnemius m.
2. Soleus m.
3. Fibula
4. Peroneus longus m.
5. Biceps femoris tendon
6. Tibialis anterior m.
7. Extensor digitorum longus m.
8. Common peroneal n.
9. Tibialis posterior m.

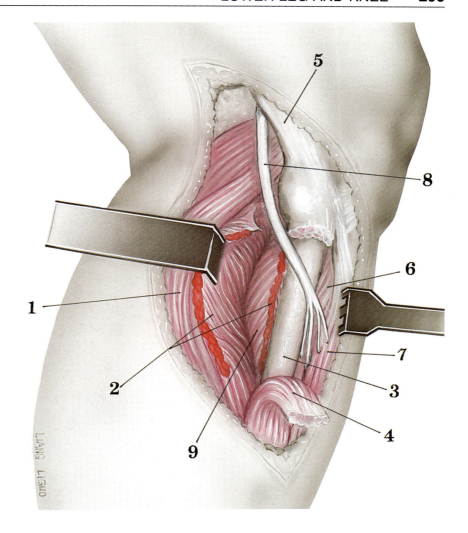

(Fig. 7-86) The shaft of the fibula is divided 8 cm below the head of the fibula with a Gigli saw. Then, the interosseous membrane, the biceps tendon, and the capsule ligaments of the upper tibiofibular joint are detached from the fibula and its head. The upper part of the fibula is then resected.

The arch of the anterior tibial artery [14] generally lies 3 to 4 cm below the articular facet [13] on the lateral condyle of the tibia. In searching for it, it is better to identify the deep peroneal nerve [15] first; this is a branch of the common peroneal nerve, joining the anterior tibial artery about 6 to 7 cm below the facet. Tracing the anterior tibial artery proximally, the arched segment can be securely exposed.

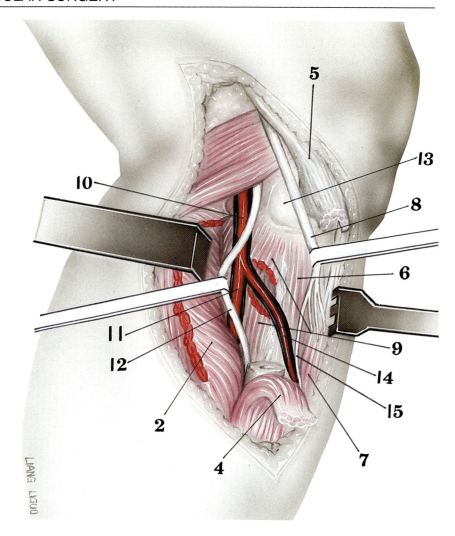

2. Soleus m.
4. Peroneus longus m.
5. Biceps femoris tendon
6. Tibialis anterior m.
7. Extensor digitorum longus m.
8. Common peroneal n.
9. Tibialis posterior m.
10. Popliteal a. and v.
11. Tibioperoneal trunk
12. Tibial n.
13. Articular facet on tibia
14. Anterior tibial a. and v.
15. Deep peroneal n.

Exposure of the Anterior Tibial Artery

(**Fig. 7-87**) A line is drawn from the anterior border of the head of the fibula to the midpoint between the lateral and medial malleoli. Any part of the anterior tibial artery of the leg can be approached, by making an incision on this line.

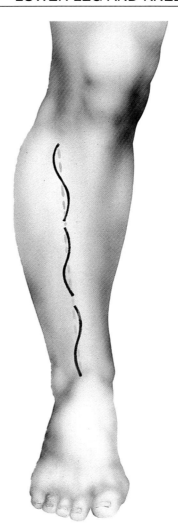

1. Anterior tibial a. and v.
2. Deep peroneal n.
3. Peroneus longus m.
4. Peroneus brevis m.
5. Extensor digitorum longus m.
6. Tibialis anterior m.
7. Interosseous membrane
8. Tibia
9. Extensor hallucis longus m.
10. Fibula

(Fig. 7-88) For exposure of the upper third, a dissection divides the deep fascia and proceeds between the tibialis anterior [6] and extensor digitorum longus [5]. Thus, the anterior tibial artery [1] with vein and the deep peroneal nerve [2] can be identified in front of the interosseous membrane [7].

1. Anterior tibial a. and v.
2. Deep peroneal n.
3. Peroneus longus m.
4. Peroneus brevis m.
5. Extensor digitorum longus m.
6. Tibialis anterior m.
7. Interosseous membrane

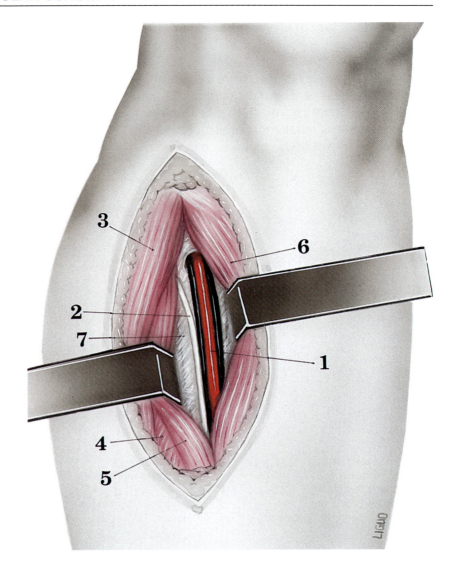

(Fig. 7-89) For exposure of the middle third, dissection divides the deep fascia and proceeds between the tibialis anterior [6] and extensor hallucis longus [9]. Then, the neurovascular bundle [1,2] can be isolated in front of the interosseous membrane [7].

1. Anterior tibial a. and v.
2. Deep peroneal n.
3. Peroneus longus m.
5. Extensor digitorum longus m.
6. Tibialis anterior m.
7. Interosseous membrane
8. Tibia
9. Extensor hallucis longus m.

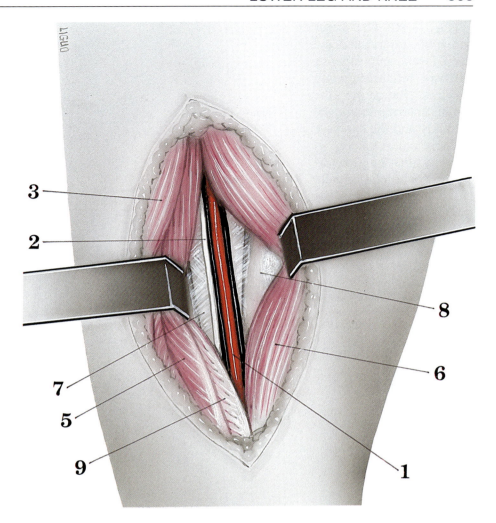

(Fig. 7-90) For exposure of the lower third, the deep fascia and superior extensor retinaculum are divided. Retracting the tibialis anterior tendon [6] medially and the extensor hallucis longus tendon [9] laterally, the anterior tibial neurovascular bundle [1,2] appears lying on the tibia [8].

1. Anterior tibial a. and v.
2. Deep peroneal n.
5. Extensor digitorum longus m.
6. Tibialis anterior m.
7. Interosseous membrane
8. Tibia
9. Extensor hallucis longus m.
10. Fibula

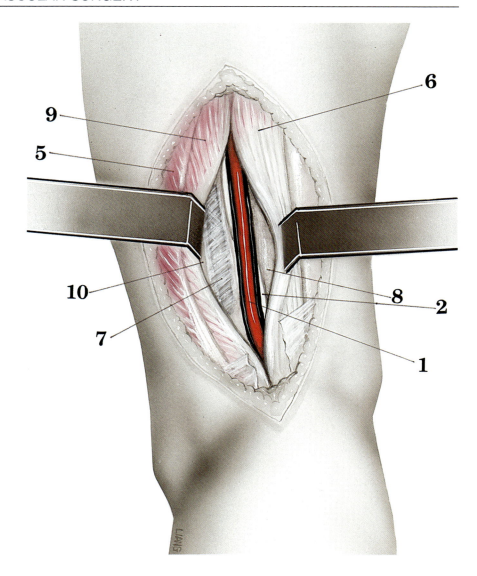

Exposure of the Posterior Tibial Artery

(**Fig. 7-91**) A line is drawn from the medial condyle of the tibia, keeping 3 cm posterior to the posteromedial edge of the tibia, and longitudinally to a point 1 cm posterior to the medial malleolus. The proximal third of this line is employed for the exposure of the tibioperoneal trunk (see sections on exposure of the tibioperoneal trunk).

1. Tibial n.
2. Posterior tibial a. and v.
3. Gastrocnemius m.
4. Soleus m.
5. Tibialis posterior m.
6. Flexor digitorum longus m.
7. Tibia
8. Flexor hallucis longus m.
9. Achilles tendon

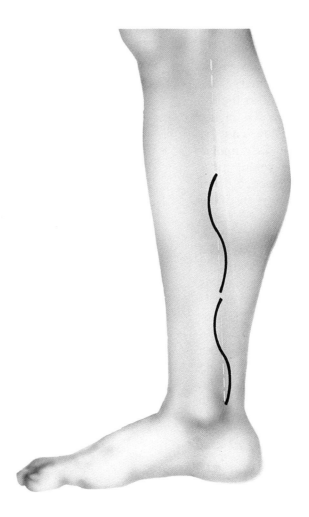

(Fig. 7-92) For exposure of the posterior tibial artery [2] at the level of the *middle third,* the deep fascia is divided and the greater saphenous vein and saphenous nerve are located anterior to the incision (not shown in the drawing). They can be protected while undermining. The soleus muscle [4] is detached from the posterior surface of the tibia [7], with care taken not to injure the neurovascular structure [1,2]. The muscle is then retracted with the gastrocnemius [3] posteriorly. The posterior tibial artery [2], accompanied by two veins, is identified behind the tibialis posterior [5], and it is isolated. The tibial nerve [1] is located deep to the artery.

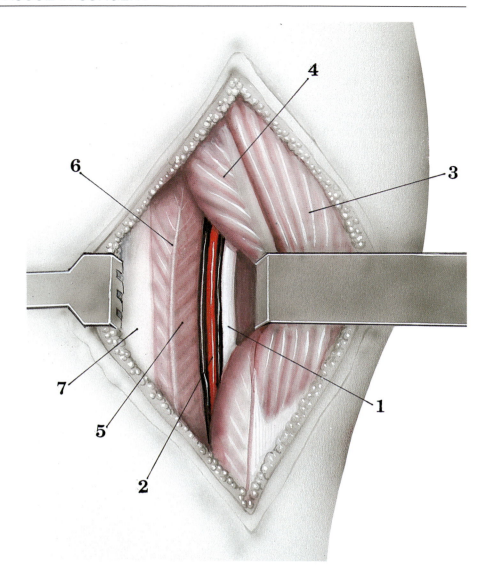

1. Tibial n.
2. Posterior tibial a. and v.
3. Gastrocnemius m.
4. Soleus m.
5. Tibialis posterior m.
6. Flexor digitorum longus m.
7. Tibia

(Fig. 7-93) For exposure of the posterior tibial artery [2] in the *distal third* of the leg, the two layers of fascia are divided, and the soleus [4] can be easily separated from the tibia; it is retracted with the Achilles tendon [9]. The posterior tibial artery [2], accompanied by two veins, lies superficially between the flexor digitorum longus [6] (anteriorly) and the flexor hallucis longus [8] (posteriorly). The tibial nerve [1] is located deep to it.

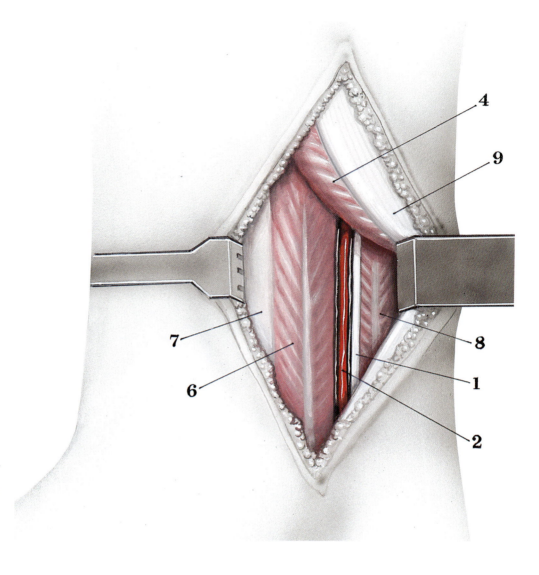

1. Tibial n.
2. Posterior tibial a. and v.
4. Soleus m.
6. Flexor digitorum longus
7. Tibia
8. Flexor hallucis longus
9. Achilles tendon

Exposure of the Peroneal Artery

(Fig. 7-94) A line is drawn longitudinally along the posterior edge of the fibula. Any portion of the peroneal artery can be exposed by making an incision on this line.

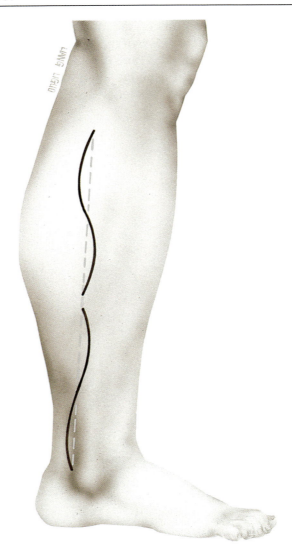

1. Lateral head of gastrocnemius m.
2. Soleus m.
3. Peroneus longus m.
4. Lateral intermuscular septum
5. Peroneal a. and v.
6. Posterior tibial a. and v. and tibial n.
7. Flexor hallucis longus m.
8. Tibialis posterior m.
9. Fibula
10. Peroneus brevis m.
11. Achilles tendon

(**Fig. 7-95**) In the *proximal portion* of the line, the skin and deep fascia are incised. The lateral intermuscular septum [4] between the soleus [2] and peroneus longus [3] is identified and entered.

1. Lateral head of gastrocnemius m.
2. Soleus m.
3. Peroneus longus m.
4. Lateral intermuscular septum

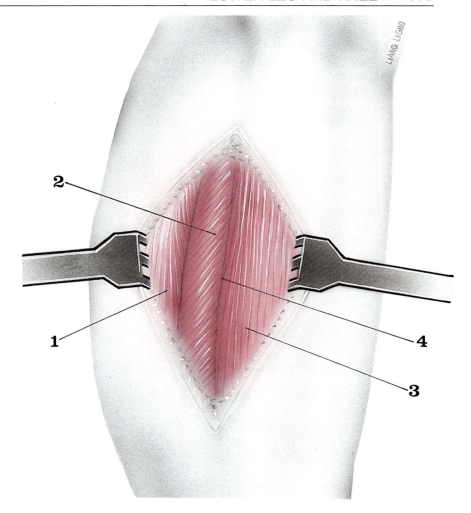

(Fig. 7-96) The soleus [2] is detached from the fibula [9] to enter the interspace between the superficial and deep groups of the posterior crural muscles. While detaching the proximal part of the soleus, care should be taken not to injure the common peroneal nerve.

Retracting the soleus [2] posteriorly, the peroneal artery [5], accompanied by two veins, appears from its origin to the proximal border of the flexor hallucis longus muscle [7]. The tibial nerve [6] is located between the peroneal vessels [5] and the posterior tibial vessels [6].

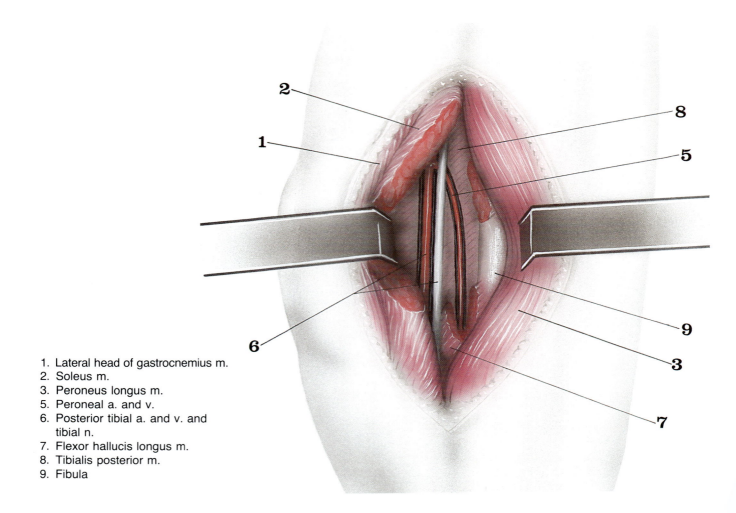

1. Lateral head of gastrocnemius m.
2. Soleus m.
3. Peroneus longus m.
5. Peroneal a. and v.
6. Posterior tibial a. and v. and tibial n.
7. Flexor hallucis longus m.
8. Tibialis posterior m.
9. Fibula

(Fig. 7-97) In the *distal portion* of the line, incising the skin and deep fascia, dissection proceeds in the lateral crural intermuscular septum. Then, the soleus with Achilles tendon [11] and peronei [3,10] are retracted posteriorly and anteriorly, respectively, to expose the flexor hallucis longus muscle [7].

3. Peroneus longus m.
7. Flexor hallucis longus m.
10. Peroneus brevis m.
11. Achilles tendon

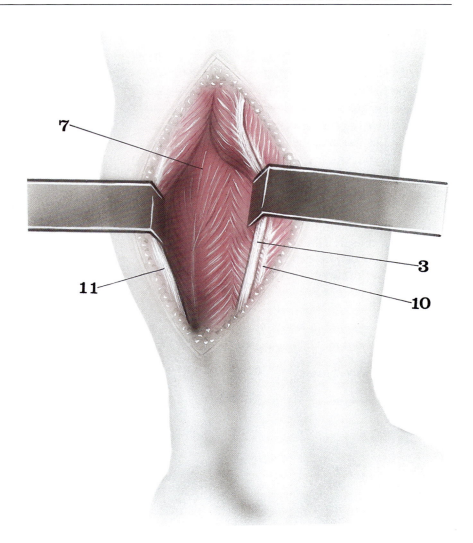

(Fig. 7-98) The peroneal artery [5] in its middle course lies deeply in a fibrous canal between the tibialis posterior and the flexor hallucis longus [7], or in the substance of the latter muscle. However, in its distal course, it lies behind the tibiofibular syndesmosis. The flexor hallucis longus [7] is therefore mobilized first, to identify the distal end of the artery. Then, tracing it and splitting the muscle fibers, the peroneal artery can be exposed from distal to proximal.

2. Soleus m.
3. Peroneus longus m.
5. Peroneal a. and v.
7. Flexor hallucis longus m.
9. Fibula
10. Peroneus brevis m.

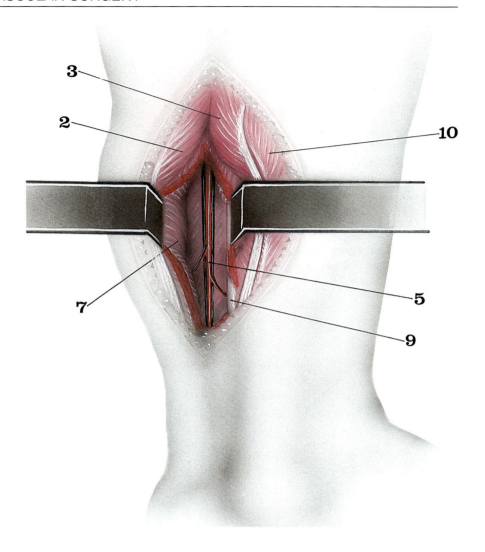

BIBLIOGRAPHY

Peroneal Flap

Baudet J, Panconi B, Caix P, et al: The composite fibula and soleus free transfer. Int J Microsurg 4:10, 1982.

Chen Z-W, Yan W: The study and clinical application of the osteocutaneous flap of fibula. Microsurgery 4:11, 1983.

Chen Y-L, Zheng B-G, Zhu J-M, et al: Microsurgical anatomy of the lateral skin flap of the leg. Ann Plast Surg 15:313, 1985.

Chan Z-W, Chen L-E, Zhang G-J, Yu H-L: Treatment of bony defect of tibia using pedicle transfer of fibula osteocutaneous flap. Chin J Surg 26:32, 1988.

Chen Z-W, Chen L-E, Zhang G-J, Yu H-L: Treatment of tibial defect with vascularized osteocutaneous pedicled transfer of fibula. J Reconstr Microsurg 2:199, 1986.

Chen ZW, Yu ZJ, Wang Y: A new method for treatment of congenital tibial pseudarthrosis: Preliminary report of free vascularized fibula transfer in 12 cases. Chin J Surg 17:147, 1979.

Fujimaki A, Yamauchi Y: Vascularized fibular grafting for treatment of aseptic necrosis of the femoral head—preliminary results in four cases. Microsurgery 4:17, 1983.

Gilbert A: Vascularized transfer of the fibular shaft. Int J Microsurg 1:100, 1979.

Gu Y-D, Wu M-M, Li H-R: Lateral lower leg skin flap. Ann Plast Surg 15:319, 1985.

Lee EH, Goh JCH, Helm R, Pho RWH: Donor site morbidity following resection of the fibula. J Bone Joint Surg 72B:129, 1990.

Pho RWH: Free vascularised fibular transplant for replacement of the lower radius. J Bone Joint Surg 61B:362, 1979.

Restrepo J, Katz D, Gilbert A: Arterial vascularization of the proximal epiphysis and the diaphysis of the fibula. Int J Microsurg 2:49, 1980.

Taylor GI: The current status of free vascularized bone grafts. Clin Plast Surg 10:185, 1983.

Taylor GI, Miller GDH, Ham FJ: The free vascularized bone graft: A clinical extension of microvascular techniques. Plast Reconstr Surg 55:533, 1975.

Wei F-C, Chen H-C, Chuang C-C, Noordhoff MS: Fibular osteoseptocutaneous flap: Anatomic study and clinical application. Plast Reconstr Surg 78:191, 1986.

Weiland AJ, Moore JR: Microvascular free transfer of fibula bone. In: Strauch B, Vasconez LO, Hall-Findlay E (eds): *Grabb's Encyclopedia of Flaps,* vol 3. Boston: Little, Brown, 1990, pp. 1802–1806.

Yoshimura M, Imura S, Shimamura K, et al: Peroneal flap for reconstruction in the extremity: Preliminary report. Plast Reconstr Surg 74:402, 1984.

Yoshimura M, Shimada T, Hosokawa M: The vasculature of the peroneal tissue transfer. Plast Reconstr Surg 85:917, 1990.

Zhang SC, Li JM, Sun KX, et al: Reconstruction of skin defects on feet and ankles using the lateral reverse island leg flap. Chin J Surg 25:353, 1987.

Gastrocnemius Flap

Aiache AE: A gastrocnemius muscle flap to fill an osteomyelitic hole in the femur. Br J Plast Surg 31:214, 1978.

Arnold PG, Mixter RC: Making the most of the gastrocnemius muscles. Plast Reconstr Surg 72:38, 1983.

Bashir AH: A gastrocnemius tenocutaneous island flap. Br J Plast Surg 35:436, 1982.

Cheng HH, Rong GW, Yin TC, et al: Coverage of wounds in the distal lower leg by advancement of an enlarged medial gastrocnemius skin flap. Plast Reconstr Surg 73:671, 1984.

Dibbell DG, Edstrom LE: The gastrocnemius myocutaneous flap. Clin Plast Surg 7:45, 1980.

Feldman JJ, Cohen BE, May JW Jr: The medial gastrocnemius myocutaneous flap. Plast Reconstr Surg 61:531, 1978.

Keller A, Allen R, Shaw W: The medial gastrocnemius muscle flap: A local free flap. Plast Reconstr Surg 73:974, 1984.

McCraw JB, Fishman JH, Sharzer LA: The versatile gastrocnemius myocutaneous flap. Plast Reconstr Surg 62:15, 1978.

Morris AM: A gastrocnemius musculocutaneous flap. Br J Plast Surg 31:216, 1978.

Salibian AH, Rogers FR, Lamb RC: Microvascular gastrocnemius muscle transfer to the distal leg using saphenous vein grafts. Plast Reconstr Surg 73:302, 1984.

Saphenous Flap

Acland RD, Schusterman M, Godina M, et al: The saphenous neurovascular free flap. Plast Reconstr Surg 67:763, 1981.

Banis JC Jr, Acland RD: Microvascular and microneurovascular transfer of the saphenous skin flap. In: Strauch B, Vasconez LO, Hall-Findlay E (eds): *Grabb's Encyclopedia of Flaps,* vol 2. Boston: Little, Brown, pp. 1114–1116.

Banis JC Jr, Acland RD: Microvascular transfer of the saphenous skin flap for simultaneous oral lining and cover. In: Strauch B, Vasconez LO, Hall-Findlay E (eds): *Grabb's Encyclopedia of Flaps,* vol 1. Boston: Little, Brown, pp. 549–555.

Guan WS, Jin YT, Huang WY, et al: Experiences in the clinical use of the medial genicular flap. J Reconstr Microsurg 1:233, 1985.

Koshima I, Endou T, Soeda S, Yamasaki M: The free or pedicled saphenous flap. Ann Plast Surg 21:369, 1988.

Posterior Leg Flap

Amarante J, Costa H, Reis J, Soares R: A new distally based fasciocutaneous flap of the leg. Br J Plast Surg 39:338, 1986.

Barclay TL, Cardoso E, Sharpe DT, Crockett DJ: Repair of lower leg injuries with fascio-cutaneous flaps. Br J Plast Surg 35:127, 1982.

Carriquiry C, Costa A, Vasconez LO: An anatomic study of the septocutaneous vessels of the leg. Plast Reconstr Surg 76:354, 1985.

Haertsch PA: The blood supply to the skin of the leg: A post-mortem investigation. Br J Plast Surg 34:470, 1981.

Hwang W-Y, Chang T-S, Cheng K-X, Gao T-M: The application of free twin flaps in one-stage treatment of severe hand deformity. Ann Plast Surg 21:430, 1988.

Morrison WA, Shen TY: Anterior tibial artery flap: Anatomy and case report. Br J Plast Surg 40:230, 1987.

Moscona AR, Govrin-Yehudain J, Hishowitz B: The island fasciocutaneous flap: A new type of flap for defects of the knee. Br J Plast Surg 38:512, 1985.

Okada T, Yasuda Y, Kitayama Y, Tsukada S: Salvage of an arm by means of a free cutaneous flap based on the posterior tibial artery. J Reconstr Microsurg 1:25, 1984.

Ponten B: The fasciocutaneous flap: Its use in soft tissue defects of the lower leg. Br J Plast Surg 34:215, 1981.

Recalde Rocha JF, Gilbert A, Masquelet A, et al: The anterior tibial artery flap: Anatomic study and clinical application. Plast Reconstr Surg 79:396, 1987.

Thatte RL, Laud N: The use of the fascia of the lower leg as a roll-over flap: Its possible clinical applications in reconstructive surgery. Br J Plast Surg 37:88, 1984.

Torii S, Namiki Y, Hayashi Y: Anterolateral leg island flap. Br J Plast Surg 40:236, 1987.

Walton RL, Bunkis J: The posterior calf fasciocutaneous free flap. Plast Reconstr Surg 74:76, 1984.

Walton RL, Petry JJ: Follow-up on the posterior calf fasciocutaneous free flap. Plast Reconstr Surg 76:149, 1985.

Wee JTK: Reconstruction of the lower leg and foot with the reverse-pedicled anterior tibial flap: Preliminary report of a new fasciocutaneous flap. Br J Plast Surg 39:327, 1986.

8 ANKLE AND FOOT

Dorsalis Pedis Flap

Arterial Anatomy (Fig. 8-1)

The *dorsalis pedis artery* [1] is the continuation of the anterior tibial artery [10], distal to the ankle joint. It passes under the extensor retinaculum [9] at the midpoint between the medial and lateral malleoli and usually across and beneath the extensor hallucis longus [8], from its medial to lateral side. After emerging at the lower border of the extensor retinaculum, it gives off the lateral and medial tarsal arteries [5,6]. The artery then proceeds under the extensor hallucis brevis [7] above the tarsal bones and toward the interspace between the bases of the first and second metatarsals. This progression takes place in a muscular arch formed by the two heads of the first dorsal interosseous muscle, where the artery, named as the deep plantar artery [4], plunges to join the plantar arch in the sole of the foot. Before this junction, the arcuate artery [2] branches out. The first dorsal metatarsal vessel [3] arises just as the dorsalis pedis artery turns into the sole.

The *lateral tarsal artery* [5] (see section on the extensor digitorum brevis flap, p. 336).

There are two or three *medial tarsal arteries* [6] on the medial border of the foot.

The *arcuate artery* [2] arises from the dorsalis pedis artery [1] on the medial cuneiform. It runs laterally over the base of the metatarsal bones and gives off the second, third, and fourth dorsal metatarsal arteries that pass distally upon each dorsal interosseous muscle. The arcuate artery is present in 51% of cases.

The *first dorsal metatarsal artery* [3] generally arises from the dorsalis pedis artery [1] after the origin of the deep plantar vessel [4]. The first dorsal metatarsal artery then runs distally, superficial or deep, to the first interosseous muscle toward the first web, where it divides into the dorsal digital arteries to the first and second toe. For its possible variations, see Figure 8-4.

In addition to the first dorsal metatarsal artery serving as a direct cutaneous artery in supplying the dorsalis pedis flap, cutaneous branches arise mainly from the dorsalis pedis artery in two other areas: beneath the retinaculum and proximal to the interspace between the first and second metatarsals.

ANKLE AND FOOT 315

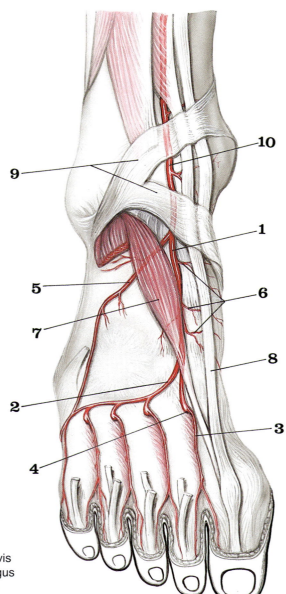

1. Dorsalis pedis a.
2. Arcuate a.
3. First dorsal metatarsal a.
4. Deep plantar a.
5. Lateral tarsal a.
6. Medial tarsal aa.
7. Extensor hallucis brevis
8. Extensor hallucis longus
9. Extensor retinaculum
10. Anterior tibial artery

Venous Drainage (Fig. 8-2)

Superficial System. The dorsal digital veins receive communications from the plantar digital veins to form dorsal metatarsal veins [3] that unite in a dorsal venous arch [2] across the proximal parts of the metatarsal bones. Then, they generally drain proximally through the lateral and medial veins that become the *lesser* and *greater saphenous veins* [5,1], respectively. In addition, oblique veins on the middle dorsum of the foot may unite to form a *median dorsal vein* [4] that normally joins the greater saphenous vein [1] several centimeters above the ankle.

Deep System. There are a pair of venae comitantes to the dorsalis pedis artery. Although the superficial system is the dominant drainage, and should be used preferentially for toe transplants, the venae comitantes alone can be adequate for an island dorsalis pedis flap.

Innervation

The *superficial peroneal nerve* [6] is a branch of the common peroneal nerve. In the distal third of the leg, it pierces the deep fascia and bifurcates to form the *medial and lateral dorsal cutaneous nerves* [8,7]. The latter are located at the front of the ankle at the anterolateral aspect of the joint. The nerves supply almost the entire dorsum of the foot, except for the first web and lateral side of the foot.

The *deep peroneal nerve* descends along the lateral side of the anterior tibial artery to the front of the ankle joint. There, it divides into lateral and medial terminal branches.

The *lateral terminal branch*, accompanying the lateral tarsal artery, passes deep to the extensor hallucis and extensor digitorum brevis and supplies them.

The *medial terminal branch*, accompanying the dorsalis pedis artery, runs forward and pierces the deep fascia at a proximal point to the first interspace of the metatarsals, supplying the first web.

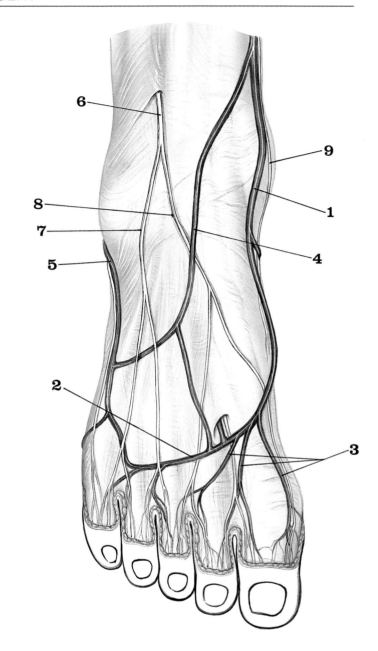

1. Greater saphenous v.
2. Dorsal venous arch
3. Dorsal metatarsal v.
4. Median dorsal v.
5. Lesser saphenous v.
6. Superficial peroneal n.
7. Lateral dorsal cutaneous n.
8. Medial dorsal cutaneous n.
9. Saphenous n.

Variations of the Dorsalis Pedis Artery (Fig. 8-3)

Type A. The artery begins as a continuation of the perforating peroneal artery in 3% of cases.

Type B. The lower end of the anterior tibial artery is in the position of the perforating peroneal artery in 1.5% of cases.

Type C. It can arise about equally from the anterior tibial and perforating peroneal arteries in 0.5% of cases.

Type D. The artery can be so reduced in size as to be considered almost absent in 12% of cases.

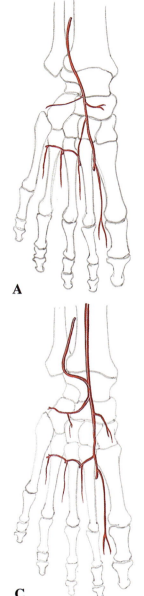
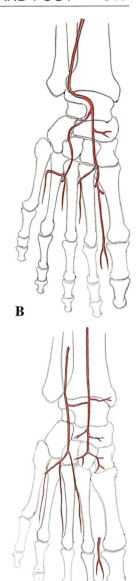

Variations of the First Dorsal Metatarsal Artery (Fig. 8-4)

Type A. (Superficial Type). In these cases, it arises from the beginning or upper part of the deep plantar artery and then intermediately turns back under a lesser muscular arch to run on the surface of the first dorsal interosseous muscle, or in this muscle at a superficial level (about 49% of cases).

Type B. (Deep Type). In these cases, it arises from the lower part of the deep plantar artery or originates from the plantar arch via a common stem with the first plantar metatarsal artery. It lies deep under the first interosseous muscle, and then runs forward and dorsally, penetrating the muscle and appearing superficial to the muscle between the heads of the first and second metatarsals. Sometimes there may be a narrow branch from the upper part of the deep plantar artery running over the interosseous muscle (about 40% of cases).

Type C. (Narrow or Absent Type). In these cases, there may be a narrow first dorsal metatarsal artery with a diameter of less than 1 mm. However, it almost disappears between the heads of the first and second metatarsals. The blood supply of the big and second toes depends on the first plantar metatarsal artery that lies under the deep transverse ligament (about 11% of cases).

Measurements

		Diameter
Dorsalis pedis	Artery	2.0–3.0 mm
	Vein	1.5–3.0 mm
First dorsal metatarsal	Artery	1.0–1.5 mm
Greater saphenous	Vein	3.0–5.0 mm
Lesser saphenous	Vein	2.2–3.0 mm
Dorsal venous arch		1.2–3.3 mm

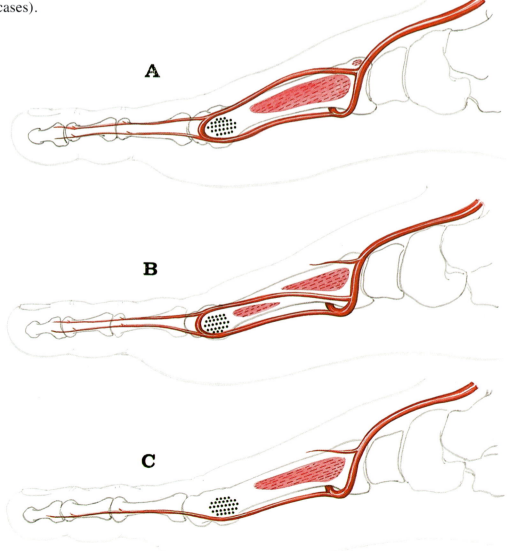

COMMENT AND INSIGHTS

The skin of the dorsum of the foot is extremely thin and pliable. It is innervated by an expendable cutaneous sensory nerve and the two-point discrimination recovered can approach about 10 mm. The size of the flap available for transfer is limited, ordinarily about 10 × 10 cm and maximally about 14 × 15 cm; the latter requires a delay procedure.

The length of the vascular pedicle is adequate for reconstruction. If necessary, the vascular pedicle can be made longer by extending it up into the lower leg. The sizes of all the relevant arteries and veins for the vascular pedicle are quite large, which makes microvascular anastomoses easy to secure.

Venous drainage of the flap is abundant and includes the greater and lesser saphenous veins, as well as the paired venae comitantes. The flap can be drained by only one vein—the greater saphenous, but, for safety, it is suggested that at least two veins should be anastomosed.

If the superficial first dorsal metatarsal artery does not exist in the subcutaneous layer, as a direct cutaneous artery between the first and second metatarsals, flap circulation (especially in the distal portion) may be in danger; sometimes unexpected failure may occur. Following investigation of the distribution of the cutaneous branches from the dorsalis pedis artery, it is advisable that the more proximally and medially the flap is designed, the more reliable the flap circulation should be.

The dorsalis pedis flap can be compounded as an osteocutaneous or tendinocutaneous flap, with the second metatarsal or extensor tendons. In addition, with the dorsalis pedis-first dorsal metatarsal arterial system, the flap can be combined with free toe transfer, first web flap, and extensor digitorum brevis muscle transfer, and so on.

The dorsalis pedis flap, including its use as a composite flap, is widely applied clinically. However, because the anatomic properties of the foot have a close resemblance to those of the hand, the flap is ideally suited for use in the hand.

Donor site sequelae from split-thickness skin grafting is not inconspicuous, but morbidity is low; few patients have any discomfort in the donor foot. Occasionally, wound healing in the first intermetatarsal space and the extensor hallucis longus tendon may be troublesome, when the skin-graft bed is not appropriately covered with the paratenon or similar vascular bed source.

DORSALIS PEDIS SKIN FLAP

(Fig. 8-5) The flap design is based on the dorsalis pedis–first dorsal metatarsal vascular axis. If the dorsalis pedis artery is not readily palpable, a Doppler flowmeter or arteriography are suggested to confirm the vasculature.

The maximum boundaries are the interdigital web space distally, the midextensor retinaculum proximally, and the area just beyond the medial and lateral margins of the venous arch. It is important to note that the distal flap (that portion distal to the dorsalis pedis pulse) may be a random-pattern extension. If there is no first dorsal metatarsal artery superficial to the interosseous muscle, delay is necessary for safe transfer. Maximum size of the average flap in adults is 14 × 15 cm.

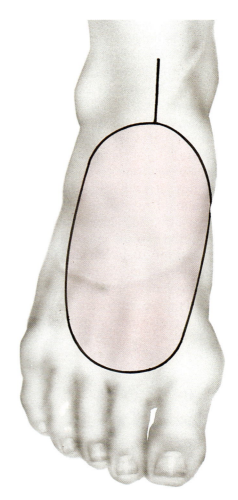

1. Extensor hallucis longus tendon
2. Extensor digitorum longus tendons
3. First dorsal metatarsal a. and deep peroneal n.
4. Dorsal metatarsal v.
5. Dorsal venous arch
6. Extensor hallucis brevis
7. Dorsalis pedis a. and v.
8. Greater saphenous v.
9. Deep plantar a.
10. Lateral and medial dorsal cutaneous n.

(Fig. 8-6) Dissection begins at the first web space, where the first dorsal metatarsal artery [3] and the deep peroneal nerve [3] are identified, since they usually lie at a superficial level. The vessel and nerve are ligated and marked. The terminal branches of the superficial peroneal nerve are divided in the second, third, and fourth web spaces.

1. Extensor hallucis longus tendon
2. Extensor digitorum longus tendons
3. First dorsal metatarsal a. and deep peroneal n.
4. Dorsal metatarsal v.

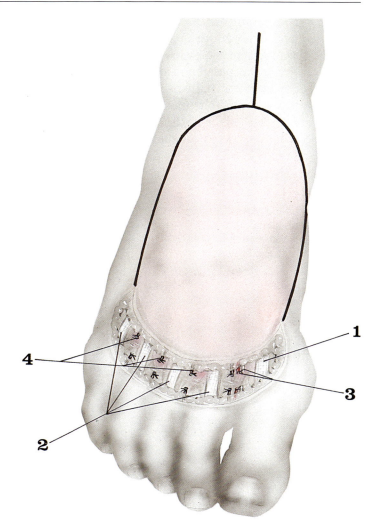

(Fig. 8-7) Keeping the first dorsal metatarsal artery [3] and deep peroneal nerve [3] intact with the flap, the flap is elevated from distal to proximal above the paratenon of all extensor tendons. The extensor hallucis brevis tendon [6] is detached, and this muscle should be included in the flap, since it passes between the dorsalis pedis-first dorsal metatarsal arterial system and the skin.

3. First dorsal metatarsal a. and deep peroneal n.
5. Dorsal venous arch
6. Extensor hallucis brevis

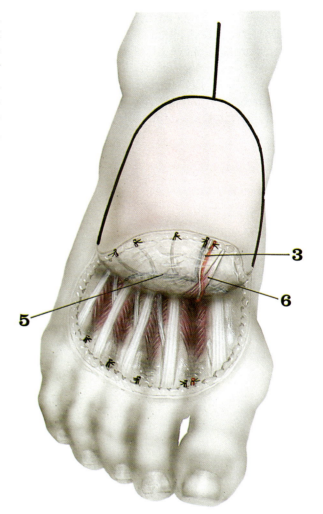

(Fig. 8-8) On the medial side, the flap is raised with the greater saphenous vein [8] maintained in the flap. Just over the extensor hallucis longus tendon, the dissection is deepened close to the lateral edge of the tendon and on the tarsal bones, to identify the dorsalis pedis vascular bundle [7] from its undersurface. The dissection proceeds between the vascular bundle and tarsal bones toward the interspace where the first dorsal metatarsal artery [3] originates and the deep plantar artery [9] plunges downward to the plantar arch. The latter is ligated deep to the takeoff of the first dorsal metatarsal artery.

3. First dorsal metatarsal a. and deep peroneal n.
6. Extensor hallucis brevis
7. Dorsalis pedis a. and v.
8. Greater saphenous v.
9. Deep plantar a.

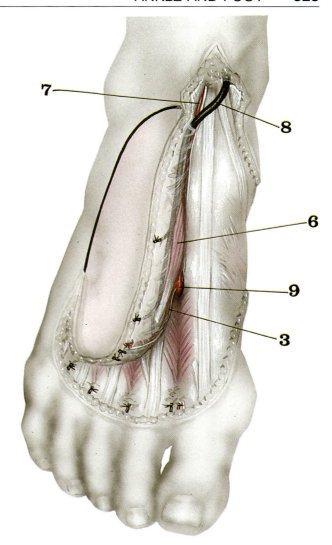

(**Fig. 8-9**) On the proximal edge of the flap and in the extension incision, the dorsalis pedis vascular bundle [7] with deep peroneal nerve is dissected further. Medial and lateral dorsal cutaneous nerves [10] (branches of the superficial peroneal nerve), greater and lesser saphenous veins [8], and the medial dorsal vein are identified and isolated. According to the venous pattern on the dorsum of the foot, a more dominant superficial vein is selected (usually the greater saphenous vein), and the other veins are ligated.

The dorsalis pedis neurovascular bundle, cutaneous nerves, and the selected vein can be dissected for adequate lengths, as required at the recipient site.

7. Dorsalis pedis a. and v.
8. Greater saphenous v.
10. Lateral and medial dorsal cutaneous n.

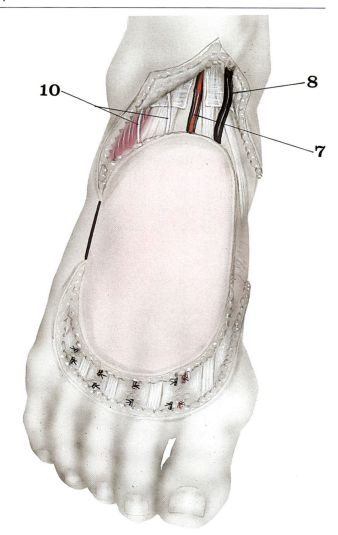

(**Fig. 8-10**) The lateral edge of the flap is elevated above the paratenon of the extensor digitorum longus tendon [2]. As soon as the medial edge of the tendon of the second toe is reached, the extensor hallucis brevis muscle [6] is divided, and the lateral tarsal artery with the arcuate artery is ligated. The muscular branch of the deep peroneal nerve is separated from its main trunk. Dissection is carried out over the periosteum of the tarsal bone. The dorsalis pedis flap, with the extensor hallucis brevis [6] and dorsalis pedis vascular bundle [7] kept intact with its undersurface, is isolated on its vascular pedicle.

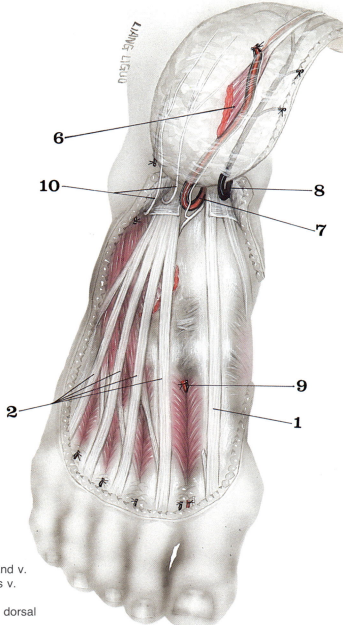

1. Extensor hallucis longus tendon
2. Extensor digitorum longus tendons
6. Extensor hallucis brevis
7. Dorsalis pedis a. and v.
8. Greater saphenous v.
9. Deep plantar a.
10. Lateral and medial dorsal cutaneous n.

DORSALIS PEDIS OSTEOCUTANEOUS FLAP WITH SECOND METATARSAL

(Fig. 8-11) The skin flap is designed with reference to the dorsalis pedis flap. It should be centralized over the base of the second metatarsal bone. This osteocutaneous flap provides a second metatarsal with a length of 7 to 8 cm.

1. Dorsalis pedis a. and v. and greater saphenous v.
2. Deep plantar a.
3. First dorsal metatarsal a.
4. Extensor hallucis brevis
5. Interosseous m.
6. Lesser saphenous v.
7. Deep transverse ligament
8. Second metatarsal bone
9. Proximal phalanx bone
10. Arcuate a.

(Fig. 8-12) After the first dorsal metatarsal artery [3] is dissected and ligated at the first web space, the flap is elevated, both laterally and medially, above the paratenon of the extensors digitorum and hallucis longus tendons, before the first and second dorsal interosseous muscles [5] are reached. The extensor hallucis brevis tendon [4] is detached, and the first dorsal metatarsal artery is dissected on its medial side, keeping it (and any musculature that lies between it and the second metatarsal) in the flap.

1. Dorsalis pedis a. and v. and greater saphenous v.
2. Deep plantar a.
3. First dorsal metatarsal a.
4. Extensor hallucis brevis
5. Interosseous m.
7. Deep transverse ligament

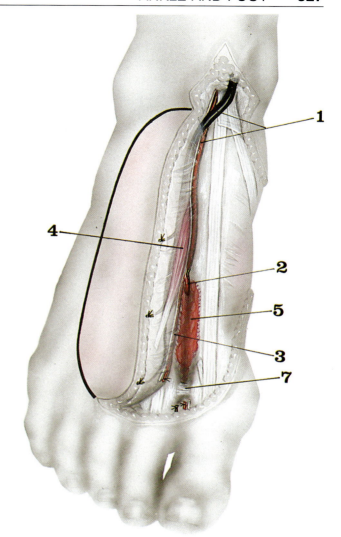

(**Fig. 8-13**) The lateral side of the flap is elevated with care in dissecting the lesser saphenous vein [6]. The interosseous muscles [5] and deep transverse metatarsal ligament [7] between the second and third metatarsals are reached and divided. The origin of the extensor hallucis brevis [4] is detached, keeping the muscle with the flap intact.

4. Extensor hallucis brevis
5. Interosseous m.
6. Lesser saphenous v.
7. Deep transverse ligament

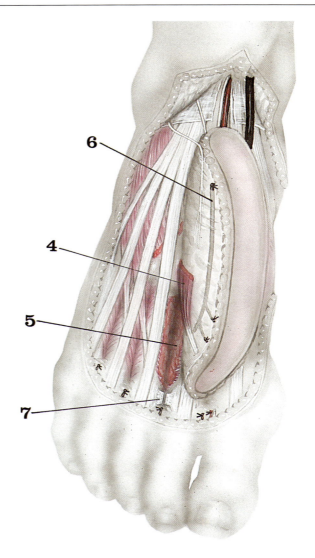

(Fig. 8-14) The extensor tendons of the second toe are divided, and the second metatarsal phalangeal joint is entered. Deep transverse metatarsal ligaments [7] and interosseous musculatures [5] are transected along the adjacent borders of the first and third metatarsals. The second metatarsal is kept intact with the flap and the first dorsal metatarsal artery.

1. Dorsalis pedis a. and v. and greater saphenous v.
5. Interosseous m.
7. Deep transverse ligament
8. Second metatarsal bone
9. Proximal phalanx bone

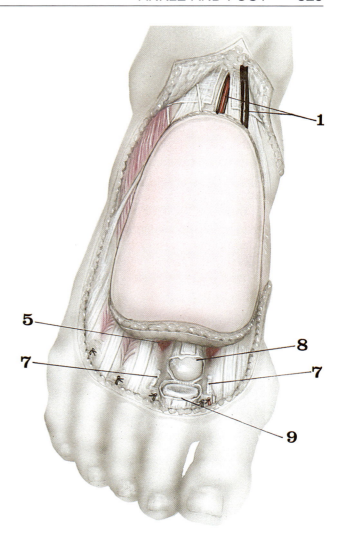

(Fig. 8-15) Proximally, the dorsalis pedis vascular bundle [1], greater and lesser saphenous veins, medial dorsal vein, and branches of the superficial peroneal nerve are dissected as already described. The proximal part of the flap is raised, including the extensor longus tendon of the second toe and extensor hallucis brevis muscles in the flap. If possible, the arcuate artery and the second dorsal metatarsal artery can also be preserved in the flap.

The dissection then proceeds to the base of the second metatarsal. Tracing the dorsalis pedis artery [1] and the first dorsal metatarsal artery, the deep plantar artery [2] is identified and ligated deep to the takeoff of the first dorsal metatarsal artery.

1. Dorsalis pedis a. and v. and greater saphenous v.
2. Deep plantar a.
7. Deep transverse ligament
8. Second metatarsal bone
9. Proximal phalanx bone

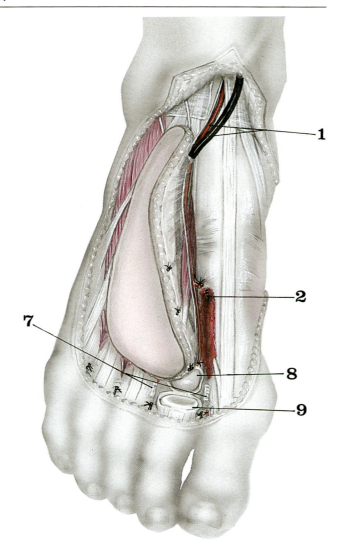

(**Fig. 8-16**) Preserving the dorsalis pedis–first dorsal metatarsal arterial system [1,3], the capsule of the joints between the second metatarsal and the cuneiforms and adjacent metatarsals are transected. Then, the dorsalis pedis osteocutaneous flap, with the second metatarsal bone, is isolated.

1. Dorsalis pedis a. and v. and greater saphenous v.
3. First dorsal metatarsal a.
5. Interosseous m.
8. Second metatarsal bone
10. Arcuate a.

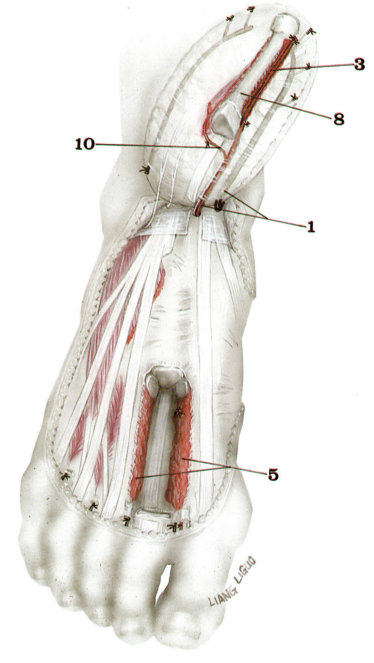

Donor Site Closure

Using heavy wire or nonabsorbable sutures, the heads of the first and third metatarsals are approximated and the second toe is amputated. The extensor hallucis longus tendon and the extensor digitorum longus tendons to the third to fifth toes are elevated from the metatarsals; they are approximated with heavy absorbable sutures to cover the residual defect of the second metatarsal. Any rents in the paratenon should be repaired with fine absorbable sutures. The defect bed is then grafted with split-thickness skin, and a tie-over dressing is applied.

DORSALIS PEDIS TENDINOCUTANEOUS FLAP WITH EXTENSOR TENDONS

The extensor digitorum longus tendons are nourished by the superior and inferior lateral tarsal arteries and the direct cutaneous branches of the dorsalis pedis artery.

(Fig. 8-17) The flap is designed as described previously. There are four tendons of the extensor digitorum longus available. If needed, the tendon of the extensor hallucis brevis can also be used, but it may be too small and short.

1. Dorsalis pedis a. and greater saphenous v.
2. First dorsal metatarsal a. and deep plantar a.
3. Extensor hallucis brevis
4. Interosseous m.
5. Extensor digitorum brevis
6. Extensor digitorum longus tendons

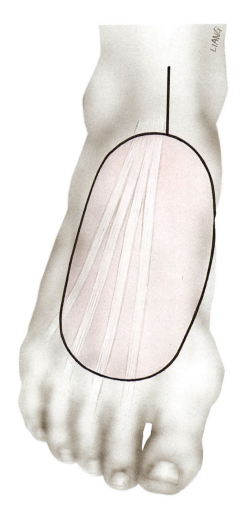

(**Fig. 8-18**) The dorsalis pedis-first dorsal metatarsal arterial system is dissected at the first web and on the medial side of the flap, and the neurovascular pedicles are isolated at the proximal border of the flap, in a fashion similar to the dorsalis pedis skin flap.

1. Dorsalis pedis a. and greater saphenous v.
2. First dorsal metatarsal a. and deep plantar a.
3. Extensor hallucis brevis
4. Interosseous m.

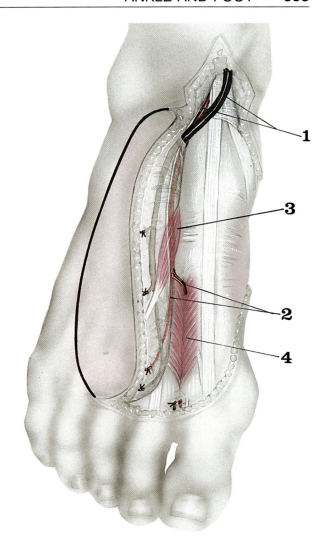

(Fig. 8-19) The distal and proximal ends of the tendons [6] are divided. The dissection proceeds between the tendons and the extensor digitorum brevis [5] or the periosteum of the metatarsals.

Preserving the extensor digitorum brevis on the foot, the extensor hallucis brevis [3] is detached and kept intact with the flap. The lateral tarsal arteries are ligated just at the medial border of the extensor digitorum brevis of the second toe.

3. Extensor hallucis brevis
5. Extensor digitorum brevis
6. Extensor digitorum longus tendons

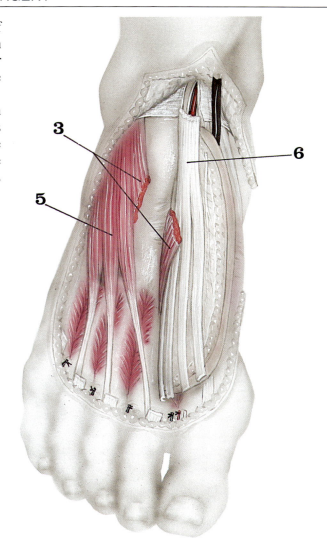

(Fig. 8-20) The dorsalis pedis tendinocutaneous flap is isolated on its neurovascular pedicles [1].

1. Dorsalis pedis a. and greater saphenous v.
5. Extensor digitorum brevis
6. Extensor digitorum longus tendons

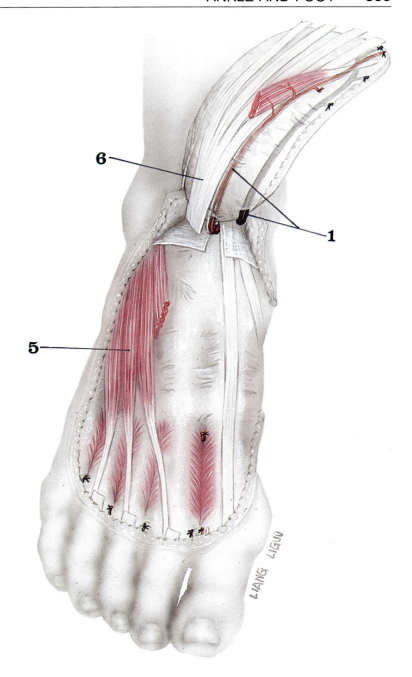

Extensor Digitorum Brevis Flap

Anatomy (Fig. 8-21)

The origin of the muscle is the superolateral surface of the calcaneus and the interosseous talocalcaneal ligament. Its insertion is usually in the form of four digitations. The first, the extensor hallucis brevis, is to the lateral aspect of the extensor hallucis longus tendon, and the other three digitations are to the lateral aspect of the extensor digitorum longus tendons to the second, third, and fourth toes.

The shape is thin, rectangular, and trapezoid, and the size of the muscle belly is 4.5 cm in width and 6.0 cm in length. Taken with the tendons, the total length can reach 13 cm.

The muscle functions, through the tendons of the extensor digitorum and hallucis longus, to aid in extension of the big, second, third, and fourth toes.

Blood Supply

There are usually two lateral tarsal arteries [2] that originate from the dorsalis pedis artery [1], 1 and 3 cm below the lower edge of the extensor retinaculum [5]. Usually, the superior artery, with a diameter of 1.8 mm, is the dominant vessel. Passing between the muscle and the tarsal bone, it branches to the undersurface of each digitation of the muscle.

Innervation

The lateral branch of the deep peroneal nerve [8] accompanies the superior lateral tarsal artery to supply each digitation. (For the anatomy of the dorsalis pedis artery and the deep peroneal nerve in detail, see the section on the dorsalis pedis flap, p. 314.)

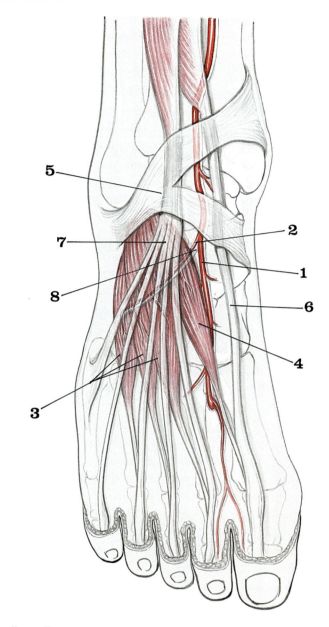

1. Dorsalis pedis a.
2. Lateral tarsal a.
3. Extensor digitorum brevis
4. Extensor hallucis brevis
5. Extensor retinaculum
6. Extensor hallucis longus tendon
7. Extensor digitorum longus tendons
8. Lateral branch of the deep peroneal n.

COMMENT AND INSIGHTS

The extensor digitorum brevis is a thin, flat, small-sized muscle. It is expendable when the extensor digitorum longus is left intact on the donor foot.

Although the dorsalis pedis artery is somewhat variable, the lateral tarsal artery and branch of the deep peroneal nerve quite constantly supply the muscle. The neurovascular pedicle can always reach a desirable length, when dissection proceeds proximally on the anterior tibial artery. Diameters of the pedicle vessels are dependably adequate for microvascular anastomosis.

The muscle flap can be transferred to the face for treatment of facial palsy, and the myocutaneous flap has been reported in reconstruction of intrinsic muscle with skin defect in hand injuries. However, the myocutaneous flap is not generally used clinically, because of the extensive soft tissue loss that results in the wide exposure of bone surface and extensor tendons, and in subsequent problems with wound healing. A muscle island flap can be used for coverage of soft tissue loss around the ankle, including the Achilles tendon, and on the lower third of the leg.

EXTENSOR DIGITORUM BREVIS MUSCLE FLAP

(Fig. 8-22) The incision is S-shaped and is made from the midline between the medial and lateral malleoli, curving smoothly laterally. It ends on the first interosseous metatarsal space. Some accessory incisions may be needed. Distally, four small transverse incisions at the metatarsal phalangeal joints of the medial four toes serve to divide the insertion of the muscle. Proximally, a longitudinal incision, anterior to the lateral malleolus, serves to detach the origin of the muscle.

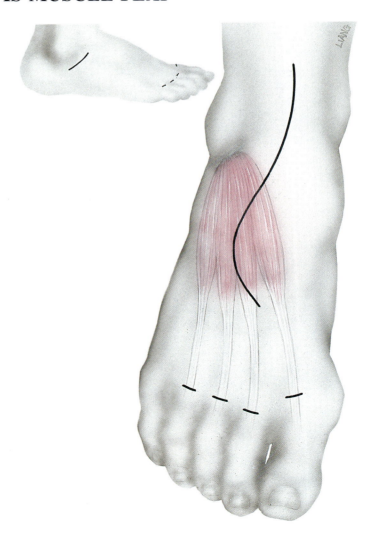

1. Dorsalis pedis a. and v.
2. Lateral tarsal a., v., and n.
3. Extensor hallucis brevis
4. Extensor digitorum brevis
5. Extensor hallucis longus tendon
6. Extensor digitorum longus tendon

(Fig. 8-23) The extensor digitorum longus tendons [6] are dissected off the underlying extensor digitorum and hallucis brevis muscles [4,3]. The dorsalis pedis vessels [1] are identified at the upper medial border of the extensor hallucis brevis [3] and dissected distally. The dorsalis pedis vessel is ligated distal to the muscle.

The extensor retinaculum is divided, and the lateral tarsal neurovascular bundle [2] is then identified, with the nerve branch separated from the main trunk of the deep peroneal nerve. The muscle, with the neurovascular bundle, is elevated from the tarsal bones.

1. Dorsalis pedis a. and v.
2. Lateral tarsal a., v., and n.
3. Extensor hallucis brevis
4. Extensor digitorum brevis
5. Extensor hallucis longus tendon
6. Extensor digitorum longus tendon

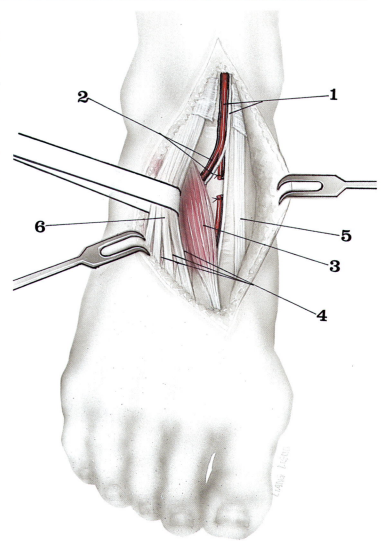

(**Fig. 8-24**) Through distal and proximal incisions, muscle insertions and origin are detached.

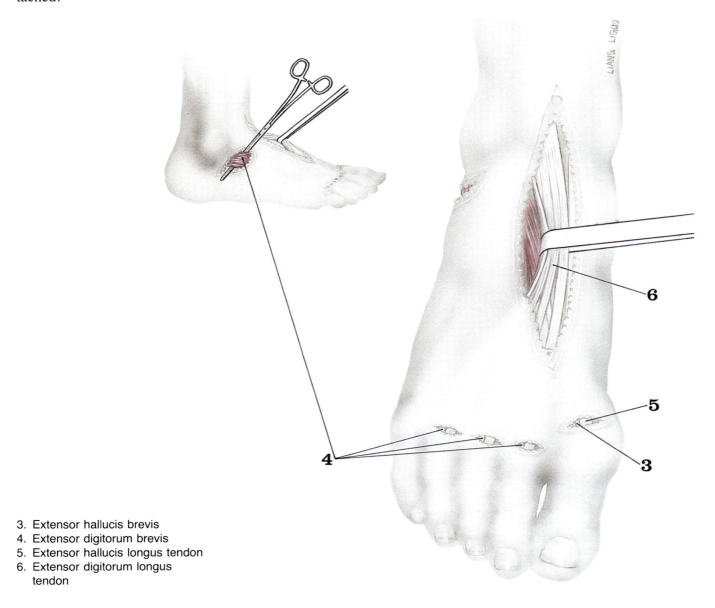

3. Extensor hallucis brevis
4. Extensor digitorum brevis
5. Extensor hallucis longus tendon
6. Extensor digitorum longus tendon

(Fig. 8-25) The extensor digitorum (and hallucis) brevis [4,3] muscle flap is raised from the dorsum of the foot on the dorsalis pedis vascular pedicle and deep peroneal nerve [1].

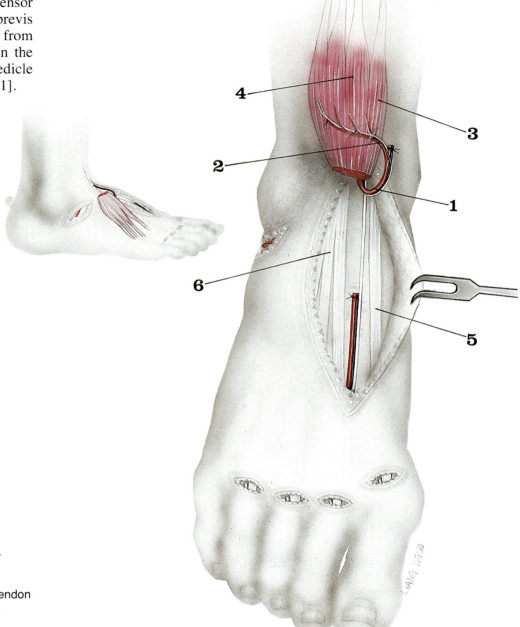

1. Dorsalis pedis a. and v.
2. Lateral tarsal a., v., and n.
3. Extensor hallucis brevis
4. Extensor digitorum brevis
5. Extensor hallucis longus tendon
6. Extensor digitorum longus tendon

Medial Plantar Flap

Anatomy (Fig. 8-26)

The nonweight-bearing region of the sole lies between the heel and the metatarsal heads. A medial plantar flap can be raised on either the medial or lateral plantar arteries [2,3], or both, based ultimately on the posterior tibial artery.

The *posterior tibial artery* [1] divides into the medial and lateral plantar arteries under the origin of the abductor hallucis [4]. The *medial plantar artery* [2], as a smaller terminal branch, runs between the abductor hallucis [4] and flexor digitorum brevis [5]. At the base of the first metatarsal bone, it passes along the medial side of the big toe and anastomoses there with the first plantar metatarsal artery. The *lateral plantar artery* [3], as a larger terminal branch, travels medially to laterally obliquely under the proximal third of the flexor digitorum brevis [5], where it supplies this muscle. It then continues distally between the flexor digitorum brevis [5] and abductor digiti minimi [6] to join the deep plantar arch.

Innervation

The *medial plantar nerve,* the larger terminal division of the tibial nerve, accompanies the medial plantar artery. Its cutaneous branches supply the medial two thirds of the sole. The *lateral plantar nerve* passes obliquely forward, accompanying the lateral plantar artery. Its cutaneous branches supply the lateral one third of the sole.

The cutaneous neurovascular branches supplying this area are given off from both medial and lateral plantar neurovascular bundles in the clefts between the abductor hallucis, flexor digitorum brevis, and abductor digiti minimi. They curve around the medial and lateral edges of the plantar fascia to the skin.

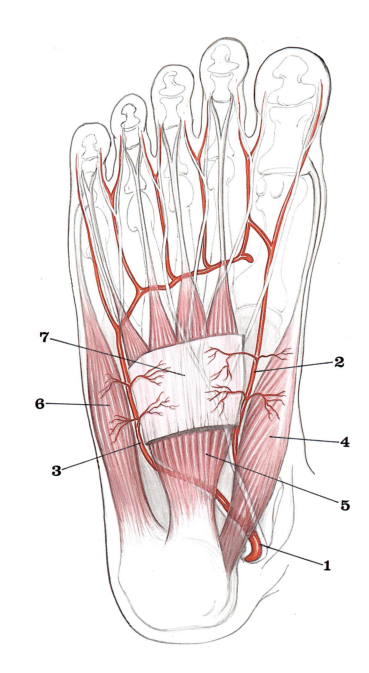

1. Posterior tibial a.
2. Medial plantar a.
3. Lateral plantar a.
4. Abductor hallucis m.
5. Flexor digitorum brevis m.
6. Abductor digitori minimi m.
7. Plantar fascia

COMMENT AND INSIGHTS

This instep skin flap has a special anatomic structure and properties; the skin is thinner but hornier. Subcutaneous tissue is dense because of the many fibrous septa that bind the skin to the plantar fascia. Flap location is in a non-weight-bearing area, and the healed defect with skin graft does not usually affect walking and weight bearing.

Since this skin flap is durable and sensitive, the donor site is ideal for reconstruction of skin defects in a weight-bearing area, such as on the heel and sole of the foot, or for reconstruction of defects of the palmar skin, even with palmar fascia. Heel defects can ordinarily be covered by an island. If both the instep and heel are lost, or either the posterior or anterior tibial artery is absent, a revascularized free flap from the contralateral foot is indicated.

The flexor digitorum brevis muscle can be included in the flap, but a muscle flap is not always suitable for reconstruction of a defect in a weight-bearing area.

Harvesting Technique

(Fig. 8-27) In designing the flap, the medial or lateral plantar artery is selected as a vascular pedicle, according to the required flap size and location; for a large flap, both arteries may be included. Usually, the medial plantar artery is chosen and designed as the flap axis. The region of the sole between the heel and the metatarsal heads, except for the lateral border overlying the fifth metatarsal, is the territory of the flap, providing a maximum area of about 10 × 10 cm.

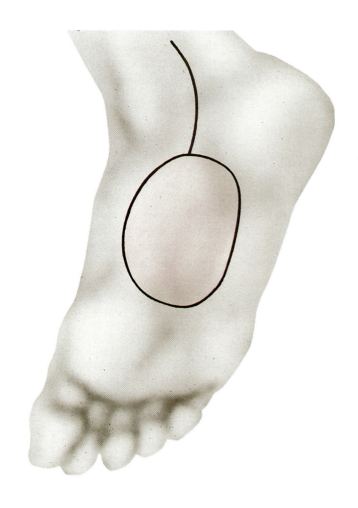

1. Medial plantar a. and n.
2. Abductor hallucis brevis m.
3. Flexor digitorum brevis m.
4. Plantar fascia
5. Posterior tibial a. and n.
6. Lateral plantar a. and n.

(Fig. 8-28) The distal edge of the flap is incised and the plantar fascia [4] is transversely divided. The medial plantar neurovascular bundle [1] is identified in the cleft between the abductor hallucis and flexor digitorum brevis [2,3], and the vessels are divided. After the vessels are separated from the medial plantar nerve [1] and kept intact with the flap, the flap is raised at the level between the plantar fascia [4] and the flexor digitorum brevis muscle [3], from distal to proximal. Attention should be paid to the cutaneous branches from the nerve to the flap, carefully peeling them off interfascicularly, and leaving the nerve trunk in the foot.

1. Medial plantar a. and n.
2. Abductor hallucis brevis m.
3. Flexor digitorum brevis m.
4. Plantar fascia

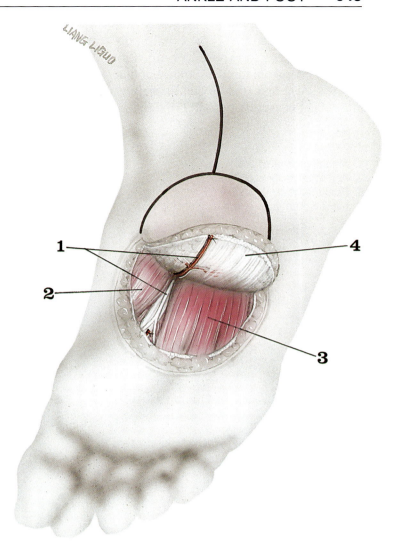

(Fig. 8-29) Tracing the medial plantar neurovascular bundle [1] proximally, dissection proceeds to expose its bifurcation with the lateral plantar neurovascular bundle [6], whereas the abductor hallucis muscle [2] is usually partially divided.

1. Medial plantar a. and n.
2. Abductor hallucis brevis m.
5. Posterior tibial a. and n.
6. Lateral plantar a. and n.

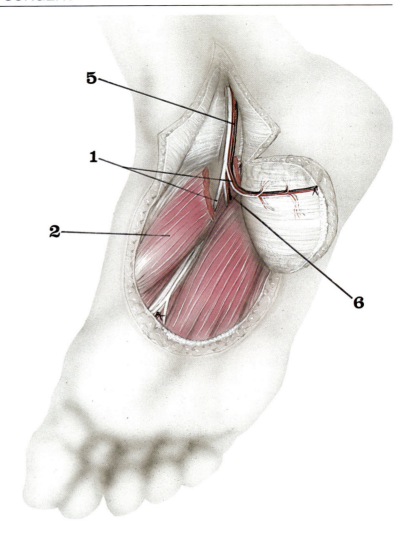

(Fig. 8-30) The flap is completed by a circumferential incision, with the plantar fascia included in the flap. If a longer and larger vascular pedicle is required, the dorsalis pedis artery should be palpated for confirmation, before ligation of the lateral plantar vessels [6] and division of the posterior tibial vessels [5].

1. Medial plantar a. and n.
2. Abductor hallucis brevis m.
5. Posterior tibial a. and n.
6. Lateral plantar a. and n.

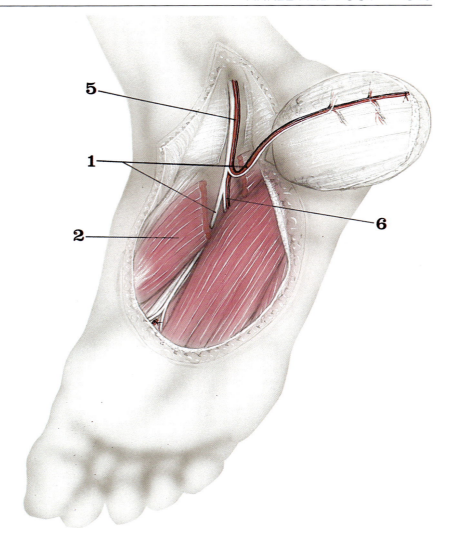

(Fig. 8-31) If the lateral plantar vessels [6] and cutaneous nerves are required for the flap, the flexor digitorum brevis [3] is divided proximally and the vascular branches to the muscle are ligated.

1. Medial plantar a. and n.
2. Abductor hallucis brevis m.
3. Flexor digitorum brevis m.
5. Posterior tibial a. and n.
6. Lateral plantar a. and n.

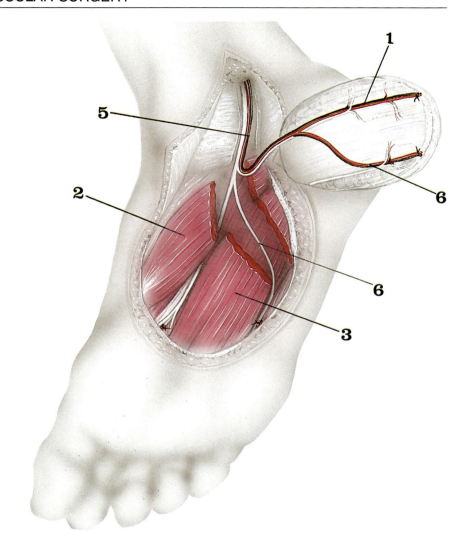

Free Toe and Toe Tissue Transfers

Arterial Anatomy (Fig. 8-32)

There are two arterial systems to supply the big and second toes, dorsal and plantar.

Dorsal Arterial System

The dorsalis pedis-first dorsal metatarsal arterial system [1,2] and its variations are described in the section on the dorsalis pedis flap.

The *first dorsal metatarsal artery* [2] courses at varying levels in relation to the interosseous muscle and gives off branches to the muscle, joints, and metatarsals. However, between the heads of the first and second metatarsals, it more constantly lies superficially over the deep transverse ligament. It then divides into two dorsal digital arteries [5] that run on adjacent sides of the big and second toes.

Plantar Arterial System

The *first plantar metatarsal artery* [10] issues from the junction between the plantar arch [9] and the *deep plantar artery* [3]. The former is a continuation of the lateral plantar artery [7], and the latter is the communicating branch of the dorsalis pedis artery [1]. In its course, the artery communicates with the *medial plantar artery* [8] between the bone and the flexor tendons, after which it passes under the deep transverse ligament and divides into two plantar arteries [11] that supply the adjacent sides of the toes.

Communication Between the Two Systems

Between the dorsal and plantar arterial systems, there are two communications in the interspace between the first and second metatarsals. Proximally, the *deep plantar artery* [3] serves as communication between the dorsalis pedis artery and the plantar arch [9] (the continuation of the lateral plantar artery). Distally, there is the *distal perforating artery* [4] just distal to the deep transverse metatarsal ligament. It joins the dorsal and plantar metatarsal arteries [2,10] near their bifurcation.

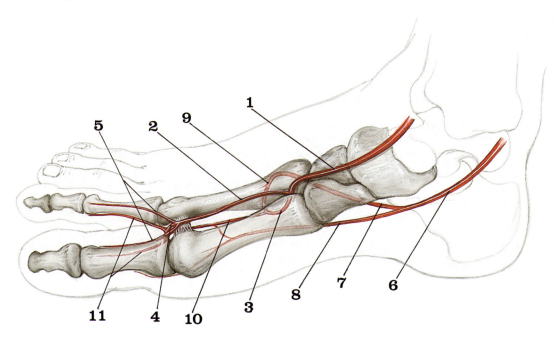

1. Dorsalis pedis a.
2. First dorsal metatarsal a.
3. Deep plantar a.
4. Distal perforating a.
5. Dorsal digital a.
6. Posterior tibial a.
7. Lateral plantar a.
8. Medial plantar a.
9. Plantar arch
10. First plantar metatarsal a.
11. Plantar digital a.

Variations of the Distal Perforating Artery (Fig. 8-33)

Type A. The distal perforating artery arises from the first dorsal metatarsal artery (FDMA) and divides into two plantar digital arteries (PDAs). The first plantar metatarsal artery (FPMA) joins into one of two PDAs (46.5% of cases).

Type B. The distal perforating artery communicates between the bifurcations of the FDMA and the FPMA (24.0% of cases).

Type C. The FPMA divides into two PDAs, and the distal perforating artery then joins into one of the two PDAs (14.5% of cases).

Type D. After the bifurcations of the FDMA and FPMA, communications occur between the dorsal digital artery (DDA) and PDA, but there is no apparent distal perforating branch in the web space.

Type E. There is no apparent communication between the FDMA and FPMA, and between the DDA and PDA.

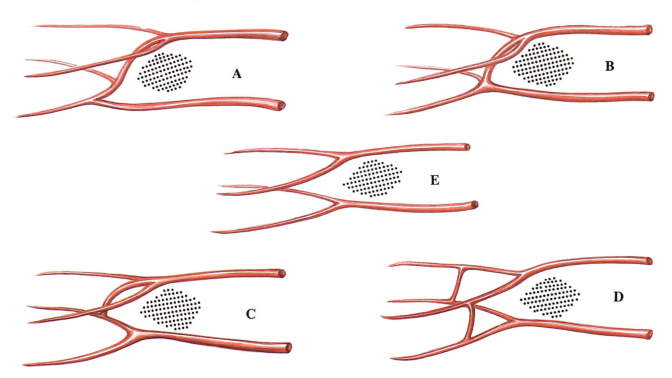

Measurements of the Arterial System of the Donor Area

Vessel	Diameter (mm)		Origin from Web Edge (cm)	
	Range	Average	Range	Average
First dorsal metatarsal a.	0.6–2.4	1.3	6.0–8.5	7.4
First plantar metatarsal a.	0.6–3.0	1.5		
Dorsal digital a. of big and second toes	0.3–1.5	0.7	1.6–3.8	2.4
Plantar digital a. of big and second toes	0.4–2.0	0.9	1.5–3.5	2.3
Distal perforating a.	0.5–2.0	1.1	1.6–3.8	2.4

Assessments of First Dorsal Metatarsal Artery

Type	Diameter (mm)	Incidence (%)
Larger	More than 1.5	26
Median	1.0–1.5	50
Narrow	Less than 1.0	19
Absent	—	5

COMMENT AND INSIGHTS

Because of a resemblance between the forefoot and hand, this donor area has become extremely useful as a multiple tissue bank in reconstructive microsurgery of the hand. There are two arterial systems available for transplantation. Although there is some variation in the dorsal system, it is still the primary choice as an arterial pedicle: it is usually superficial, more easily accessible, and a fairly long pedicle length can be obtained. The superficial venous system is usually more consistent and reliable.

If the first dorsal metatarsal artery is absent or narrow, the following procedures can be used as alternates: (1) the deep transverse metatarsal ligament is divided, and the first plantar metatarsal and deep plantar arteries are dissected out in continuity with the dorsalis pedis artery as the vascular pedicle; (2) the dorsalis pedis-second dorsal metatarsal artery can be used as the pedicle for the second toe; or (3) only the first plantar metatarsal artery can be used as the pedicle.

In the development and refinement of thumb reconstruction, free toe transfer has been a milestone. It provides a reconstructed thumb with good appearance, function, sensibility, stability, and cold tolerance. If the surgical procedures are successful, patient acceptance is high.

Using microsurgical techniques, the thumb can be reconstructed with several optional procedures, each with advantages and disadvantages. The big toe transfer involves two phalanges and a large nail, similar to a normal thumb, but it is excessively large. Also, loss of the big toe may impair appearance of the foot to a certain extent. However, grip strength, using reconstruction of the thumb with a big toe, is much stronger than with a second toe. This procedure is usually indicated for a male patient who is engaged in heavy manual work.

The second toe transfer involves a digit that is smaller than the big toe, although it has three phalanges. If the proximal and distal interphalangeal (PIP and DIP) joints are maintained in varying degrees of flexion, the second toe transfer may have a more pleasing cosmetic effect. In societies where sandals are standard footwear, surgeons and patients prefer to sacrifice the second toe, rather than the big toe, for thumb reconstruction. Currently, the total number of cases reported for thumb reconstruction, using vascularized second toe, is much larger than that for vascularized big toe.

Contrasted with the disadvantages of size and appearance of big or second toe transfer for thumb reconstruction, the wrap-around flap reconstructs a thumb almost identical in size to the original. This particular procedure is ideal for function and cosmesis of a degloved thumb, where skeleton and tendon remain intact. Combined with an iliac bone graft, this procedure is indicated for reconstruction of a thumb loss distal to the metacarpophalangeal (MCP) joint; however, no interphalangeal joint is present.

Currently, the modified wrap-around, rather than the original, flap is more commonly applied in thumb reconstruction. In the original wrap-around flap, there almost always were wound-healing problems on the dorsum of the distal phalanx of the toe, as well as painful hyperkeratosis on the plantar surface of the skin graft at the donor site. Also, there would frequently be resorption and fracture of the iliac bone graft, as well as problems with toenail growth resulting from harvesting damaged skin matrix, occurring in the reconstructed thumb at the recipient site. Usually, the partial or even whole distal phalanx would be resected and discarded, so that the plantar surface could be covered properly by an intact medial flap.

With the modified wrap-around flap, the distal phalanx that would have been discarded is included in the flap, keeping it intact with the toenail, so that damage to the nail bed and matrix is avoided. In addition, the iliac bone graft becomes an interposition between the distal and proximal phalanx or metacarpal, thus decreasing the length and degree of resorption of the graft.

Removing the bulging condyles at the base of the distal phalanx, the modified wrap-around flap can be tailored to the exact size of the lost thumb.

Neither traditional nor modified wrap-around flaps are applicable for children, because there is no growth plate in the bony components.

Although the first web skin flap provides a limited amount of tissue, the glabrous skin texture and excellent recovered sensibility are ideal for skin coverage to the hand. In addition, following its special shape in the first web space and matching the texture and color of dorsal skin, the flap can be properly applied in reconstruction of the upper and lower eyelids.

Each toe is composed of several components, viz., nail, pulp, bones, joints, epiphysis, and tendons. To meet the requirements for reconstruction of a recipient site, various techniques have been designed for selective transfer of parts from the big or second toe, or both. The procedure can be a single transfer (pulp) or a combination of composite tissue transfers.

To the present time, vascularized joint transfer reported for autograft has been donated from the PIP and metatarsophalangeal (MTP) joints of the second toe, applied for reconstruction of the PIP and MCP joints of the hand. The PIP joint of the second toe is preferably applied in adults for both MCP and PIP reconstruction, because of its greater flexion range, lateral stability, size match, and smaller secondary defect. In children, the PIP joint provides only a single growth plate. The MTP joint, including both growth centers, should be used for replacing the hand joint, so that the reconstructed finger can keep up growth rate with the adjacent digits.

Because of greater hyperextensibility and less flexion of the MTP joint of the second toe, reverse insetting into the recipient site is recommended.

The second and third toes can be transferred en bloc to the hand. Indications for this technique are limited to special cases, when all fingers have been amputated.

If microsurgically transferred skin flaps or toes in the donor area are used and if vessels and nerves are successfully anastomosed, recovery of postoperative sensibility in the hand can be excellent. Surprisingly, these flaps or toes often develop better two-point discrimination in the hand than was ever present in the foot.

FREE BIG TOE TRANSFER

(Fig. 8-34) The ipsilateral big toe is commonly used in reconstruction of the thumb.

A curvilinear incision is made on the dorsum of the foot between the dorsalis pedis artery and the greater saphenous vein, down to the first web. There, the incision is turned circumferentially around the big toe at about the MTP joint level.

The procedure should be carried out under tourniquet application, without exsanguination, to allow the vessels to be more visible.

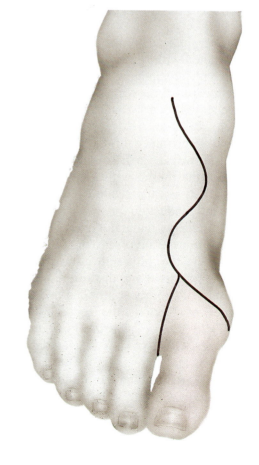

1. Dorsalis pedis a., greater saphenous v., deep peroneal n.
2. First dorsal metatarsal a.
3. Extensor hallucis brevis
4. Extensor hallucis longus tendon
5. Deep transverse metatarsal ligament
6. Plantar digital a. and n.
7. Flexor hallucis tendon
8. Dorsal metatarsal v.
9. Deep plantar a.
10. Interosseous m.

ANKLE AND FOOT 351

(**Fig. 8-35**) The incision on the plantar aspect is illustrated.

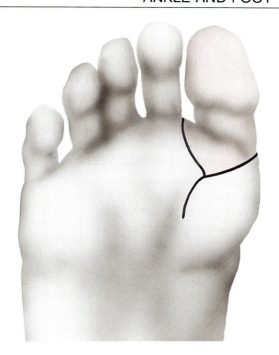

(**Fig. 8-36**) The dorsal metatarsal veins [8] that drain the big toe, the dorsal venous arch, and the greater saphenous vein [1] are dissected. After the branches to the second toe and the communicating branch to the deep vein are ligated, this superficial venous system is isolated.

1. Greater saphenous v.
3. Extensor hallucis brevis
4. Extensor hallucis longus tendon
8. Dorsal metatarsal v.

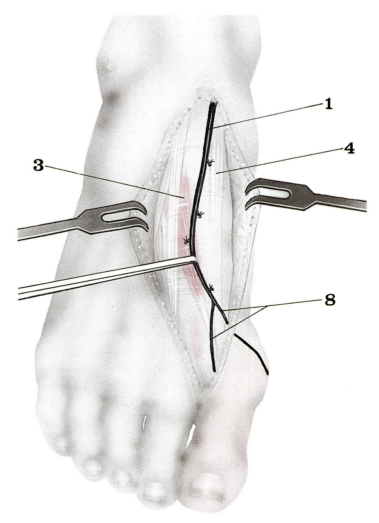

352 ATLAS OF MICROVASCULAR SURGERY

(Fig. 8-37) Then, the extensor hallucis brevis tendon [3] is identified at the lateral side of the extensor hallucis longus tendon [4]. The extensor hallucis brevis tendon is divided, and this muscle is turned proximally to expose the dorsalis pedis vessels [1] and the deep peroneal nerve [1]. The vessels are dissected and traced to identify the first dorsal metatarsal artery [2] at the proximal end of the first intermetatarsal space.

If the first dorsal metatarsal artery is superficial and adequate in caliber (more than 1 mm), the dissection proceeds to the first web space.

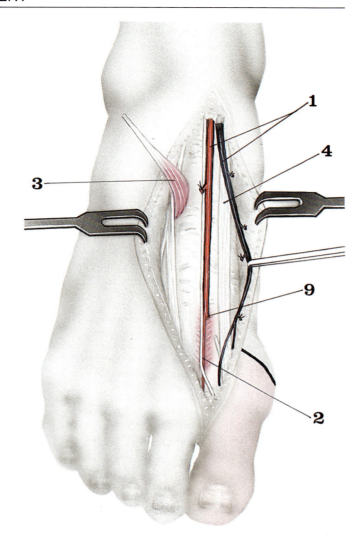

1. Dorsalis pedis a., greater saphenous v., deep peroneal n.
2. First dorsal metatarsal a.
3. Extensor hallucis brevis
4. Extensor hallucis longus tendon
9. Deep plantar a.

ANKLE AND FOOT

(**Fig. 8-38**) If there is no adequate superficial first dorsal metatarsal artery or if it takes off deeply from the deep plantar artery [9] or the first plantar metatarsal artery, the dissection turns toward the first web space, between the heads of the first and second metatarsals, where the first dorsal metatarsal artery usually lies quite superficially over the deep transverse metatarsal ligament. Then, dividing the interosseous muscle [10], the dissection proceeds proximally to isolate the artery [2].

1. Dorsalis pedis a., greater saphenous v., deep peroneal n.
2. First dorsal metatarsal a.
9. Deep plantar a.
10. Interosseous m.

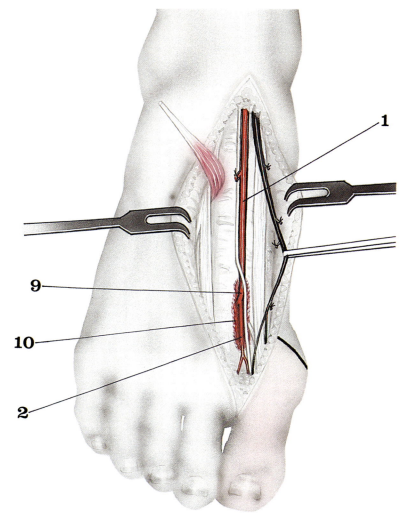

(Fig. 8-39) After isolating the dorsalis pedis artery [1] and the first dorsal metatarsal artery [2], the deep plantar artery [9] is carefully ligated distal to the takeoff of the first dorsal metatarsal artery [2]. The extensor tendon [4] of the big toe is divided as proximally as possible.

The vessels supplying the second toe should be ligated, and the deep transverse metatarsal ligament [5] on the lateral side of the MTP joint of the big toe is carefully divided.

1. Dorsalis pedis a., greater saphenous v., deep peroneal n.
2. First dorsal metatarsal a.
3. Extensor hallucis brevis
4. Extensor hallucis longus tendon
5. Deep transverse metatarsal ligament
9. Deep plantar a.

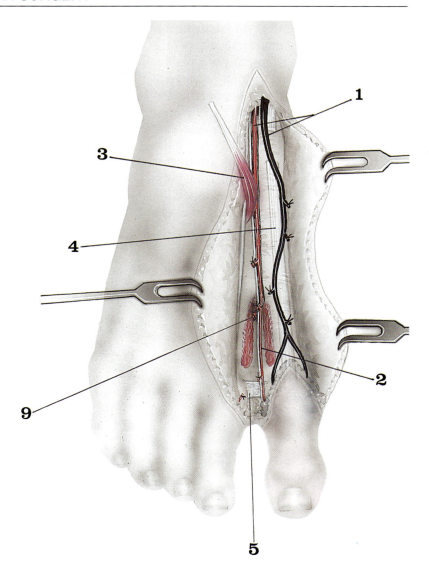

(Fig. 8-40) Through a longitudinal incision on the plantar aspect, the lateral and medial plantar digital nerves [6] and flexor hallucis longus tendon [7] are exposed and dissected for an adequate length, and then divided.

5. Deep transverse metatarsal ligament
6. Plantar digital a. and n.
7. Flexor hallucis tendon

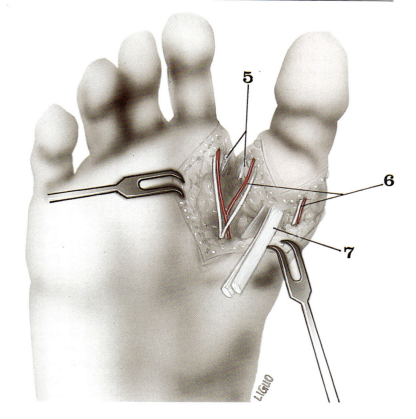

(Fig. 8-41) The metatarsophalangeal joint is disarticulated and, after releasing the tourniquet, its circulation is assessed. The big toe is now ready for transfer.

1. Dorsalis pedis a., greater saphenous v., deep peroneal n.
4. Extensor hallucis longus tendon
6. Plantar digital a. and n.
7. Flexor hallucis tendon

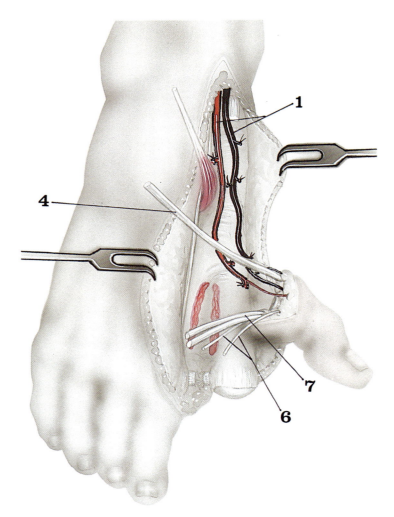

FREE SECOND TOE TRANSFER

(**Fig. 8-42**) It is suggested that the contralateral second toe be selected in reconstructions of the thumb, especially if there is a contracture of the first web on the hand that needs release.

A curvilinear incision is made between the greater saphenous vein and the dorsalis pedis artery, from the ankle to the head or neck of the second metatarsal. There, the incision forks toward the first and second webs, and then merges at the plantar aspect of the MTP joint. To meet recipient site requirements, a dorsalis pedis flap or first web space flap can be combined with a second toe transfer.

The procedure should be carried out under tourniquet application to allow the vessels to be more visible without exsanguination.

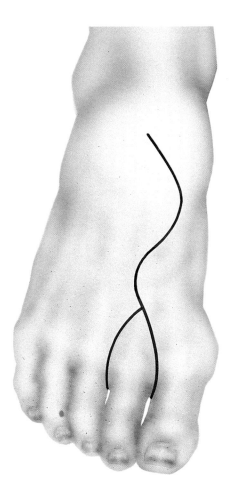

1. Greater saphenous v.
2. Extensor hallucis brevis
3. Extensor hallucis longus tendon
4. Dorsal metatarsal v.
5. Dorsalis pedis a. and deep peroneal n.
6. Deep plantar a.
7. First dorsal metatarsal a.
8. Interosseous m.
9. Extensor tendons
10. Deep transverse metatarsal ligament
11. Flexor tendon
12. Plantar digital a. and n.

(**Fig. 8-43**) The incision is shown in a plantar view.

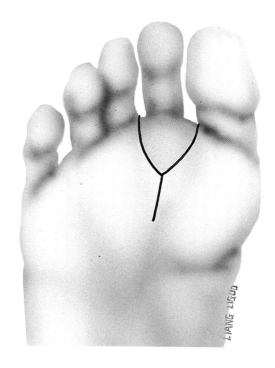

(**Fig. 8-44**) The dorsal metatarsal veins [4] that drain the second toe, the dorsal venous arch, and the greater saphenous vein [1] are dissected. After the branches to the adjacent toes and the communicating branch to the deep vein are ligated, this superficial venous system is isolated.

1. Greater saphenous v.
2. Extensor hallucis brevis
3. Extensor hallucis longus tendon
4. Dorsal metatarsal v.
9. Extensor tendons

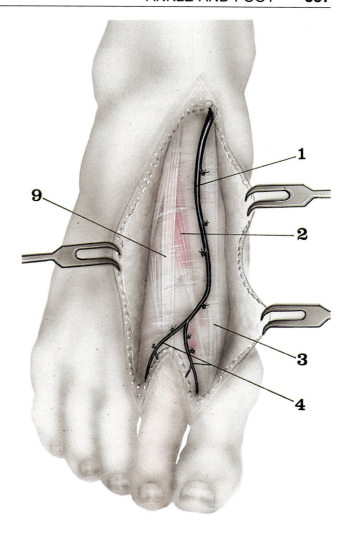

(Fig. 8-45) Then, the extensor hallucis brevis tendon [2] is identified at the lateral side of the extensor hallucis longus tendon. The extensor hallucis brevis tendon is divided, and this muscle is turned proximally to expose the dorsalis pedis vessels [5] and the deep peroneal nerve [5]. The vessels are dissected and traced, to identify the first dorsal metatarsal artery [7] at the proximal end of the first intermetatarsal space.

If the first dorsal metatarsal artery is superficial and adequate in caliber (more than 1 mm), the dissection proceeds to the first web space.

2. Extensor hallucis brevis
5. Dorsalis pedis a. and deep peroneal n.
6. Deep plantar a.
7. First dorsal metatarsal a.
9. Extensor tendons

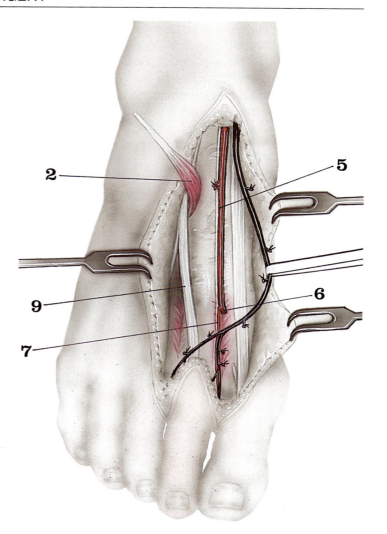

(Fig. 8-46) If there is no adequate superficial first dorsal metatarsal artery or if it takes off deeply from the deep plantar artery or the first plantar metatarsal artery, the dissection turns toward the first web space, between the heads of the first and second metatarsals, where the first dorsal metatarsal artery usually lies quite superficially over the deep transverse metatarsal ligament. Then, dividing the interosseous muscle [8], the dissection proceeds proximally to isolate the artery.

5. Dorsalis pedis a. and deep peroneal n.
6. Deep plantar a.
7. First dorsal metatarsal a.
8. Interosseous m.

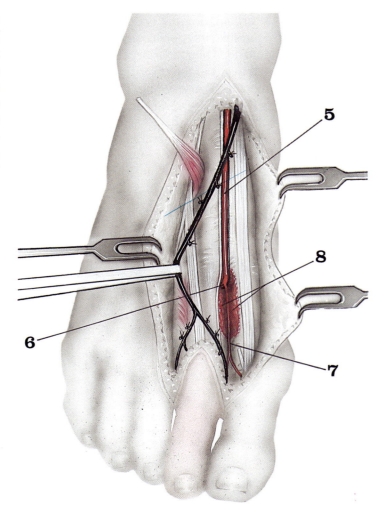

(Fig. 8-47) After isolating the dorsalis pedis artery [5] and the first dorsal metatarsal artery [7], the deep plantar artery [6] is carefully ligated distal to the takeoff of the first dorsal metatarsal artery [7]. The extensor tendons [9] of the second toe are divided as proximally as possible.

The vessels supplying the big and third toes should be ligated, and the deep transverse metatarsal ligaments [10] on both sides of the second MTP joint are carefully divided.

5. Dorsalis pedis a. and deep peroneal n.
6. Deep plantar a.
7. First dorsal metatarsal a.
8. Interosseous m.
9. Extensor tendons
10. Deep transverse metatarsal ligament

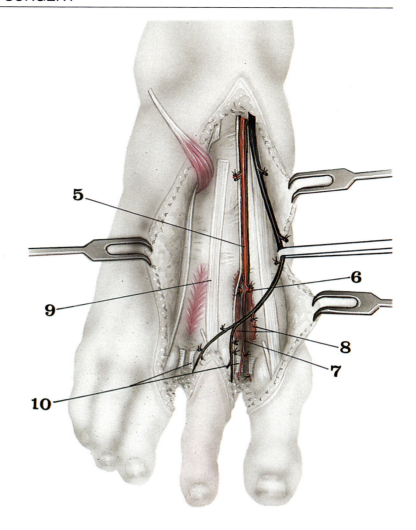

(Fig. 8-48) Plantar dissection is carried out to identify the plantar digital nerves [12] and to separate them from the lateral and medial plantar digital nerves of the big and third toes, respectively. The flexor longus and flexor brevis [11] are exposed, and all flexor tendons and plantar digital nerves are divided as proximally as possible, usually at the middle sole.

10. Deep transverse metatarsal ligament
11. Flexor tendon
12. Plantar digital a. and n.

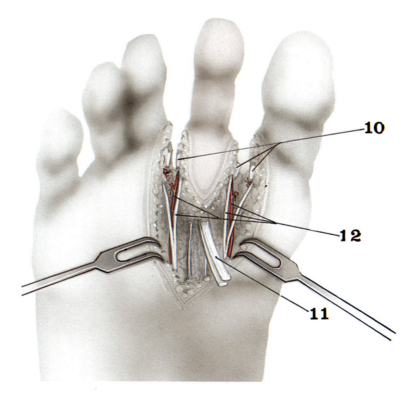

(Fig. 8-49) With great attention to protect all the soft tissues from injury, including the vascular pedicle, nerves, and tendons, the MTP joint is disarticulated. The second toe is then isolated only on the dorsalis pedis-first dorsal metatarsal artery [5,7] and the greater saphenous vein [1]. If metacarpal reconstruction with thumb or finger reconstruction is needed at the same time, the second metatarsal bone is divided with a Gigli saw at a proper level (instead of disarticulating it). The distal part of the second metatarsal should be removed, to allow primary donor site closure.

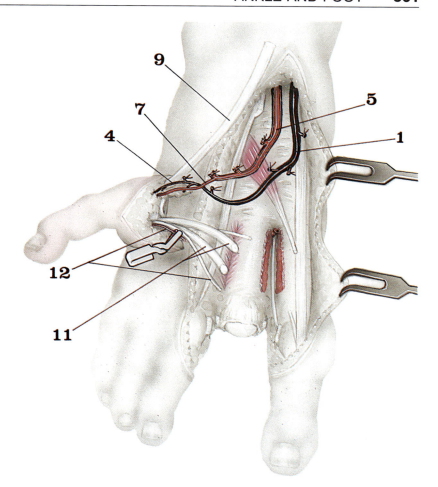

1. Greater saphenous v.
4. Dorsal metatarsal v.
5. Dorsalis pedis a. and deep peroneal n.
7. First dorsal metatarsal a.
9. Extensor tendons
11. Flexor tendon
12. Plantar digital a. and n.

FIRST WEB SPACE SKIN FLAP

(Fig. 8-50) A standard first web space skin flap is comprised of four parts, each part providing a separate dimension: the lateral side of the big toe (5 × 3 cm), the medial side of the second toe (4 × 3 cm), the dorsal aspect of the web (4 × 3 cm), and the plantar aspect of the web (3 × 3 cm). The total area can reach a size of 7 × 7 cm, and the flap can be combined with a dorsalis pedis flap, the second toe, or other designs.

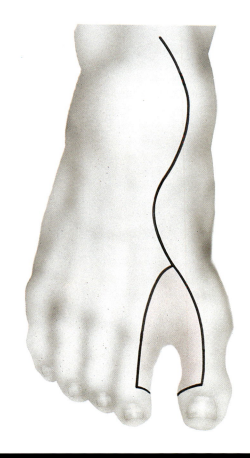

1. Dorsalis pedis a., greater saphenous v.
2. Extensor hallucis brevis
3. Extensor hallucis longus tendon
4. Common plantar digital a. and n.
5. Deep transverse metatarsal ligament
6. Flexor tendons
7. Deep peroneal n.

(Fig. 8-51) The incision on the plantar aspect is shown.

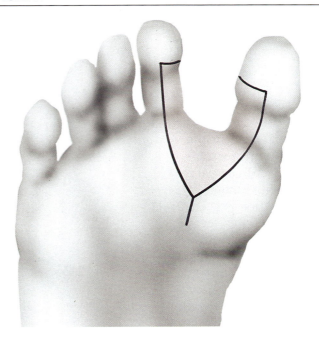

(Fig. 8-52) The greater saphenous vein and the dorsalis pedis-first dorsal metatarsal artery [1] are dissected out through an incision on the dorsum of the foot. The deep peroneal nerve [7] is preserved for inclusion in the flap.

1. Dorsalis pedis a., greater saphenous v.
2. Extensor hallucis brevis
3. Extensor hallucis longus tendon
7. Deep peroneal n.

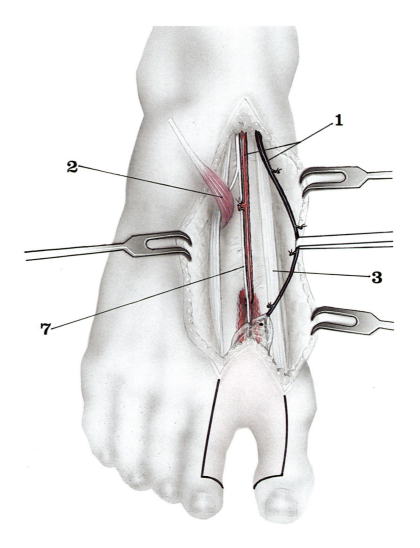

(**Fig. 8-53**) Through the incision on the plantar aspect, the common plantar digital nerve [4] is dissected for some length and cut.

4. Common plantar digital a. and n.
6. Flexor tendons

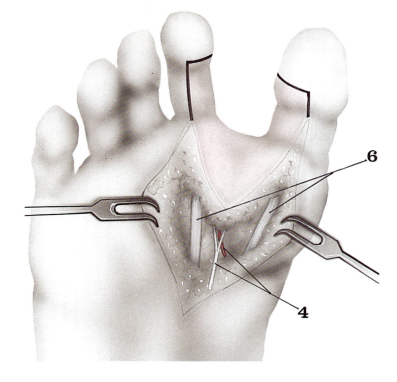

(**Fig. 8-54**) The skin flap is dissected away from the fascia of the two toes and then isolated. The defect is covered with a split-thickness skin graft.

1. Dorsalis pedis a., greater saphenous v.
2. Extensor hallucis brevis
4. Common plantar digital a. and n.
5. Deep transverse metatarsal ligament

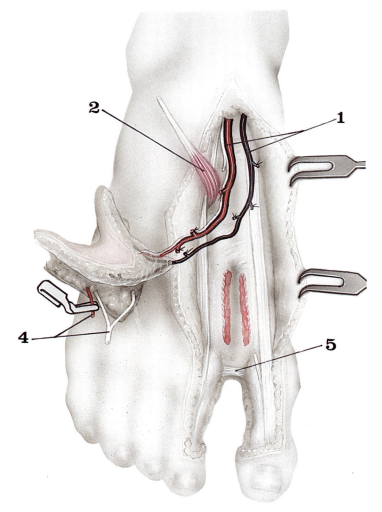

WRAP-AROUND FLAP

(**Fig. 8-55**) The ipsilateral big toe is selected, and the circumference and length of the opposite, normal thumb are measured. A template is made for marking the flap on the donor big toe.

A medial skin bridge, extending around the tip, is preserved, with its width just the difference between the circumferences of the thumb and the toe. It usually measures 1.0 to 1.5 cm at its base. Since the nail of the big toe is wider than that of the thumb, the medial margin of the flap on the dorsum is placed on the medial third of the toenail and its matrix.

1. Dorsalis pedis a., deep peroneal n., greater saphenous v.
2. Extensor hallucis brevis
3. Extensor hallucis longus tendon
4. Common plantar digital a. and n.
5. Deep transverse metatarsal ligament
6. Flexor tendon
7. Medial plantar digital a. and n.
8. Distal perforator a.

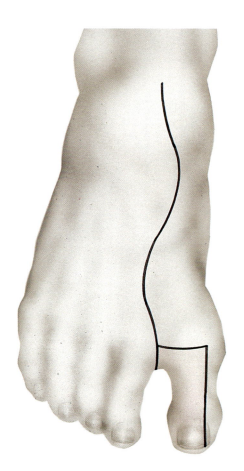

(**Fig. 8-56**) The incision is shown in an oblique-lateral view.

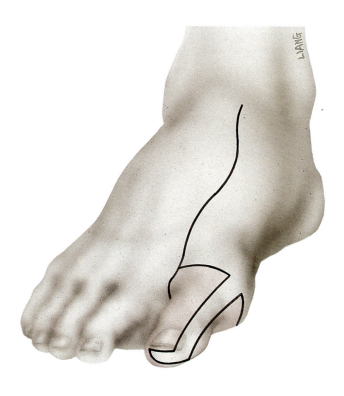

(**Fig. 8-57**) The greater saphenous vein, dorsalis pedis-first dorsal metatarsal artery, and deep peroneal nerve [1] are dissected out through the incision on the dorsum of the foot. Branches to the second toe are ligated. The flap over the dorsum of the toe is raised medially over the paratenon of the extensor tendon [3], with the dissection below the nail proceeding subperiosteally, to avoid damage to the germinal matrix. If necessary, a fine sliver of bone may be included, further to ensure integrity.

1. Dorsalis pedis a., deep peroneal n., greater saphenous v.
2. Extensor hallucis brevis
3. Extensor hallucis longus tendon

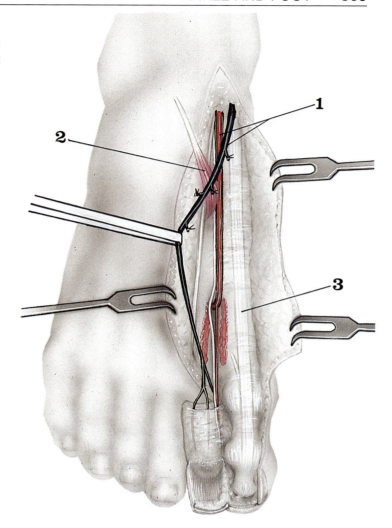

(**Fig. 8-58**) The medial plantar digital artery and nerve [7] are preserved on the plantar aspect for the medial skin flap. The lateral plantar digital artery and nerve [4] are dissected, the artery is ligated, and the nerve is separated from the nerve of the second toe and divided to the proper length. Then, the plantar part of the flap is raised toward the first web, with care taken to include the lateral plantar digital neurovascular bundle [4] in the flap.

4. Common plantar digital a. and n.
6. Flexor tendon
7. Medial plantar digital a. and n.

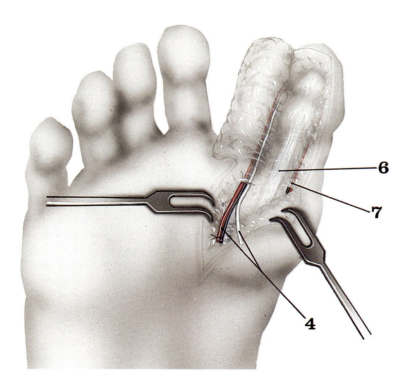

(**Fig. 8-59**) During dissection in the first web, attention should be paid to the distal edge of the deep transverse ligament [5], so that the distal perforating artery is not injured and keeps its communication between the dorsal and plantar arteries. Then, the flap is isolated on the dorsalis pedis-first dorsal metatarsal artery and greater saphenous vein [1]

1. Dorsalis pedis a., deep peroneal n., greater saphenous v.
4. Common plantar digital a. and n.
5. Deep transverse metatarsal ligament
8. Distal perforator a.

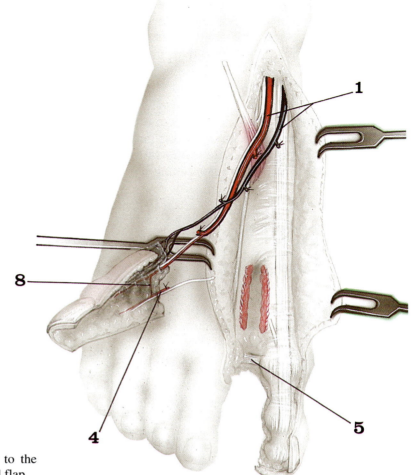

Note. For donor site closure, please refer to the following section on the modified wrap-around flap.

MODIFIED WRAP-AROUND FLAP

(Fig. 8-60) The ipsilateral big toe is selected, and the circumference and length, as well as the nail width, of the opposite, normal thumb are measured. A template is made for marking the flap on the donor big toe.

A medial skin bridge, extending around the tip, is preserved, with its width just the difference between the circumferences of the thumb and the toe. It usually measures 1.0 to 1.5 cm at its base. Since the nail of the big toe is wider than that of the thumb, the medial margin of the flap on the dorsum is placed on about the medial third of the toenail and its matrix, to match the nail width of the normal thumb.

1. Dorsalis pedis a., deep peroneal n., greater saphenous v.
2. Extensor hallucis brevis
3. Extensor hallucis longus tendon
4. Lateral plantar digital a. and n.
5. Deep transverse metatarsal ligament
6. Flexor tendon
7. Medial plantar digital a. and n.
8. Distal perforating a.

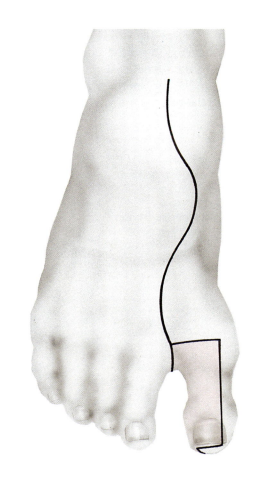

(Fig. 8-61) The incision is shown in an oblique-lateral view.

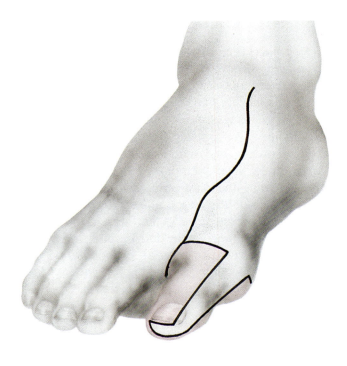

(**Fig. 8-62**) The greater saphenous vein, dorsalis pedis – first dorsal metatarsal artery system, and deep peroneal nerve [1] are dissected out through the incision on the dorsum of the foot. Branches of the superficial veins and deep peroneal nerve to the second toe are ligated and divided, except the arterial branch to the second toe.

1. Dorsalis pedis a., deep peroneal n., greater saphenous v.
2. Extensor hallucis brevis
3. Extensor hallucis longus tendon

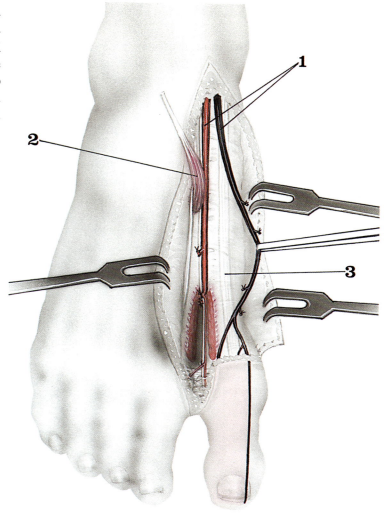

(**Fig. 8-63**) The dissection is turned to the plantar aspect. The medial plantar digital artery and nerve [7] are preserved for the medial skin flap. The lateral plantar digital artery and nerve [4] are dissected, and the nerve is separated from the nerve of the second toe and divided to the proper length. Then, the plantar part of the flap is raised toward the first web, with care taken to include the lateral plantar digital neurovascular bundle [4] in the flap.

After assessment that the dorsalis pedis-first dorsal metatarsal arterial system is capable of blood supply to the big toe, the lateral plantar digital artery is ligated as far as possible proximally.

4. Lateral plantar digital a. and n.
6. Flexor tendon
7. Medial plantar digital a. and n.

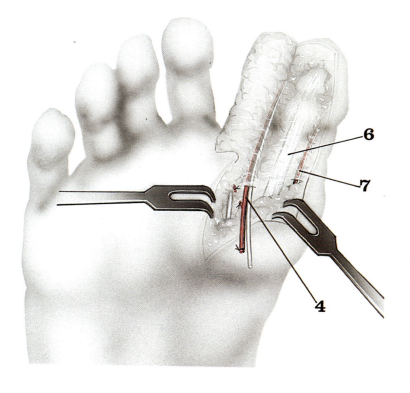

(**Fig. 8-64**) During dissection in the first web, attention should be paid to the distal edge of the deep transverse ligament [5], so that the distal perforating artery [8] is not injured and keeps its communication between the dorsal and plantar arteries [1,4], before ligating the dorsal and plantar digital arteries to the second toe.

1. Dorsalis pedis a., deep peroneal n., greater saphenous v.
4. Lateral plantar digital a. and n.
5. Deep transverse metatarsal ligament
8. Distal perforating a.

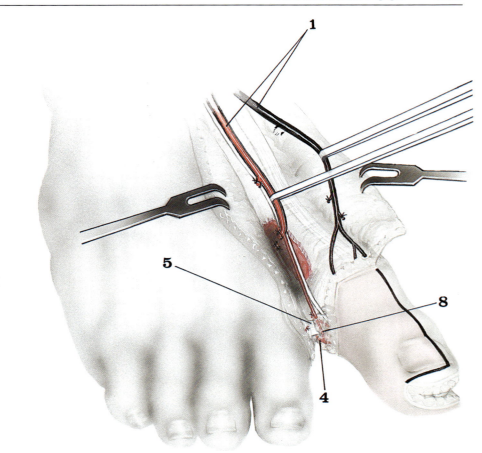

(**Fig. 8-65**) The medial excess portion of the toenail with its bed and germinal matrix is resected. The medial flap of the toe is elevated from the tip of the distal phalanx proximally, until reaching the middle portion of the proximal phalanx. Then, the skin flap over the dorsum of the proximal phalanx is raised over the paratenon of the extensor tendon distally until reaching the interphalangeal joint, with care to protect the arterial and venous system of the wrap-around flap.

1. Dorsalis pedis a., deep peroneal n., greater saphenous v.
3. Extensor hallucis longus tendon
7. Medial plantar digital a. and n.

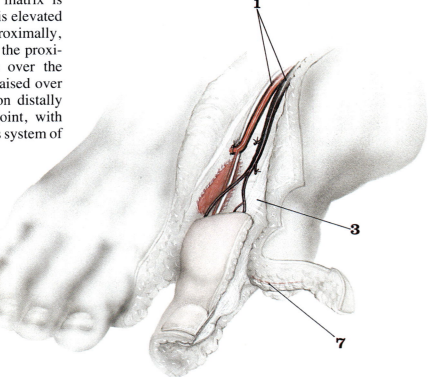

(Fig. 8-66) The extensor and flexor tendons [3] are divided, and the interphalangeal joint is disarticulated. At this point, the modified wrap-around flap, with nail and distal phalanx intact together, is isolated on the dorsalis pedis-first dorsal metatarsal artery and greater saphenous vein [1].

1. Dorsalis pedis a., deep peroneal n., greater saphenous v.
2. Extensor hallucis brevis
3. Extensor hallucis longus tendon
4. Lateral plantar digital a. and n.
8. Distal perforating a.

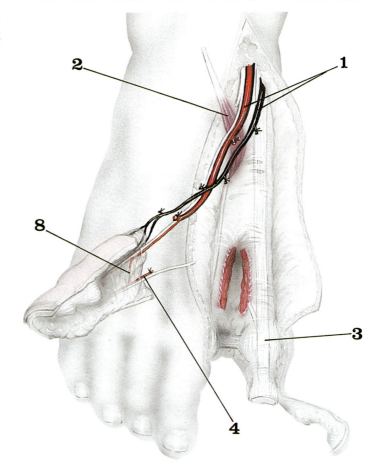

(Fig. 8-67) Both the medial and lateral condyles of the distal phalanx are resected with a rongeur in order to lessen the bulge on the base and to match the normal size of the contralateral thumb.

After the articular cartilage is removed, a customized iliac bone graft of the proper size, shape, and length (referring to the normal thumb), is fixed on the base of the distal phalanx. Usually, the distal half of the proximal phalanx is resected for proper donor closure.

1. Dorsalis pedis a., deep peroneal n., greater saphenous v.
4. Lateral plantar digital a. and n.
8. Distal perforating a.

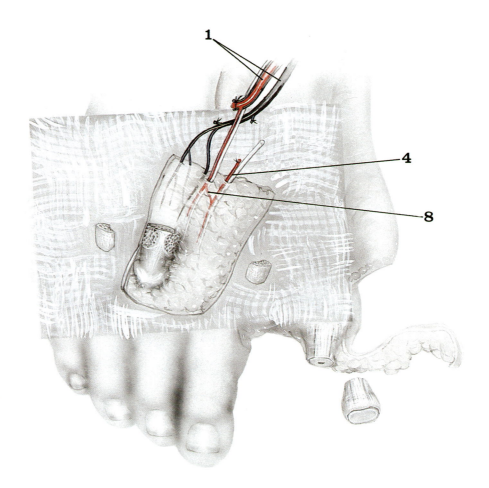

(**Fig. 8-68**) The plantar portion of the wrap-around flap is brought back and advanced mediodorsally for closure of the tip and medial margin of the nail. After the interpositional iliac bone graft is fixed to the distal phalanx by Kirschner wires, the proximal portion of the flap is wrapped around it.

1. Dorsalis pedis a., deep peroneal n., greater saphenous v.
4. Lateral plantar digital a. and n.

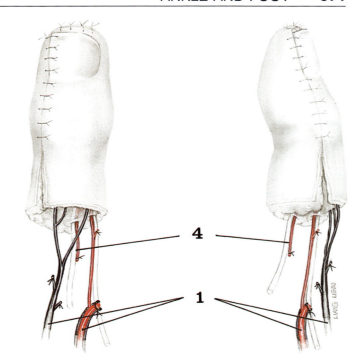

(**Fig. 8-69**) At the donor site, the end of the proximal phalanx and the plantar wound of the big toe are covered by the medial flap, and the dorsal wound is covered with a split-thickness skin graft.

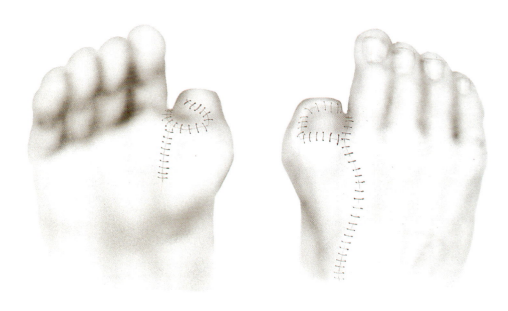

FREE PULP FLAP

(Fig. 8-70) The first choice of donor is the big toe, which provides a larger flap area; the second toe is the next choice. For reconstruction of the thumb pulp, the ipsilateral foot is selected; for the index finger, the contralateral foot is chosen, to afford better sensibility to the ulnar side of the thumb and the radial side of the index. The dimensions and location of the flap vary according to requirements in the recipient finger.

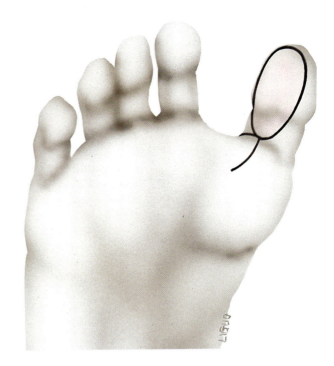

1. Dorsalis pedis a. and v., deep peroneal n., greater saphenous v.
2. Plantar digital a. and n.
3. Extensor hallucis brevis

(Fig. 8-71) The dorsal superficial vein and the dorsalis pedis-first dorsal metatarsal artery [1] are dissected out, for lengths meeting the requirements of the recipient vessels. If there is no adequate dorsal artery, the plantar arterial system [2] can be used. When the flap is elevated, the distal perforating artery and the lateral digital nerve [2] should be included in the flap.

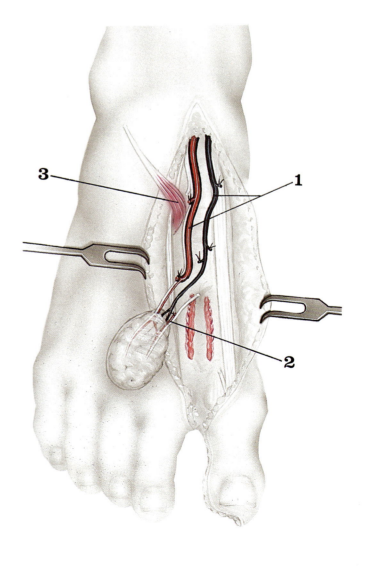

1. Dorsalis pedis a. and v., deep peroneal n., greater saphenous v.
2. Plantar digital a. and n.
3. Extensor hallucis brevis

Note. Based on the same arteriovenous pedicles, the pulp flap can be tailored and developed, by combining the toenail bed, the distal phalanx, the interphalangeal joint, or even the distal segment of the toe, to meet requirements in the recipient hand.

VASCULARIZED JOINT TRANSFER

Arterial Anatomy of the Proximal Interphalangeal and Metatarsophalangeal Joints (Fig. 8-72)

The PIP joint [8] or MTP joint [7] of the second toe are chosen as donors for transfer.

The PIP joint [8] of the second toe is supplied by the transverse branch [4] of the digital artery. It is a hinge joint, and its normal range of motion (ROM) is between 0° in extension and 90° in flexion.

The MTP joint [7] of the second toe is supplied by the articular branch [3] originating from the first dorsal metatarsal artery [1]. It is an ellipsoid joint, and its normal ROM is between 45° in hyperextension and 30° in flexion. Ordinarily, the PIP joint is preferable to the MTP joint.

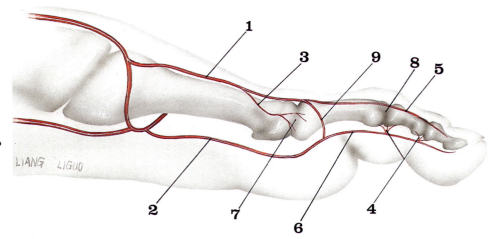

1. First dorsal metatarsal a.
2. First plantar metatarsal a.
3. Articular branch of the MTP
4. Transverse a.
5. Dorsal digital a.
6. Plantar digital a.
7. MTP joint
8. PIP joint
9. Distal perforating a.

Free Proximal Interphalangeal Joint Transfer of the Second Toe

(Fig. 8-73) A skin island is designed over the dorsum of the PIP joint as a monitor of graft circulation or as a graft for repair of the skin defect in the recipient site.

1. First dorsal metatarsal a. and deep peroneal n.
2. Dorsal digital a.
3. Greater saphenous v.
4. Distal perforating a.
5. Plantar digital a. and n.
6. MTP joint
7. PIP joint

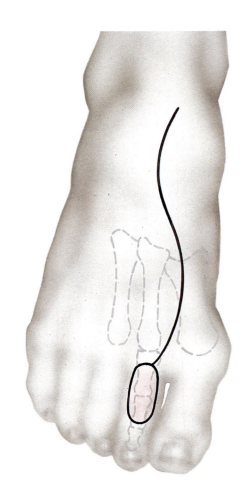

(Fig. 8-74) In a majority of cases, the greater saphenous vein and the dorsalis pedis-first dorsal metatarsal artery [3,1] are dissected through an incision on the dorsum of the foot, as described before.

The medial neurovascular bundle is divided at the DIP joint, taking care to preserve the distal perforating branch [4] and the articular branches to the PIP joint.

1. First dorsal metatarsal a. and deep peroneal n.
2. Dorsal digital a.
3. Greater saphenous v.
4. Distal perforating a.
5. Plantar digital a. and n.

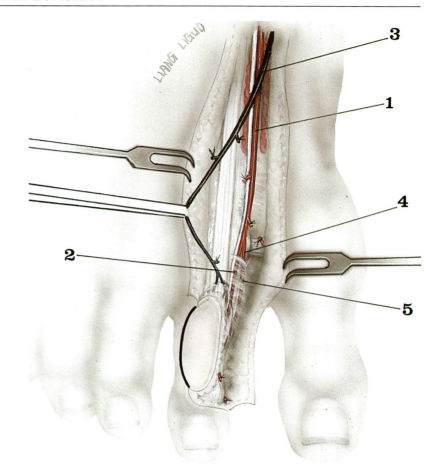

(**Fig. 8-75**) The lateral skin with the lateral neurovascular bundle is separated from the digital bones and joint. Both ends of the extensor tendon are divided. Usually, the extensor and flexor tendons can be included in the graft. The PIP joint [7] with vascular pedicles [1,3] is then isolated by disarticulation through the DIP joint and osteotomy through the proximal phalanx.

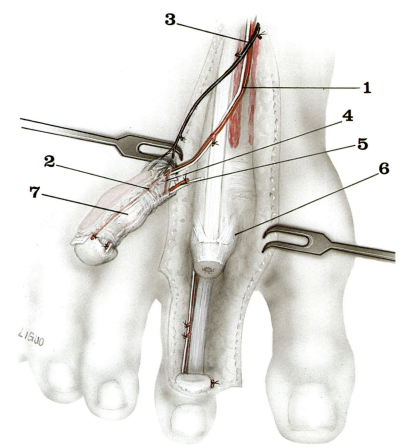

1. First dorsal metatarsal a. and deep peroneal n.
2. Dorsal digital a.
3. Greater saphenous v.
4. Distal perforating a.
5. Plantar digital a. and n.
6. MTP joint
7. PIP joint

Note. The defect resulting from removal of the joint can be treated by either arthroplasty or, preferably, by fusion, using bone removed from the hand. In the event that two PIP joints are needed, the second plantar metatarsal artery is used as an arterial pedicle for the donor second and third toes.

Free Metatarsophalangeal Joint Transfer of the Second Toe

(Fig. 8-76) A skin paddle is designed over the dorsum of the MTP joint.

1. First dorsal metatarsal a. and deep peroneal n.
2. Dorsal digital a.
3. Greater saphenous v.
4. Distal perforating a.
5. Plantar digital a. and n.
6. MTP joint
7. PIP joint

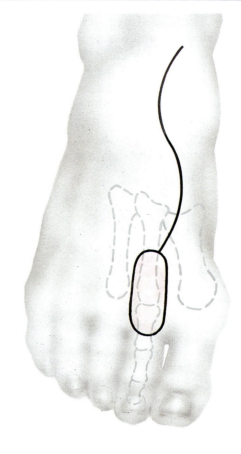

(Fig. 8-77) During the dissection of the first dorsal metatarsal artery [1] in the interosseous muscle, the articular branch to the MTP joint should be carefully protected from damage. While dividing the first deep transverse metatarsal ligament and ligating the digital artery of the big toe, attention should be paid to preserving the distal perforating branch to the joint, to keep it communicating with the dorsal and plantar arterial nets around the medial aspect of the MTP joint.

1. First dorsal metatarsal a. and deep peroneal n.
2. Dorsal digital a.
3. Greater saphenous v.
7. PIP joint

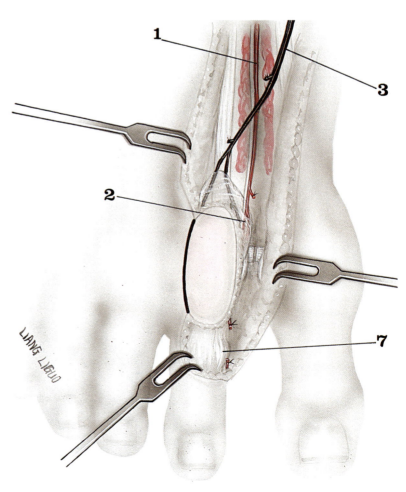

(Fig. 8-78) Both ends of the extensor tendon, the metatarsal and proximal phalanx bones, and the second deep transverse metatarsal ligament are divided. The MTP joint [6], with the overlying skin and extensor tendon, is isolated. If needed, the flexor tendon can be included in the graft.

1. First dorsal metatarsal a. and deep peroneal n.
2. Dorsal digital a.
3. Greater saphenous v.
4. Distal perforating a.
5. Plantar digital a. and n.
6. MTP joint
7. PIP joint

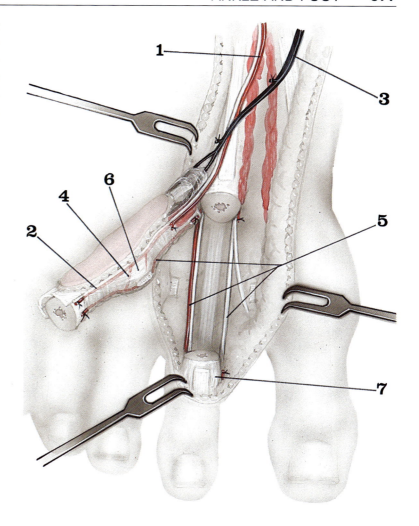

SECOND AND THIRD TOE TRANSFER EN BLOC

(**Fig. 8-79**) In order to obtain a better blood supply to the third toe, the second dorsal metatarsal artery [5] should be included in the arterial pedicle, if one exists. However, if the arcuate artery [4] is absent, the first dorsal metatarsal artery [3] is usually able to supply the third toe, with its lateral circulation through the second toe and web space.

1. Dorsalis pedis a. and v., and deep peroneal n.
2. Greater saphenous v.
3. First dorsal metatarsal a.
4. Arcuate a.
5. Second dorsal metatarsal a.
6. Extensor tendons
7. Flexor tendons
8. Plantar digital n.

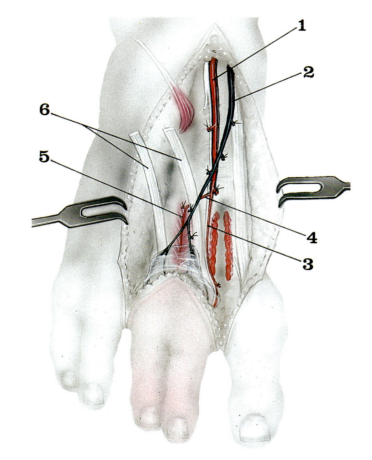

(**Fig. 8-80**) After dividing the first and third deep transverse metatarsal ligaments and disarticulating the second and third MTP joints or osteotomy of their metatarsals, the second and third toes are isolated en bloc with their sensory nerves [8] and extensor [6] and flexor [7] tendons, on the greater saphenous vein and the dorsalis pedis-first and second dorsal metatarsal arterial system [1,2].

1. Dorsalis pedis a. and v. and deep peroneal n.
2. Greater saphenous v.
6. Extensor tendons
7. Flexor tendons
8. Plantar digital n.

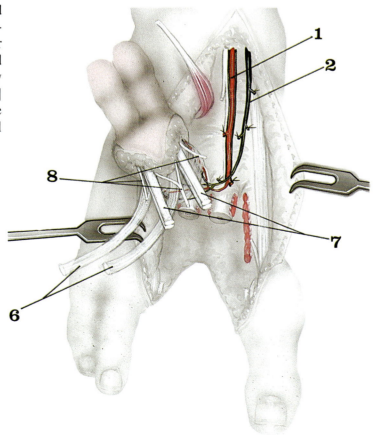

Closure of the Donor Defect

The distal halves of the second and third metatarsal bones are removed. Then, the heads of the first and fourth metatarsals are approximated as closely as possible. The ends of the metatarsal bones are covered with local interosseous muscles, and the whole site is covered with a split-thickness skin graft.

RECIPIENT SITE EXPOSURES

Exposure of the Dorsalis Pedis Artery

(Fig. 8-81) An incision is made from the midpoint between the medial and lateral malleoli, to the proximal end of the first metatarsal interspace.

1. Extensor hallucis brevis m.
2. Extensor hallucis longus tendon
3. Inferior extensor retinaculum
4. Extensor digitorum longus tendon
5. Dorsalis pedis a. and v. and deep peroneal n.
6. Lateral tarsal a. and v.
7. Tarsal branch of deep peroneal n.

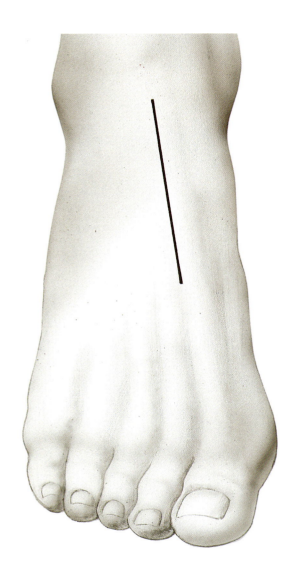

(Fig. 8-82) The deep fascia and inferior extensor retinaculum [3] are divided, and the extensor hallucis brevis muscle [1] and extensor hallucis longus tendon [4] are then exposed.

1. Extensor hallucis brevis m.
2. Extensor hallucis longus tendon
3. Inferior extensor retinaculum
4. Extensor digitorum longus tendon

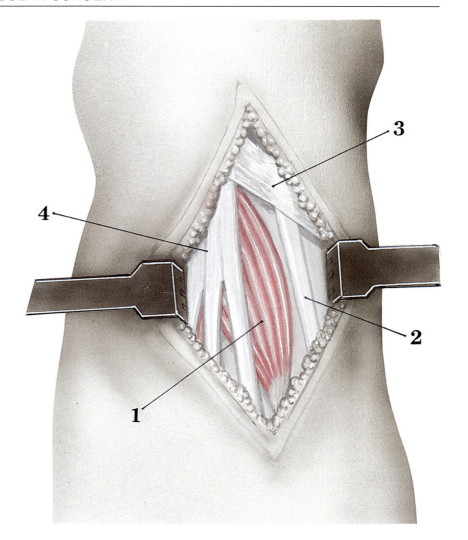

(**Fig. 8-83**) The extensor hallucis brevis muscle [1] is mobilized and retracted laterally. The dorsalis pedis artery [5], accompanied by two veins, can subsequently be identified lying on the tarsal bones, and isolated. The deep peroneal nerve [5] lies lateral to the artery.

1. Extensor hallucis brevis m.
2. Extensor hallucis longus tendon
3. Inferior extensor retinaculum
5. Dorsalis pedis a., v., and deep peroneal n.
6. Lateral tarsal a. and v.
7. Tarsal branch of deep peroneal n.

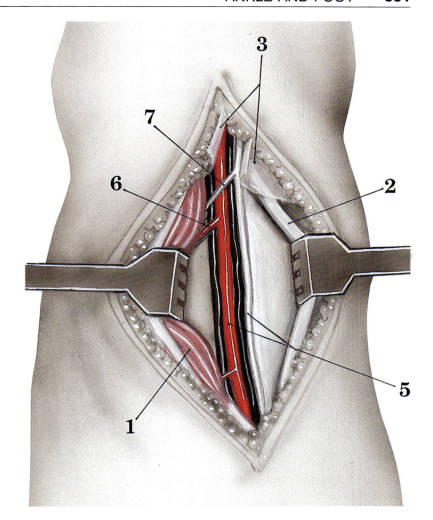

Exposure of the Posterior Tibial Artery Behind the Medial Malleolus

(Fig. 8-84) A curved incision begins midway between the medial malleolus and Achilles tendon, keeping 1 cm posterior to the medial malleolus and running distally and anteriorly toward the tuberosity of the navicular bone.

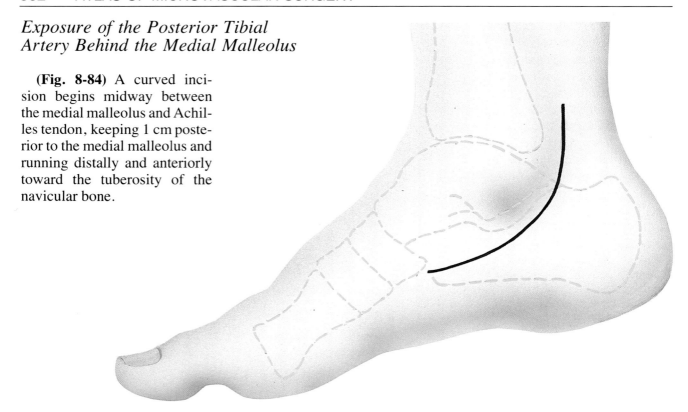

1. Posterior tibial a. and v.
2. Tibial n.
3. Achilles tendon
4. Laciniate ligament
5. Tibialis posterior tendon
6. Flexor digitorum longus tendon
7. Flexor hallucis longus tendon
8. Medial malleolus
9. Tuberosity of navicular bone
10. Abductor hallucis m.

(Fig. 8-85) Dividing the deep fascia and laciniate ligament [4], which forms a bridge between the medial malleolus [8] and calcaneus, the posterior tibial artery [1], accompanied by two veins, is identified between the flexor digitorum longus [6] and flexor hallucis longus [7] tendons. The tibial nerve [2] lies posterior to the vessels. Under the origin of the abductor hallucis [10], the posterior tibial artery divides into medial and lateral plantar arteries.

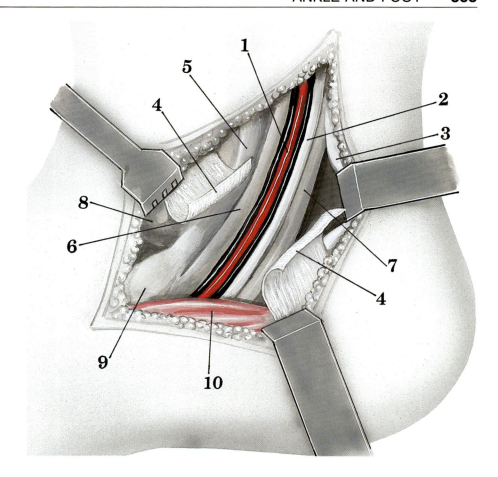

1. Posterior tibial a. and v.
2. Tibial n.
3. Achilles tendon
4. Laciniate ligament
5. Tibialis posterior tendon
6. Flexor digitorum longus tendon
7. Flexor hallucis longus tendon
8. Medial malleolus
9. Tuberosity of navicular bone
10. Abductor hallucis longus

384 ATLAS OF MICROVASCULAR SURGERY

Exposure of the Medial Plantar Artery and its Bifurcation with the Lateral Plantar Artery

(Fig. 8-86) A curvilinear incision is made from the medial aspect of the head of the first metatarsal via the tuberosity of the navicular bone to the medial prominence of the calcaneus.

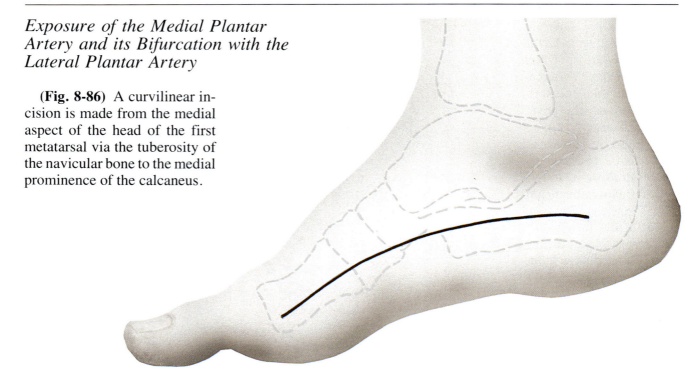

1. Medial plantar a., v., and n.
2. Lateral plantar a., v., and n.
3. Posterior tibial a. and v. and tibial n.
4. Abductor hallucis m.
5. Flexor hallucis longus tendon
6. Flexor digitorum longus tendon
7. Tibialis posterior tendon
8. Calcaneus
9. Tuberosity of navicular bone

(**Fig. 8-87**) Dividing the deep fascia and laciniate ligament, the abductor hallucis muscle and tendon [4] are exposed. Using the tendon as a guide, the less distinctive margin of the belly is separated from the tuberosity of the navicular bone [9] and laciniate ligament.

Detaching the abductor hallucis from the medial side of the calcaneus [8], it is retracted plantarly, taking care to save a pair of branches from the medial plantar nerve to the abductor hallucis. Now, the medial plantar artery [1] and its bifurcation with the lateral plantar artery [2] are identified distal to the medial malleolus, and 5 cm behind the tuberosity of the navicular bone [9], under the abductor hallucis [4].

Then, the medial plantar artery [1] runs distally between the abductor hallucis and flexor digitorum brevis, while the lateral plantar artery [2] goes under the flexor digitorum brevis, obliquely toward the base of the fifth metatarsal. The medial plantar nerve [1] is lateral to the artery.

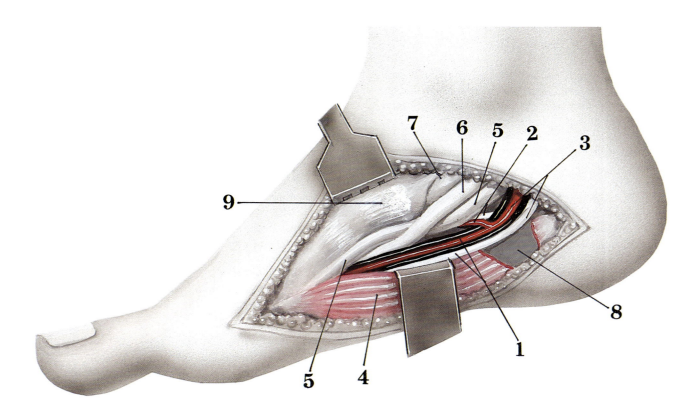

1. Medial plantar a., v., and n.
2. Lateral plantar a., v., and n.
3. Posterior tibial a., v., and tibial n.
4. Abductor hallucis m.
5. Flexor hallucis longus tendon
6. Flexor digitorum longus tendon
7. Tibialis posterior tendon
8. Calcaneus
9. Tuberosity of navicular bone

BIBLIOGRAPHY

Dorsalis Pedis Flap

Caffee HH, Hoefflin SM: The extended dorsalis pedis flap. Plast Reconstr Surg 64:807, 1979.

Cheng XX, Lu JZ, Ying DQ, et al: Reconstruction of deep-degree electric burns using the dorsalis pedis skin flap transfer. Chin J Surg 18:136, 1980.

Daniel RK, Terzis J, Midgley RD: Restoration of sensation to an anesthetic hand by a free neurovascular flap from the foot. Plast Reconstr Surg 57:275, 1976.

Daniel RK, Terzis JK, May JW Jr: Neurovascular free flaps. In: Serafin D, Buncke HJ (eds): *Microsurgical Composite Tissue Transplantation*. St. Louis:

CV Mosby, 1979, pp 285–316.
Duncan MJ, Manktelow RT, Zuker RM, Rosen IB: Mandibular reconstruction in the irradiated patient: The role of osteocutaneous free tissue transfers. Plast Reconstr Surg 76:820, 1985.
Franklin JD, Withers EH, Madden JJ Jr, Lynch JB: Use of the free dorsalis pedis flap in head and neck repairs. Plast Reconstr Surg 63:195, 1979.
Gilbert A: Composite tissue transfers from the foot: Anatomic basis and surgical technique. In: Daniller AI, Strauch B (eds): *Symposium on Microsurgery*. St. Louis: CV Mosby, 1976, pp 230–242.
Guyuron B, Labandter HP: Dorsalis pedis free flap for eye socket reconstruction. In: Strauch B, Vasconez LO, Hall-Findlay E (eds): *Grabb's Encyclopedia of Flaps*, vol. I. Boston: Little, Brown, 1990, pp 130–134.
Huber JF: The arterial network supplying the dorsum of the foot. Presented at the Fifty-fourth Annual Session, American Association of Anatomists, Pittsburgh, April 14, 1938.
Ling T, Wang XL, Tong JQ, et al: Clinical significance of dorsalis pedis vessels for transfers of toes and skin flaps. Chin J Surg 19:297, 1981.
MacLeod AM, Robinson DW: Reconstruction of defects involving the mandible and floor of mouth by free osteocutaneous flaps derived from the foot. Br J Plast Surg 35:239, 1982.
Man D, Acland RD: The microarterial anatomy of the dorsalis pedis flap and its clinical applications. Plast Reconstr Surg 65:419, 1980.
May JW Jr, Chait LA, Cohen BE, O'Brien BMcC: Free neurovascular flap from the first web of the foot in hand reconstruction. J Hand Surg 2B:387, 1977.
McCraw JB, Furlow JT Jr: The dorsalis pedis arterialized flap. Plast Reconstr Surg 55:177, 1975.
O'Brien BMcC, Morrison WA, MacLeod AM, Dooley BJ: Microvascular osteocutaneous transfer using the groin flap and iliac crest and the dorsalis pedis flap and second metatarsal. Br J Plast Surg 32:188, 1979.
Ohmori K: Microvascular free transfer of a compound dorsalis pedis skin flap with second metatarsal bone. In: Strauch B, Vasconez LO, Hall-Findlay E (eds): *Grabb's Encyclopedia of Flaps*, vol I. Boston: Little, Brown, 1990, pp 254–257.
Ohmori K, Harii K: Free dorsalis pedis sensory flap to the hand, with microneurovascular anastomoses. Plast Reconstr Surg 58:546, 1976.
Robinson DW: Microsurgical transfer of the dorsalis pedis neurovascular island flap. Br J Plast Surg 29:209, 1976.
Robinson DW: Dorsalis pedis flap. In: Serafin D, Buncke HJ (eds): *Microsurgical Composite Tissue Transplantation*. St. Louis: CV Mosby, 1979, pp 257–284.
Sharzer LA: Microvascular free transfer of a dorsalis pedis flap for intraoral lining. In: Strauch B, Vasconez LO, Hall-Findlay E (eds): *Grabb's Encyclopedia of Flaps*, vol I. Boston: Little, Brown, 1990, pp 546–548.
Sharzer LA: Microneurovascular transfer of a dorsalis pedis flap to the heel. In: Strauch B, Vasconez LO, Hall-Findlay E (eds): *Grabb's Encyclopedia of Flaps*, vol III. Boston: Little, Brown, 1990, pp 1797–1800.
Strauch B, Shafiroff BB: The foot: A versatile source of donor tissue. In: Serafin D, Buncke HJ (eds): *Microsurgical Composite Tissue Transplantation*. St. Louis: CV Mosby, 1979, pp. 345–356.
Taylor GI, Corlett RJ: Microvascular free transfer of a dorsalis pedis skin flap with extensor tendons. In: Strauch B, Vasconez LO, Hall-Findlay E (eds): *Grabb's Encyclopedia of Flaps*, vol II. Boston: Little, Brown, 1990, pp 1109–1111.
Taylor GI, Townsend: Composite free flap and tendon transfer: An anatomical study and a clinical technique. Br J Plast Surg 32:170, 1979.
Vila-Rovira R, Ferreira BJ, Guinot A: Transfer of vascularized extensor tendons from the foot to the hand with a dorsalis pedis flap. Plast Reconstr Surg 76:421, 1985.
Zuker RM, Manktelow RT: Microvascular transfer of the compound dorsalis pedis skin flap with second metatarsal for mandible and floor of mouth reconstruction. In: Strauch B, Vasconez LO, Hall-Findlay E (eds): *Grabb's Encyclopedia of Flaps*, vol I. Boston: Little, Brown, 1990, pp 583–588.
Zuker RM, Manktelow RT: The dorsalis pedis free flap: Technique of elevation, foot closure, and flap application. Plast Reconstr Surg 77:93, 1986.

Extensor Digitorum Brevis Flap

Landi A, Soragni O, Monteleone M: The extensor digitorum brevis muscle island flap for soft-tissue loss around the ankle. Plast Reconstr Surg 75:892, 1985.
Leitner DW, Gordon L, Buncke HJ: The extensor digitorum brevis as a muscle island flap. Plast Reconstr Surg 76:777, 1985.
Tolhurst DE, Bos KE: Free revascularized muscle grafts in facial palsy. Plast Reconstr Surg 69:760, 1982.

Medial Plantar Flap

Amarante J, Martins A, Reis J: A distally based median plantar flap. Ann Plast Surg 20:468, 1988.
Baker GL, Newton ED, Franklin JD: Fasciocutaneous island flap based on the medial plantar artery: Clinical applications for leg, ankle, and forefoot. Plast Reconstr Surg 85:47, 1990.
Gao XS, Yuan XB, He QL, et al: Reconstruction of soft-tissue defects on the heel using the medial plantar island flap. Chin J Surg 23:104, 1985.

Hartrampf CR, Scheflan M, Bostwick J III: The flexor digitorum brevis muscle island pedicle flap: A new dimension in heel reconstruction. Plast Reconstr Surg 66:264, 1980.

Hidalgo DA, Shaw WW: Anatomic basis of plantar flap design. Plast Reconstr Surg 78:627, 1986.

Hwang W-Y, Chang T-S, Cheng K-X, Gao T-M: The application of free twin flaps in one-stage treatment of severe hand deformity. Ann Plast Surg 21:430, 1988.

Ikuta Y, Murakami T, Yoshioka K, Tsuge K: Reconstruction of the heel pad by flexor digitorum brevis musculocutaneous flap transfer. Plast Reconstr Surg 74:86, 1984.

Masquelet AC, Romana MC: The medialis pedis flap: A new fasciocutaneous flap. Plast Reconstr Surg 85:765, 1990.

Morrison WA, Crabb DMcK, O'Brien BMcC, Jenkins A: The instep of the foot as a fasciocutaneous island and as a free flap for heel defects. Plast Reconstr Surg 72:56, 1983.

Reiffel RS, McCarthy JG: Coverage of heel and sole defects: A new subfascial arterialized flap. Plast Reconstr Surg 66:250, 1980.

Shanahan RE, Gingrass RP: Medial plantar sensory flap for coverage of heel defects. Plast Reconstr Surg 64:295, 1979.

Shaw WW, Hidalgo DA: Anatomic basis of plantar flap design: Clinical applications. Plast Reconstr Surg 78:637, 1986.

Free Toe and Toe Tissue Transfers

Biemer E: Microvascular transplantation en bloc of the second and third toes. In: Strauch B, Vasconez LO, Hall-Findlay (eds): *Grabb's Encyclopedia of Flaps*, vol II. Boston: Little, Brown, 1990, pp 1001–1005.

Buncke HJ: Free toe-to-hand transfers. In: Daniller AI, Strauch B (eds.): *Symposium on Microsurgery*, vol 14. St. Louis: CV Mosby, 1976, pp 216–229.

Buncke HJ Jr, McLean DH, George PT, Creech BJ, Chater NL, Commons GW: Thumb replacement: Great toe transplantation by microvascular anastomosis. Br J Plast Surg 26:194, 1973.

Buncke HJ, Rose EH: Free toe-to-fingertip neurovascular flaps. Plast Reconstr Surg 63:607, 1979.

Chait LA: Microvascular free transfer of a first web space skin flap of the foot to reconstruct the upper and lower eyelids. In: Strauch B, Vasconez LO, Hall-Findlay E (eds): *Grabb's Encyclopedia of Flaps*, vol I. Boston: Little, Brown, 1990, pp 126–129.

Chen ZW, Wang Y: Reconstruction of total hand loss using free toe transfer. Chin J Surg 19:7, 1981.

Cobbett JR: Free digital transfer: Report of a case of transfer of a great toe to replace an amputated thumb. J Bone Joint Surg 51B:677, 1969.

Foucher G, Braun FM, Smith DJ Jr: Custom-made free vascularized compound toe transfer for traumatic dorsal loss of the thumb. Plast Reconstr Surg 87:310, 1991.

Foucher G, Hoang P, Citron N, Merle M, Dury M: Joint reconstruction following trauma: Comparison of microsurgical transfer and conventional methods: A report of 61 cases. J Hand Surg 11B:388, 1986.

Foucher G, Merle M, Maneaud M, Michon J: Microsurgical free partial toe transfer in hand reconstruction: A report of 12 cases. Plast Reconstr Surg 65:616, 1980.

Foucher G, Van Genechten F: Microneurovascular partial toe transfer. In: Strauch B, Vasconez LO, Hall-Findlay E (eds): *Grabb's Encyclopedia of Flaps*, vol II. Boston: Little, Brown, 1990, pp 1010–1017.

Gu Y-D, Wu M-M, Zheng Y-L, Yang D-Y, Li H-R: Vascular variations and their treatment in toe transplantation. J Reconstr Microsurg 1:227, 1985.

Kuo E-T, Ji Z-L, Zhao Y-C, Zhang M-L: Reconstruction of metacarpophalangeal joint by free vascularized autogenous metatarsophalangeal joint transplant. J Reconstr Microsurg 1:65, 1984.

Kutz JE, Klein HW: Microvascular free transfer of a toe phalangeal joint. In: Strauch B, Vasconez LO, Hall-Findlay E (eds): *Grabb's Encyclopedia of Flaps*, vol II. Boston: Little, Brown, 1990, pp 1018–1022.

Lister GD: Microvascular free transfer of the nail. In: Strauch B, Vasconez LO, Hall-Findlay E (eds): *Grabb's Encyclopedia of Flaps*, vol II. Boston: Little, Brown, 1990, pp 898–901.

Lister GD, Kalisman M, Tsai T-M: Reconstruction of the hand with free microneurovascular toe-to-hand transfer: Experience with 54 toe transfers. Plast Reconstr Surg 71:372, 1983.

Logan A, Elliot D, Foucher G: Free toe pulp transfer to restore traumatic digital pulp loss. Br J Plast Surg 38:497, 1985.

May JW Jr, Savage RC: Microneurovascular free transfer of the great toe. In: Strauch B, Vasconez LO, Hall-Findlay E (eds): *Grabb's Encyclopedia of Flaps*, vol. II. Boston: Little, Brown, 1990, pp 988–997.

May JW Jr, Smith RJ, Peimer CA: Toe-to-hand free tissue transfer for thumb construction with multiple digit aplasia. Plast Reconstr Surg 67:205, 1981.

Morrison WA: Wrap-around toe flap. In: Strauch B, Vasconez LO, Hall-Findlay E (eds): *Grabb's Encyclopedia of Flaps*, vol II. Boston: Little, Brown, 1990, pp 1006–1009.

Morrison WA, O'Brien BMcC, MacLeod AM: Thumb reconstruction with a free neurovascular wrap-around flap from the big toe. J Hand Surg 5B:575, 1980.

Nakayama Y, Iino T, Uchida A, Kiyosawa T, Soeda S: Vascularized free nail grafts nourished by arterial inflow from the venous system. Plast Reconstr Surg 85:239, 1990.

O'Brien BMcC, Gould JS, Morrison WA, Russell RC, MacLeod AM, Pribaz JJ: Free vascularized small joint transfer to the hand. J Hand Surg 9B:634, 1984.

Steichen JB: Thumb reconstruction by great toe microvascular wraparound flap. In: Urbaniak JR (ed): *Microsurgery for Major Limb Reconstruction.* St. Louis: CV Mosby, 1987, pp 86–111.

Strauch B, Hall-Findlay EJ: Microneurovascular transfer on a first web space skin flap. In: Strauch B, Vasconez LO, Hall-Findlay E: *Grabb's Encyclopedia of Flaps,* vol II. Boston: Little, Brown, 1990, pp 1053–1058.

Strauch B, Hall-Findlay EJ: Microneurovascular free transfer of the second toe. In: Strauch B, Vasconez LO, Hall-Findlay E (eds): *Grabb's Encyclopedia of Flaps,* vol II. Boston: Little, Brown, 1990, pp 996–1000.

Strauch B, Tsur H: Restoration of sensation to the hand by a free neurovascular flap from the first web space of the foot. Plast Reconstr Surg 62:361, 1978.

Tamai S, Hori Y, Tatsumi Y, Okuda H: Hallux-to-thumb transfer with microsurgical technique: A case report in a 45-year-old woman. J Hand Surg 2B:152, 1977.

Tsai T-M, Jupiter JB, Kutz JE, Kleinert HE: Vascularized autogenous whole joint transfer in the hand—a clinical study. J Hand Surg 7B:335, 1982.

Tsai T-M, Singer R, Elliott E, Klein H: Immediate free vascularized joint transfer from second toe to index finger proximal interphalangeal joint: A case report. J Hand Surg 10B:85, 1985.

Yoshimura M: Toe-to-hand transfer. Plast Reconstr Surg 66:74, 1980.

Part Three
TRUNK

9 THORAX

Pectoralis Major Flap

Anatomy (Fig. 9-1)

The muscle origin consists of three subunits: a clavicular segment [1] from the medial half of the clavicle, a sternocostal segment [2] from the sternum and anterior surface of the upper six costal cartilages, and an abdominal segment [3] from the anterior rectus sheath. There is usually a distinct intermuscular septum with loose connective tissue between the clavicular and sternocostal segments. The abdominal segment, which has a width of about 2 to 4 cm, is commonly fused morphologically to the sternocostal segment. It often has an independent neurovascular supply, but its vascular supply is somewhat variable.

Muscle insertion is on the lateral lip of the intertubercular sulcus of the humerus, with a flat tendon of 5 cm in width. The anterior layer of insertion is from the fibers of the clavicular segment and the middle portion of the sternocostal segment. The posterior layer of insertion is from the lower portion of the pectoralis major.

The muscle is broad, flat, and fan-shaped. Its function is adduction and medial rotation of the arm. On average, the total width is 27.5 cm (the muscle belly, 22.7 cm; the tendon, 4.9 cm); its total length is 16 cm, and its approximate thickness is 1.5 cm.

Blood Supply

The source of blood supply to the muscle includes: the thoracoacromial artery [5], the lateral thoracic artery [10], the internal mammary artery, and the intercostal artery. Among these vessels, the dominant blood supply is from the *thoracoacromial artery* [5], which arises from the second part of the axillary artery. It courses along the medial edge of the pectoralis minor for 1.5 to 3 cm before piercing the clavipectoral fascia and dividing into four branches: pectoral [6], acromial [8], clavicular [9], and deltoid [7].

The *pectoral branch* [6] descends between the pectoralis major and minor muscles. It enters the sternocostal portion of the pectoralis major 5 to 6 cm below the midpoint of the clavicle, or 3 to 5 cm after its takeoff from the thoracoacromial trunk [5], and about 5.5 cm lateral to the edge of the sternum. The sternocostal and abdominal portions of the muscle [2,3] (the lower four fifths) can be nourished by this branch.

The *deltoid branch* [7] usually arises with the acromial branch [8] and runs laterally with the cephalic vein, crossing over the pectoralis minor to supply the deltoid muscle. In its course, it gives off one or two major branches to supply the clavicular portion of the pectoralis major [1], and a fasciocutaneous perforator running through the deltopectoral groove to supply the overlying skin of the clavicular portion of the pectoralis major and of the deltoid muscle.

The *acromial branch* [8] and *clavicular branch* [9] are much smaller and less important. The former runs laterally over the coracoid process and under the deltoid, while the latter goes medially to the sternoclavicular joint and the subclavius.

The *lateral thoracic artery* [10] descends along the lateral border of the pectoralis minor to the side of the chest and runs to the serratus anterior, subscapularis, and breast. In over 70% of cases, it gives off a branch with a diameter of about 1 mm, entering the abdominal portion of the pectoralis major [3] about 5 cm inferior to its origin from the axillary artery and about 1.5 cm medial to the lateral edge of the muscle.

Innervation

The *lateral pectoral nerve* arises from the lateral cord of the brachial plexus and then crosses the axillary artery and vein anteriorly. After piercing the clavipectoral fascia, it divides into several branches to supply the clavicular portion and the upper part of the sternocostal portion of the pectoralis major. It also forms a loop with the medial pectoral nerve to supply the pectoralis minor.

The *medial pectoral nerve* arises from the medial cord of the brachial plexus and runs forward between the axillary artery and vein under the deep surface of the pectoralis minor. It then divides into several branches. One or two supply the pectoralis minor; two or three pierce the pectoralis minor to supply the lower part of the sternocostal portion of the pectoralis major; another passes around the lateral border of the pectoralis minor to supply the abdominal portion of the pectoralis major.

Measurements

		Diameter (mm)
Thoracoacromial (trunk)	Artery	3.2
	Vein	3.5
Pectoral branch	Artery	2.0
	Vein	3.0
Deltoid branch	Artery	2.0
	Vein	3.0
Acromial branch	Artery	1.4
	Vein	2.0
Clavicular branch	Artery	1.2
	Vein	1.6
Lateral thoracic	Artery	1.6
	Vein	2.0

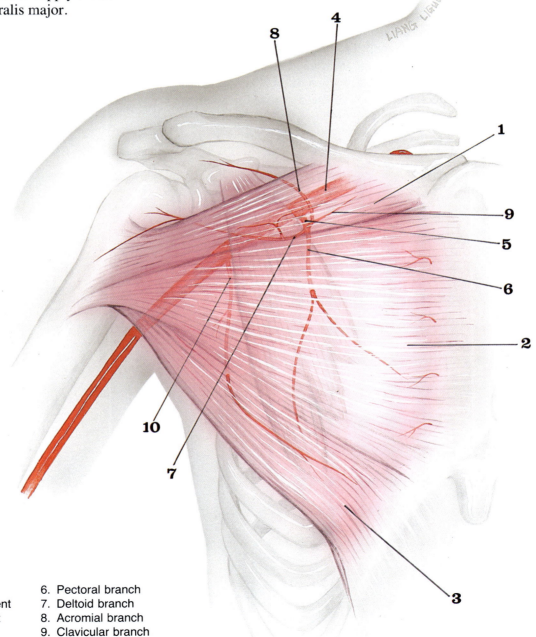

1. Clavicular segment
2. Sternocostal segment
3. Abdominal segment
4. Axillary a.
5. Thoracoacromial a.
6. Pectoral branch
7. Deltoid branch
8. Acromial branch
9. Clavicular branch
10. Lateral thoracic a.

COMMENT AND INSIGHTS

Based on experience with local transfer for restoration of elbow flexion, the pectoralis major muscle flap was one of the revascularized muscle transfers developed comparatively early. Because of cosmetic disadvantages (such as its proximity to the breast) and its short neurovascular pedicle, the pectoralis major flap has not ordinarily been selected for free transfer. However, it is frequently used for reconstruction of the neck, face, oral cavity, or mandible, using local transfer, as a myocutaneous flap or as an osteomyocutaneous flap, because of its particular anatomic location.

The abdominal segment of the muscle is not always reliable for free transfer, since the vascular pedicle from the lateral thoracic artery is somewhat variable. Generally, the sternocostal and abdominal segments are combined to provide a muscle flap of large or medium size based on the pectoral branch of the thoracoacromial artery. This type of muscle or myocutaneous flap was first reported in application for functional reconstruction of the flexor musculature in Volkmann's ischemic contracture.

The clavicular segment can be independently isolated based on the deltoid branch of the thoracoacromial artery to provide a muscle flap of small size for free transfer. The medial anterior half of the clavicle is available for inclusion in the muscle flap. This procedure was first reported in application for intraoral reconstruction and extremity reconstruction.

Clinical experience has indicated that the loss of the pectoralis major muscle has minimal functional consequences, particularly if one segment is preserved, either the clavicular segment or another. The donor scar is somewhat conspicuous and all the described procedures should be used prudently, especially for young women.

PECTORALIS MAJOR MUSCLE FLAP

Sternocostal and Abdominal Segments Combined

This procedure may provide at maximum a muscle flap 20 cm wide, 15 cm long, and 1.5 cm thick when it includes both segments. If the vascular anatomy of the lateral thoracic artery is adequate (in about 70% of cases), the abdominal segment with a width of 4 cm at minimum can be independently isolated for vascularized transfer.

(**Fig. 9-2**) An incision is made from the coracoid process, running along the deltopectoral groove and the lateral border of the pectoralis major toward the xiphoid.

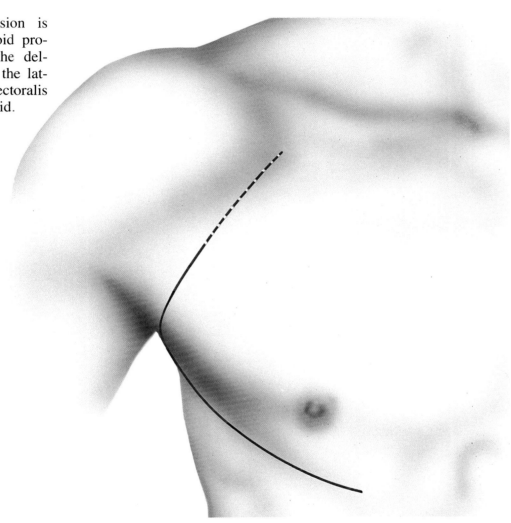

1. Pectoralis major m.
2. Serratus anterior m.
3. External oblique m.
4. Clavicular head
5. Pectoralis minor m.
6. Deltoid m.
7. Lateral thoracic a. and v. and medial pectoral n.
8. Thoracoacromial a. and v. and lateral pectoral n.

(**Fig. 9-3**) The lateral border of the muscle [1] is identified and the skin flap over the muscle is raised with undermining and turned medially to expose the anterior surface of the muscle [1].

1. Pectoralis major m.
2. Serratus anterior m.
3. External oblique m.
4. Clavicular head

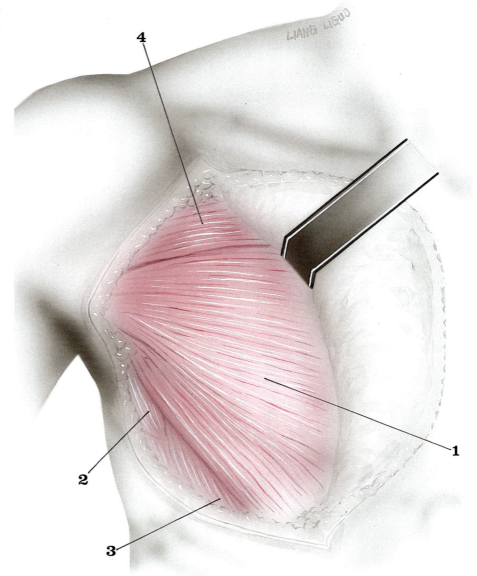

(**Fig. 9-4**) The origins of the muscle are detached from the anterior rectus sheath, the sternum, and the ribs, according to the width requirements of the muscle flap. However, detachment is usually limited below the level of the sternal angle, since the muscle fibers over this level are dominantly supplied by the clavicular branch on occasion.

The upper part of the anterior rectus abdominis sheath can be included in the muscle flap, since it serves to secure the flap to the tendons at the recipient site. As the flap is raised from the chest wall proximally, the neurovascular bundles of the pectoral vessels [8] and the lateral thoracic vessels [7] are gradually displayed in the undersurface of the muscle.

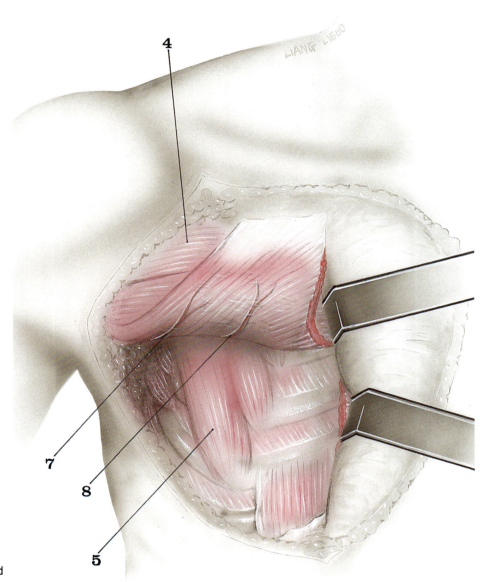

4. Clavicular head
5. Pectoralis minor m.
7. Lateral thoracic a. and v. and medial pectoral n.
8. Thoracoacromial a. and v. and lateral pectoral n.

(Fig. 9-5) The posterior layer and a part of the anterior layer of the muscle insertion are detached. Dissection and evaluation of the neurovascular pedicles [7,8], the lateral thoracic vessels [7], the medial pectoral nerve [7], the pectoral vessels [8], and the lateral pectoral nerve [8] follow at the lateral and medial borders of the pectoralis minor [5] and in front of it. Subsequently, the entrances of these neurovascular pedicles are defined.

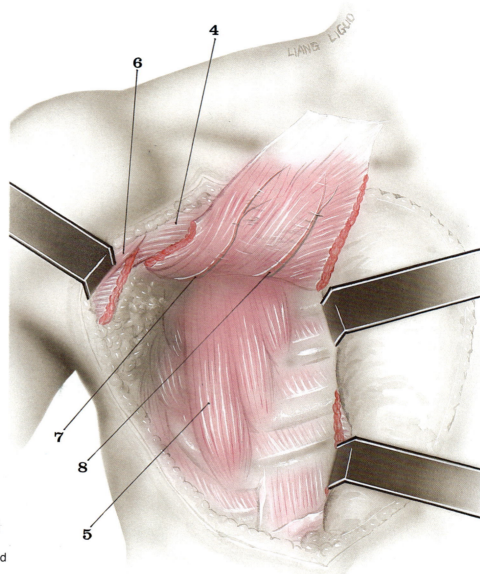

4. Clavicular head
5. Pectoralis minor m.
6. Deltoid m.
7. Lateral thoracic a. and v. and medial pectoral n.
8. Thoracoacromial a. and v. and lateral pectoral n.

(Fig. 9-6) With care taken to protect these neurovascular bundles, the muscle fibers are split at the proposed level of the pectoralis major muscle and the flap (with sternocostal and abdominal segments combined) is raised from the chest wall. The vascular pedicles can be dissected to their parent trunks—the lateral thoracic vessels and thoracoacromial vessels—obtaining pedicle lengths of 3 to 4 cm.

As mentioned previously, it is usual for the pectoral artery to nourish both sternocostal and abdominal segments dominantly. Although an abdominal segment only about 4 cm wide is needed, the lateral thoracic artery [7] should also be carefully evaluated. Flap innervation may be determined by electrically stimulating each of the branches.

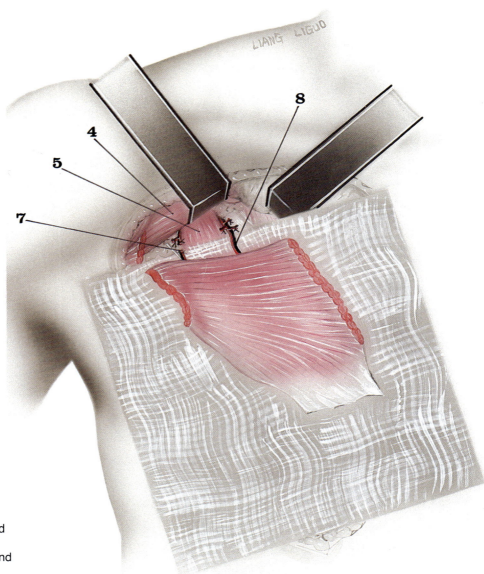

4. Clavicular head
5. Pectoralis minor m.
7. Lateral thoracic a. and v. and medial pectoral n.
8. Thoracoacromial a. and v. and lateral pectoral n.

PECTORALIS MAJOR MYOCUTANEOUS FLAP

(Fig. 9-7) The location, size, and shape of the skin paddle can be variably designed. To avoid the breast, the territory of the skin paddle is usually defined below the nipple-areola in men or the inframammary fold in women, above the costal margin, lateral to the costochondral line, and medial to the anterior axillary line.

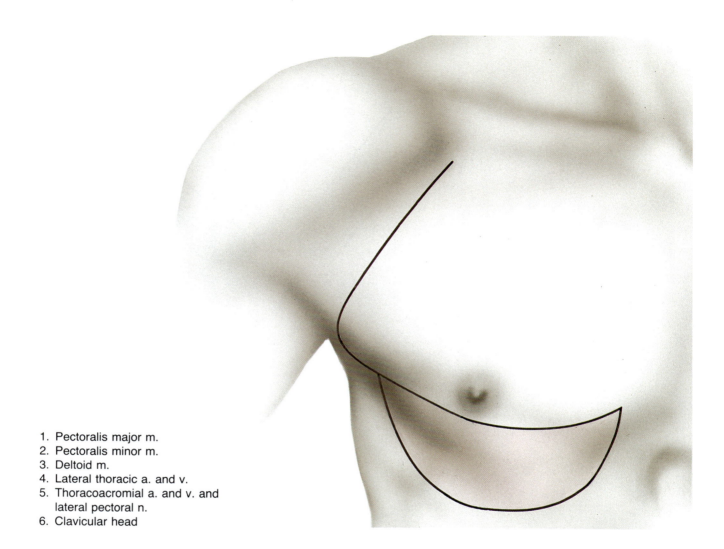

1. Pectoralis major m.
2. Pectoralis minor m.
3. Deltoid m.
4. Lateral thoracic a. and v.
5. Thoracoacromial a. and v. and lateral pectoral n.
6. Clavicular head

(Fig. 9-8) The pectoralis major myocutaneous flap can be harvested following the principles of the muscle flap procedure.

1. Pectoralis major m.
2. Pectoralis minor m.
3. Deltoid m.
4. Lateral thoracic a. and v.
5. Thoracoacromial a. and v. and lateral pectoral n.
6. Clavicular head

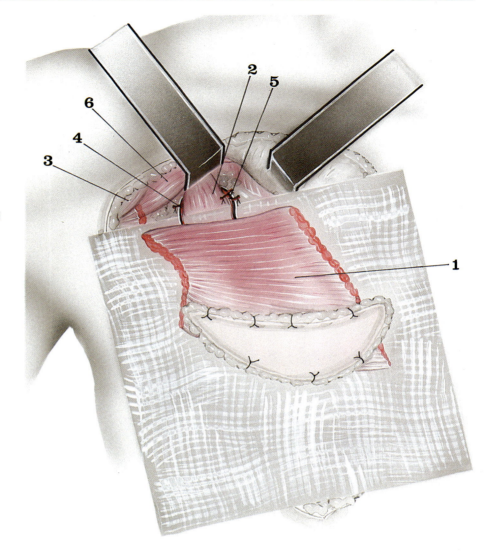

PECTORALIS MAJOR OSTEOMYOCUTANEOUS FLAP

(Fig. 9-9) Commonly, the fifth rib is selected for inclusion in the flap. The proposed skin paddle and fifth rib are marked.

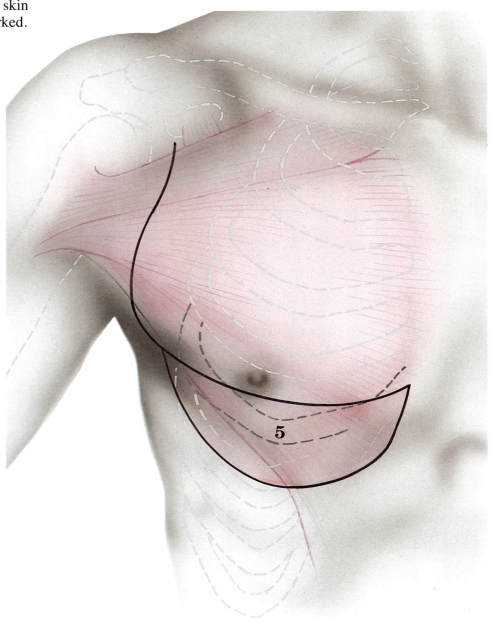

1. Pectoralis major m.
2. Pectoralis minor m.
3. Fifth rib
4. Lateral thoracic a. and v. and medial pectoral n.
5. Thoracoacromial a. and v. and lateral pectoral n.
6. Clavicular head
7. Deltoid m.
8. Pleura
9. Intercostal muscles

(**Fig. 9-10**) The intercostal muscles [9] of the fifth rib space are divided down to the pleura [8] along the upper border of the sixth rib. The pleura is then carefully separated from the fifth costal segment and both ends of the rib are cut to the designed length. The intercostal muscles of the fourth rib space are divided from their deep surface and the pectoralis major [1] with the skin paddle and fifth rib [3] are lifted off the chest wall according to the principles of the muscle flap procedure.

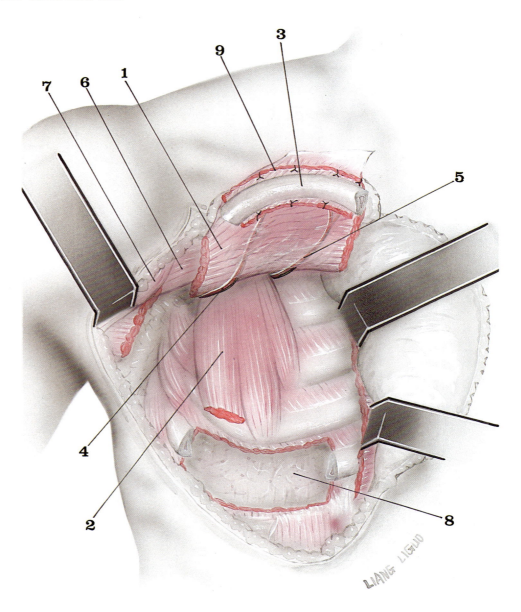

1. Pectoralis major m.
2. Pectoralis minor m.
3. Fifth rib
4. Lateral thoracic a. and v. and medial pectoral n.
5. Thoracoacromial a. and v. and lateral pectoral n.
6. Clavicular head
7. Deltoid m.
8. Pleura
9. Intercostal m.

CLAVICULAR SEGMENT OF THE PECTORALIS MAJOR MUSCLE FLAP

The clavicular segment provides a flap with a length of 12 cm, a width of 5 to 6 cm, and a thickness of 0.8 cm.

(Fig. 9-11) An incision is made from the sternoclavicular joint via the midpoint of the clavicle and then running along the deltopectoral groove.

1. Deltoid m.
2. Sternocostal head
3. Clavicular head
4. Cephalic v.
5. Clavicle
6. Thoracoacromial a. and v. and lateral pectoral n.
7. Pectoralis minor m.
8. Deltoid a. and v.

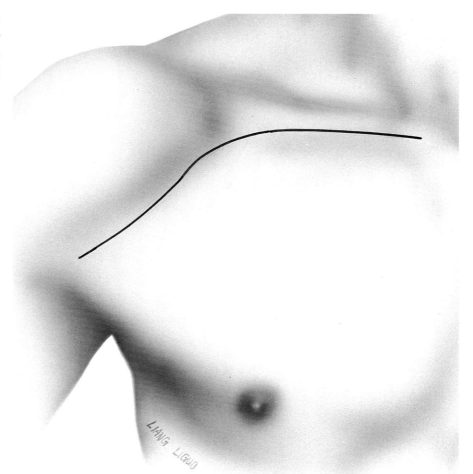

(Fig. 9-12) The skin is undermined to expose the cephalic vein [4] in the groove and the interseptum between the clavicular [3] and sternocostal [2] portions of the muscle. The latter can be identified from the sternoclavicular joint to its insertion and it is then carefully split.

1. Deltoid m.
2. Sternocostal head
3. Clavicular head
4. Cephalic v.

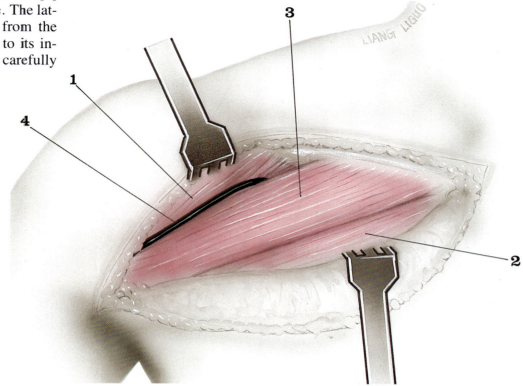

(Fig. 9-13) The cephalic vein [4] is isolated and traced to find the deltoid artery [8] which accompanies the vein. Then the insertion of the clavicular portion [3] is divided. Tracing the deltoid artery from distal to proximal, the neurovascular branches from the artery to the lateral pectoral nerve [6] are identified and the deltoid artery [8] is then ligated distal to these branches.

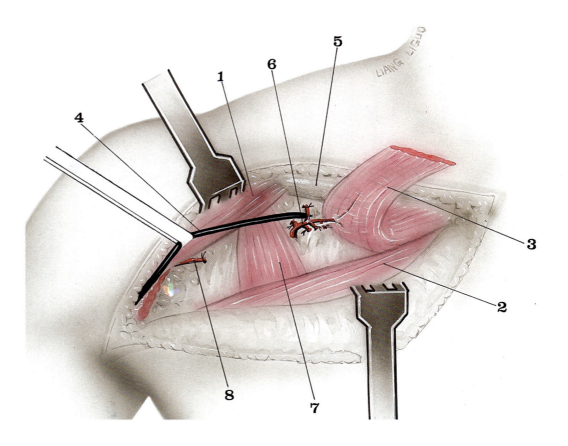

1. Deltoid m.
2. Sternocostal head
3. Clavicular head
4. Cephalic v.
5. Clavicle
6. Thoracoacromial a. and v. and lateral pectoral n.
7. Pectoralis minor m.
8. Deltoid a. and v.

(**Fig. 9-14**) Gradually turning the detached insertion medially, the deltoid artery is dissected further in the clavipectoral fascia to the thoracoacromial trunk [6], ligating the acromial, clavicular, and pectoral arteries. Its pedicle can be 4 to 6 cm. If a longer pedicle is required, the pectoral artery can be dissected and included with the deltoid artery for reverse flow in the pedicle. The cephalic vein [4] is also available for a vein graft.

The origin of this portion of the muscle is detached from the clavicle and the clavicular segment [3] of the pectoralis major muscle flap is raised, based on the deltoid artery and the lateral pectoral nerve.

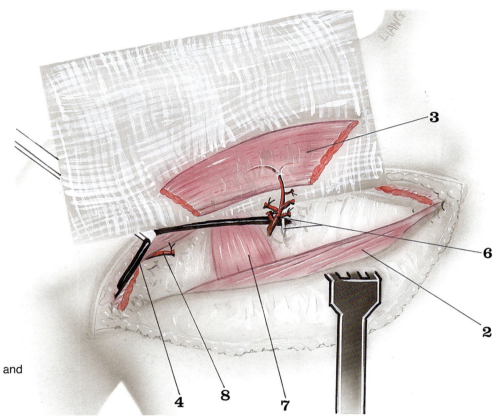

2. Sternocostal head
3. Clavicular head
4. Cephalic v.
6. Thoracoacromial a. and v. and lateral pectoral n.
7. Pectoralis minor m.
8. Deltoid a. and v.

(Fig. 9-15) If an osteomuscular flap is required, the anteroinferior half of the clavicle [5] is divided with an oscillating saw, including in the flap the attachment of the muscle [3] and leaving the posterosuperior half of the clavicle [5] intact to support the shoulder.

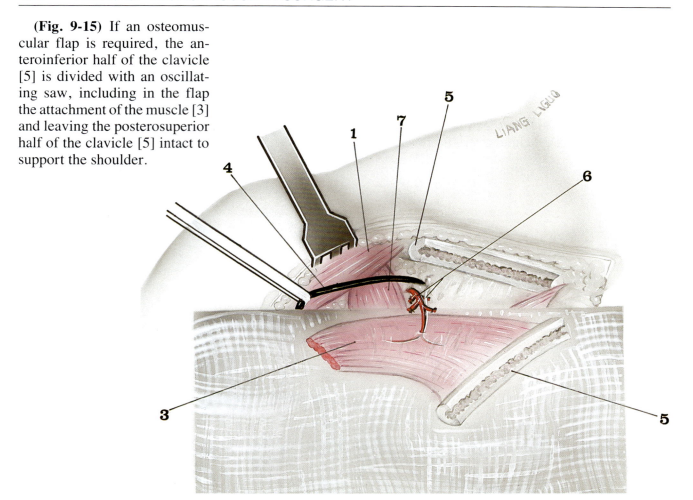

1. Deltoid m.
3. Clavicular head
4. Cephalic v.
5. Clavicle
6. Thoracoacromial a. and v. and lateral pectoral n.
7. Pectoralis minor m.

(Fig. 9-16) If a myocutaneous flap is required, a skin paddle is outlined on or slightly over the territory of the muscle portion that is defined by three points as a triangle—the sternoclavicular joint, the midpoint of the clavicle, and the muscle insertion.

The myocutaneous flap is raised as previously described.

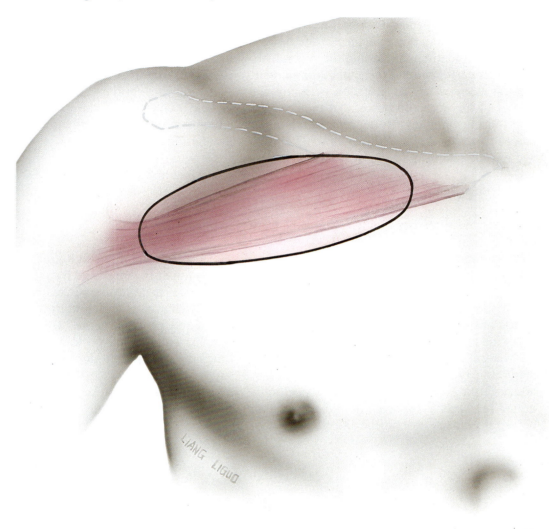

Pectoralis Minor Muscle Flap

Anatomy (Fig. 9-17)

The origin of the pectoralis minor muscle is the upper margins and outer surface of the third to fifth ribs (sometimes including the second rib) near their cartilage, and the aponeurosis covering the intercostals. Its insertion is the medial border of the coracoid process of the scapula. The muscle functions to depress the shoulder and to rotate the scapula downward. The average muscle length is 12 cm in adults.

Blood Supply

The arterial supply is variable and may be from three arterial trunks: the lateral thoracic artery [3], the direct branch [6] of the axillary artery, and the pectoral branch [5] of the thoracoacromial artery [4]. Usually, the branch from the lateral thoracic artery [3] appears predominant. If it is absent or too slender, the direct branch [6] of the axillary artery can be a second choice. The lateral thoracic artery [3] arises from the beginning of the third portion of the axillary artery [2]. It gives off a branch to the pectoralis minor [1] with a diameter of 0.5 to 0.9 mm before it courses around the lateral margin of the muscle. The direct branch [6] of the axillary artery arises from the second arterial portion behind the muscle.

(For the arterial anatomy of the thoracoacromial artery, refer to section on the details of the pectoralis major, p. 390.)

A branch supplying the upper part of the muscle comes from the pectoral artery [5], which then courses around the medial margin of the muscle.

Venous drainage is variable; there are several veins including venae comitantes and a direct vein.

Innervation

The lower two or three digitations of the muscle are dominantly innervated by a major branch of the medial pectoral nerve, whereas the uppermost digitation is supplied by a tiny branch of the lateral pectoral nerve. However, a larger branch of the lateral pectoral nerve also penetrates the muscle (but does not innervate it), to supply the pectoralis major. Usually, the two nerves join loosely before entering the pectoralis minor muscle.

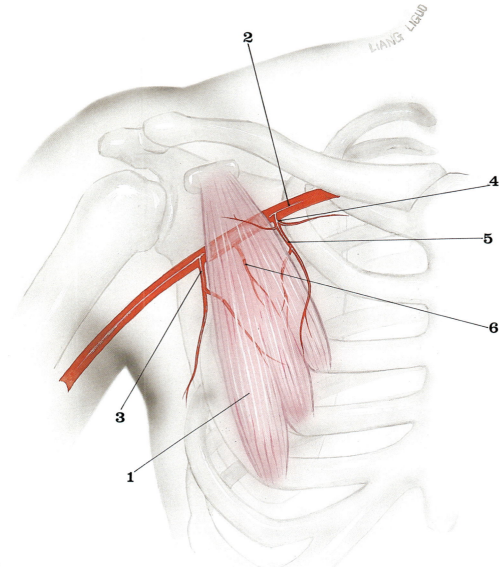

1. Pectoralis minor m.
2. Axillary a.
3. Lateral thoracic a.
4. Thoracoacromial a.
5. Pectoral branch
6. Direct branch of axillary a.

COMMENT AND INSIGHTS

Although the vascular structure supplying the pectoralis minor is variable, the dominant vascular pedicle can usually be clarified. Generally, the lateral thoracic vessels are chosen as the dominant pedicle, but pedicle length is limited to less than 3 cm. The muscle and its neurovascular structures are deeply located, making the harvesting procedure somewhat difficult and complicated.

Clinically, the pectoralis minor muscle flap has been reported in functional reconstruction of the facial musculature for reanimation in facial palsy. Because of its adequate shape, small size, flatness, and thickness, this muscle flap is ideally suited for use in the face, especially because its dual nerve supply allows for independent movement of the upper and lower portions.

The function of the pectoralis minor is not significantly important and there is no disability following its removal. The donor scar is relatively inconspicuous.

Harvesting Technique

(Fig. 9-18) With the patient in a supine position, an incision is made from the coracoid process along the lateral edge of the pectoralis major to a point below the breast.

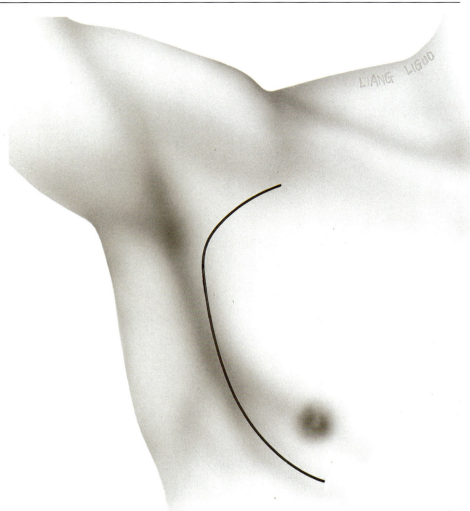

1. Pectoralis minor m.
2. Pectoralis major m.
3. Serratus anterior m.
4. Lateral thoracic a. and v.
5. Medial pectoral n.
6. Thoracoacromial a. and v.
7. Pectoral branch
8. Lateral pectoral n.
9. Axillary a. and v. and brachial plexus
10. Direct branch of axillary a. and v.

(**Fig. 9-19**) The lateral edge of the pectoralis major muscle [2] is exposed and retracted medially and anteriorly. Then, the lateral thoracic vessels [4] are identified and isolated under the lateral part of the pectoralis major. Ligating the branches to the pectoralis major [2] and serratus anterior [3] muscles, the lateral thoracic vessels [4] are traced to the undersurface of the pectoralis minor [1].

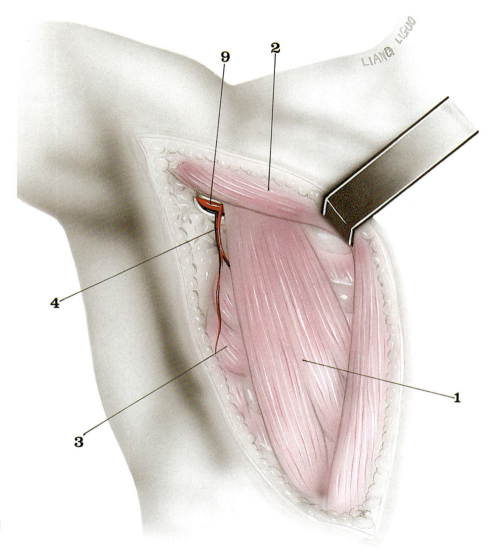

1. Pectoralis minor m.
2. Pectoralis major m.
3. Serratus anterior m.
4. Lateral thoracic a. and v.
9. Axillary a. and v. and brachial plexus

(Fig. 9-20) The insertion of the pectoralis minor is then divided from the coracoid process and retracted downward with a holding suture, displaying and assessing the neurovascular structures. It is sometimes necessary partially to divide the pectoralis major [2] at its insertion to gain greater access.

The dominant arterial and venous supplies are clarified, and the medial and lateral pectoral nerves [5,8] and their communicating loop are identified and dissected.

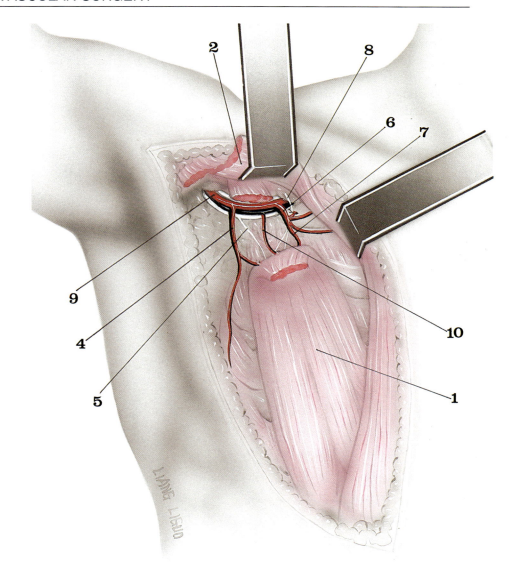

1. Pectoralis minor m.
2. Pectoralis major m.
4. Lateral thoracic a. and v.
5. Medial pectoral n.
6. Thoracoacromial a. and v.
7. Pectoral branch
8. Lateral pectoral n.
9. Axillary a. and v. and brachial plexus
10. Direct branch of axillary a. and v.

(**Fig. 9-21**) Detaching the muscle origin from the third to fifth ribs, the pectoralis minor muscle flap [1] is raised from the chest wall, based on the dominant neurovascular pedicle [4], which can be dissected up to the axillary vessels [9], providing a pedicle length of 2 to 3 cm.

1. Pectoralis minor m.
2. Pectoralis major m.
4. Lateral thoracic a. and v.
9. Axillary a. and v. and brachial plexus

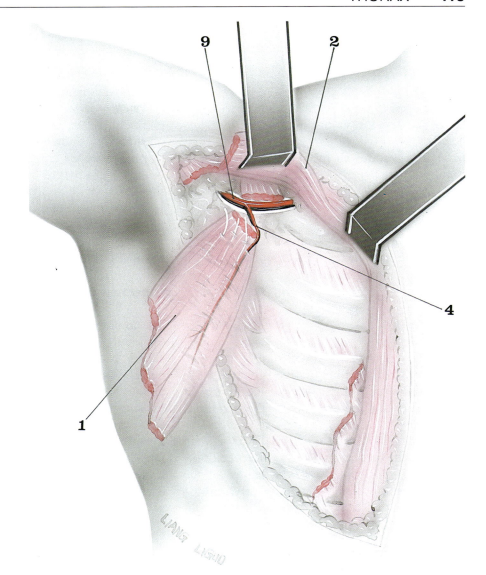

Serratus Anterior Flap

Anatomy (Fig. 9-22)

Muscle origin: outer surfaces and superior border of the upper eight or nine ribs.

Insertion: ventral surface of vertebral border of the scapula [8].

Shape: broad, flat.

Function: moves the scapula forward away from spine and fixes the scapula against the chest wall.

Blood Supply

The muscle receives its blood supply from two sources: the upper four or five digitations are from the lateral thoracic artery, and the lower five or six digitations are from the thoracodorsal artery.

The *lateral thoracic artery,* [6] as a main trunk (see the section on details of the pectoralis major flap), follows the lower border of the pectoralis minor and runs inferiorly on the surface of the anterior part of the upper digitations of the muscle. It gives off multiple branches to them.

The *thoracodorsal artery* [4] (see Chapter 11 on details of the latissimus dorsi flap) gives off one to three branches [5] to the serratus anterior. In 66% of cases, there is only a single branch 5 cm before the entrance to the latissimus dorsi, with an average diameter of 2 mm. In 32% of cases, there are two branches, 4 and 7 cm before the entrance, with diameters of 1 mm. In 2% of cases, there are three or four branches to the muscle.

Innervation

The long thoracic nerve [7] formed by the 5th, 6th, and 7th cervical nerves, pierces the substance of the scalenus medius and descends behind the brachial plexus and the axillary artery. It reaches the upper border of the serratus anterior at the apex of the axillary fossa, and then runs downward on the lateral surface of the muscle between the middle and posterior axillary line. It joins the serratus branch of the thoracodorsal artery at the level of the sixth digitation. In its course, the long thoracic nerve gives off branches to supply each digitation.

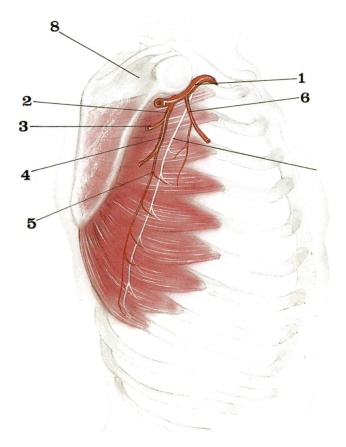

1. Axillary a.
2. Subscapular a.
3. Circumflex scapular a.
4. Thoracodorsal a.
5. Branch to serratus anterior
6. Lateral thoracic a.
7. Long thoracic n.
8. Scapular bone

COMMENT AND INSIGHTS

This is a medium-sized muscle flap with a long pedicle. The outstanding advantage of the flap is in its possible combination with vascularized ribs or latissimus dorsi flaps. Following the latissimus dorsi flap, this muscle flap was one of the earliest applied flaps. However, it has not been widely used, even though its vascular anatomy is constant and reliable. Surgeons prefer the latissimus dorsi donor site to that of the serratus anterior.

The serratus anterior flap has been applied in reanimation of facial paralysis, coverage of hands or feet with cutaneous flaps or skin grafts, reconstruction of the mandible with an osteomyocutaneous flap, and chest-wall reconstruction with local transfer. The donor scar is acceptable and the skin defect after myocutaneous flap transfer can usually be closed directly.

To prevent a "winging" scapula and limitations in arm movement resulting from loss of muscle function, maximal preservation of the upper digitations and their innervation is suggested. The use of the middle or lower portion (four or five digitations) as the donor is advisable.

SERRATUS ANTERIOR MUSCLE FLAP

(Fig. 9-23) The patient is placed in the lateral decubitus position. An incision is made from the posterior axillary fold on the lateral chest wall along the anterior border of the latissimus dorsi. It then turns anteriorly along the 8th rib. The digitations from the 5th to the 10th ribs can be taken for transfer. Usually, the digitations from the 5th to the 8th ribs are chosen, because the 9th and 10th digitations are sometimes not reliable.

1. Axillary a. and v.
2. Subscapular a. and v.
3. Thoracodorsal a. and v.
4. Thoracodorsal n.
5. Branch to serratus anterior
6. Serratus anterior m.
7. Latissimus dorsi m.
8. Long thoracic n.
9. Pectoralis major m.

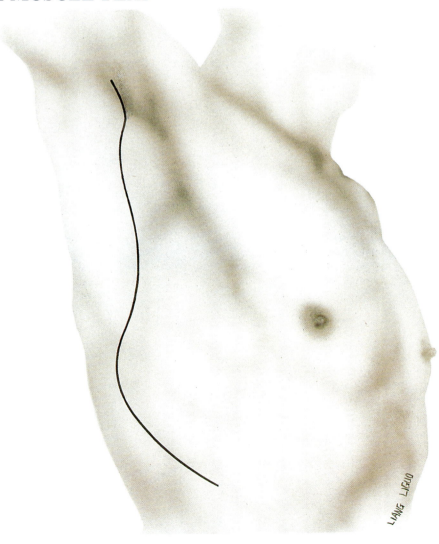

(**Fig. 9-24**) The anterior border of the latissimus dorsi [7] and the anterior part of the serratus anterior [6] are exposed. Retracting the proximal portion of the latissimus dorsi dorsally, the main trunk of the thoracodorsal neurovascular bundle [3] is identified between the serratus anterior [6] and latissimus dorsi [7]. Careful dissection of the vessels leads to finding one or two branches [5] to the serratus anterior that arise from the thoracodorsal vessel 3 to 6 cm cephalad to the entrance of the latissimus dorsi. The long thoracic nerve [8] can be found on the surface of the muscle joining the vascular bundle at the level of the 6th rib.

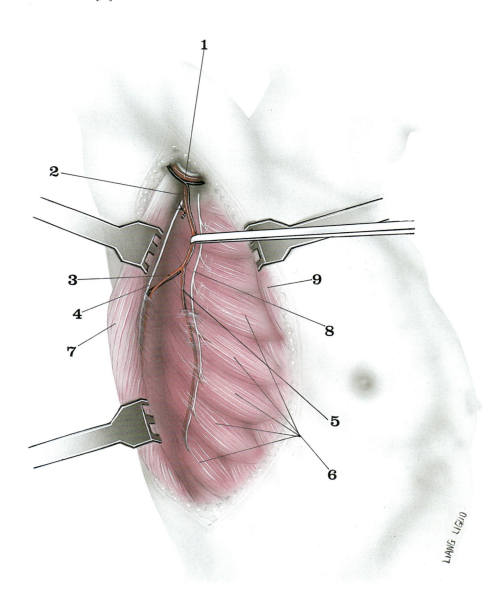

1. Axillary a. and v.
2. Subscapular a. and v.
3. Thoracodorsal a. and v.
4. Thoracodorsal n.
5. Branch to serratus anterior
6. Serratus anterior m.
7. Latissimus dorsi m.
8. Long thoracic n.
9. Pectoralis major m.

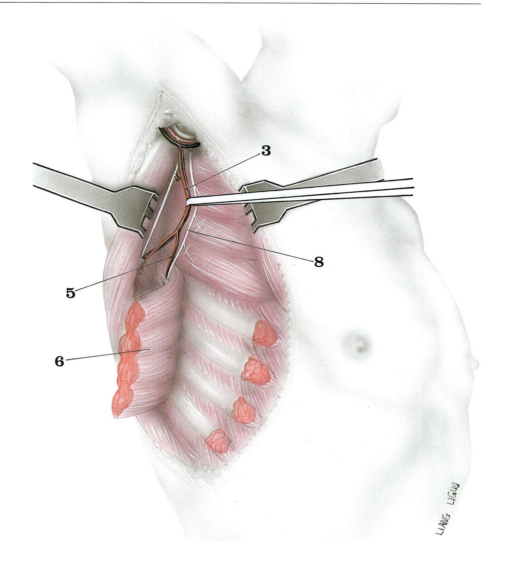

(Fig. 9-25) The 5th to 8th digitations of the serratus anterior [6] are mobilized from the chest wall by carefully dividing attachments on the ribs with a cautery. The upper and lower portion with their innervation should be preserved, in order to prevent a winging scapula and limitation of arm movement.

3. Thoracodorsal a. and v.
5. Branch to serratus anterior
6. Serratus anterior m.
8. Long thoracic n.

(Fig. 9-26) The branch to the latissimus dorsi [7] is ligated, preserving the thoracodorsal nerve. Then, the latissimus dorsi [7] is retracted posteriorly. Dissection between the muscle and subscapularis exposes its insertion as far as possible.

3. Thoracodorsal a. and v.
5. Branch to serratus anterior
6. Serratus anterior m.
7. Latissimus dorsi m.
8. Long thoracic n.

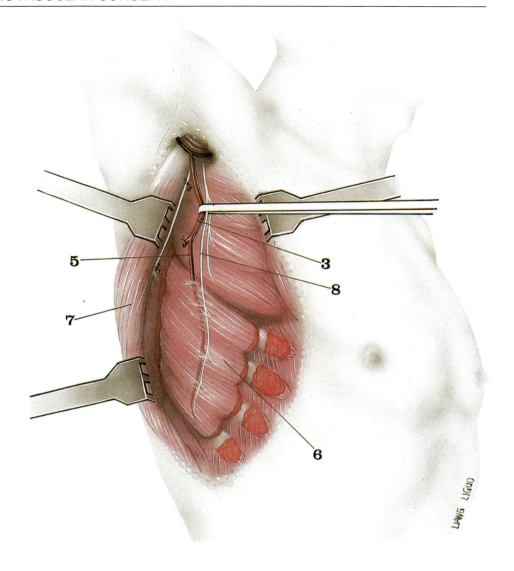

(**Fig. 9-27**) After dividing the muscle from its scapular attachment by cautery, the serratus anterior muscle flap [5] is raised.

5. Branch to serratus anterior
6. Serratus anterior m.
8. Long thoracic n.

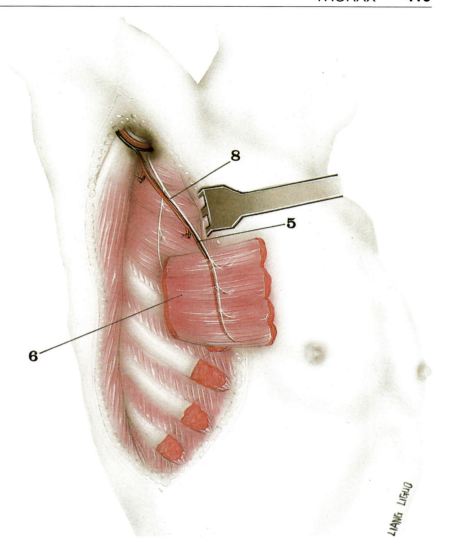

SERRATUS ANTERIOR MYOCUTANEOUS FLAP

(Fig. 9-28) The skin territory comprises: posteriorly, to the lateral border of the latissimus dorsi muscle; anteriorly, to the anterior line of the axilla. The skin paddle usually lies over the 4th to 7th ribs.

1. Thoracodorsal a. and v.
2. Long thoracic n.
3. Serratus anterior m.

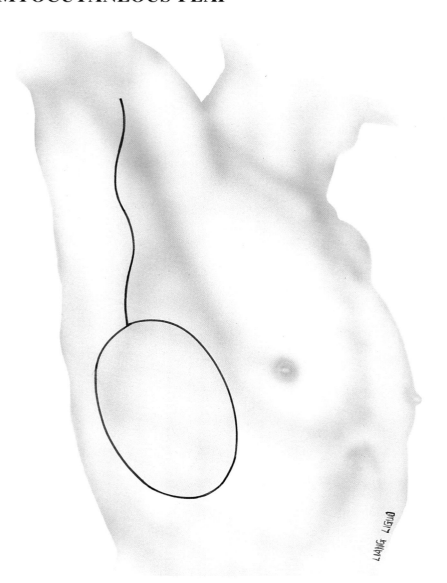

(Fig. 9-29) Dissection starts with a posterior incision. While dissecting the thoracodorsal vessels [1], attention should be paid to preserve the muscular and cutaneous branches from the vessels to the serratus anterior and its overlying skin. Keeping the skin paddle intact with the 4th to 7th digitations of the muscle [3], the serratus anterior myocutaneous flap is elevated, following similar procedures described for the muscle flap.

1. Thoracodorsal a. and v.
2. Long thoracic n.
3. Serratus anterior m.

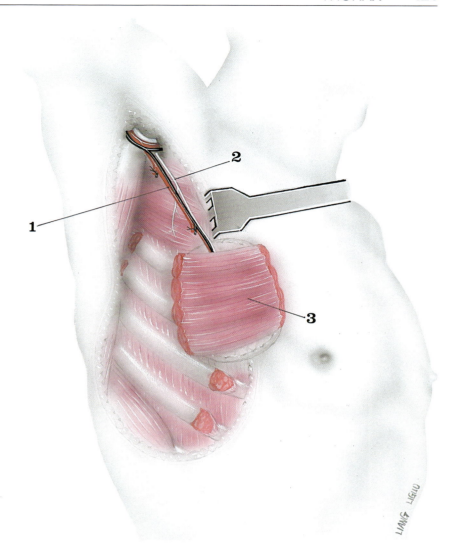

COMPOSITE SERRATUS-LATISSIMUS MUSCLE FLAP

(Fig. 9-30) The latissimus dorsi and serratus anterior muscles can be isolated on a common vascular pedicle of the thoracodorsal artery and can be transferred together. The incision is demonstrated in the illustration.

1. Thoracodorsal a., v., and n.
2. Branch to serratus m.
3. Long thoracic n.
4. Serratus anterior m.
5. Latissimus dorsi m.

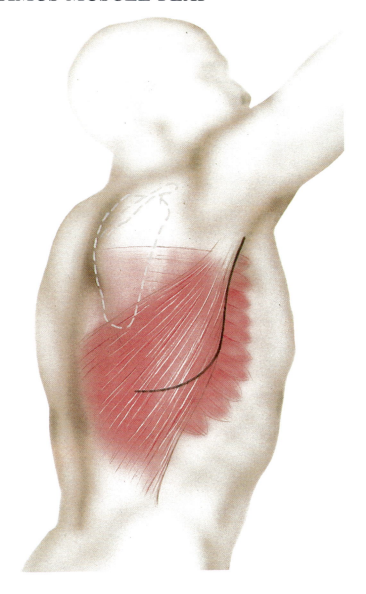

(Fig. 9-31) After identification of the thoracodorsal artery [1] and its branches [2] to these two muscles, the latissimus dorsi flap [5] is raised and reflected cranially. The serratus anterior [4] is then detached from the ribs and scapula. (See the techniques detailed in the sections on both of these muscles.)

1. Thoracodorsal a., v., and n.
2. Branch to serratus m.
3. Long thoracic n.
4. Serratus anterior m.
5. Latissimus dorsi m.

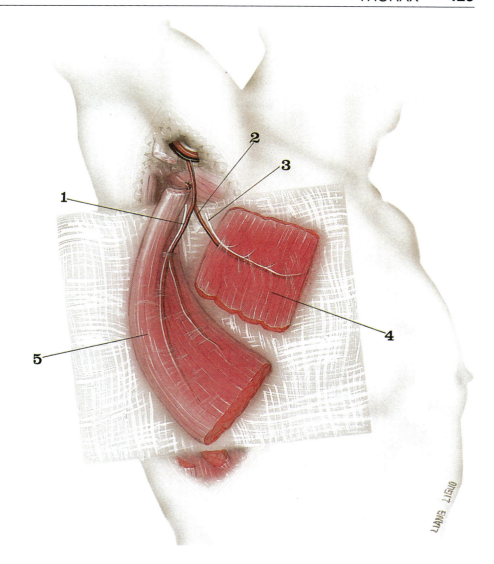

SERRATUS ANTERIOR COSTO-OSTEOMUSCULAR FLAP

(Fig. 9-32) Any of the 5th to 8th ribs is available for combination with the serratus anterior muscle flap, but the 6th rib is usually selected.

1. Thoracodorsal a. and v.
2. Long thoracic n.
3. Serratus anterior m.
4. Intercostal m.
5. Sixth rib

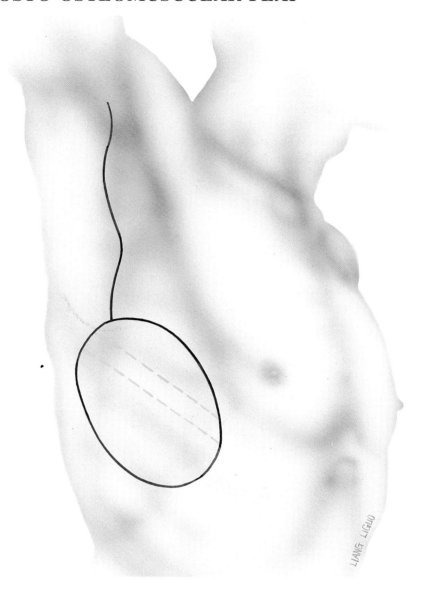

(**Fig. 9-33**) After dissection of the thoracodorsal vessels [1] and branches to the serratus anterior [3], the digitations of the muscle are separated from all other ribs except the 6th. All connections between the muscle and the 6th rib [5] are preserved. Both ends of the rib are transected, according to length requirements. The blood supply to the bone can be maintained through the periosteal circulation.

1. Thoracodorsal a. and v.
2. Long thoracic n.
3. Serratus anterior m.
4. Intercostal m.
5. Sixth rib

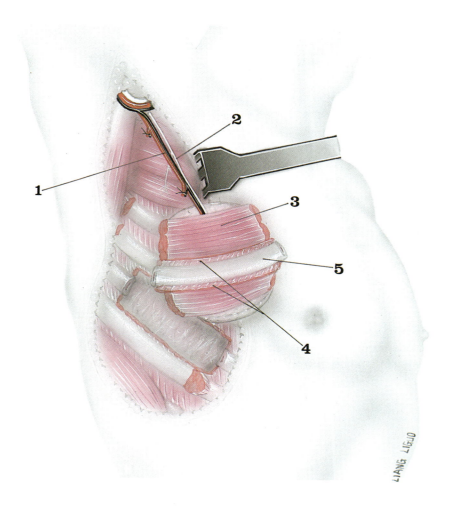

Revascularized Costal Bone Graft and Intercostal Flap

Arterial Anatomy (Fig. 9-34)

The *posterior intercostal artery* [2] arises directly from the aorta [1] and soon gives off the dorsal branch to the paraspinal muscle and spinal cord. It then goes upward in the costal groove of the rib above, continuing anteriorly. The nutrient artery [6] of the rib arises from the posterior intercostal artery and enters the nutrient foramen just distal to the tubercle. The diameter of the posterior intercostal artery [2] is about 2.0 mm up to the nutrient artery and about 1.5 mm beyond the nutrient artery.

For the lower three intercostal spaces, the *lateral cutaneous perforator* [3] arises from the posterior intercostal artery [2] in the distal part of the costal groove, accompanied by a vein and nerve branch. It reaches the subcutaneous level a short distance in front of the anterior edge of the latissimus dorsi muscle. At or before this point, it divides into two branches—a small posterior branch and a large anterior branch.

The *anterior intercostal artery* [4] arises from the internal mammary artery [5], ultimately communicating with the posterior intercostal artery [2] at the anteromiddle third of the rib. The diameter of this artery is about 1.0 mm.

The *internal mammary artery* [5] descends along the internal surface of the anterior part of the rib cage, about 1 to 2 cm lateral to the margin of the sternum. Below the third costal cartilage, it is separated from the parietal pleura by the transverse thoracic muscle. The diameter is about 2.0 to 3.0 mm.

The anterior perforator to supply the skin and pectoralis muscle is directly derived from the internal mammary artery. Its diameter is about 0.5 to 1.0 mm.

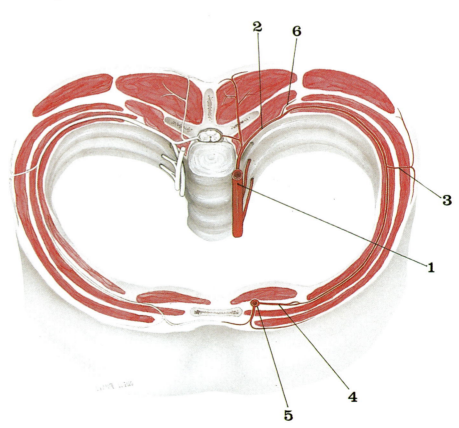

1. Aorta
2. Posterior intercostal a.
3. Lateral cutaneous perforator
4. Anterior intercostal a.
5. Internal mammary a.
6. Nutrient a.

COMMENT AND INSIGHTS

Because the anatomic relationships between the ribs, neurovascular bundles, and intervening structures are constant, harvesting the vascularized rib or osteocutaneous flap is not too difficult. The donor sites can either singly or as a composite provide vascularized rib bone, sensitive skin, and intercostal nerve for grafting. Also, the natural curvature of the rib is particularly suited for mandibular reconstruction, although it is generally too weak structurally to be used in the lower extremity.

The literature has reported some cases of venous congestion, particularly in skin or costal osteocutaneous flaps based on the posterior intercostal vessels. While incising the skin of the flap, it is therefore advisable to preserve a subcutaneous vein for subsequent anastomosis.

Removing the posterior rib from its costovertebral joint and including the nutrient vessels are technically quite difficult and may endanger the blood supply to the spinal cord. Without the nutrient vessel, the revascularized rib receives its circulation only through periosteal pathways.

Experience in thoracic surgery is recommended for these techniques, because the pleura may be ruptured during flap harvesting. Postoperative pulmonary complications may occur, including pleural effusion, atelectasis, pneumonia, and empyema. For these reasons, the use of vascularized costal bone grafts and osteocutaneous flaps is limited in clinical practice. They can be only a second choice, following iliac and fibular revascularized bone grafts.

VASCULARIZED RIB GRAFT (Based on the Posterior Intercostal Artery)

(Fig. 9-35) The 7th to 10th ribs can be utilized as donors. More commonly, however, the 8th or 9th rib would commonly be selected.

An incision is placed directly over the selected rib (the 8th rib), beginning posteriorly 5.0 cm from the midline and extending as far as is necessary.

1. Latissimus dorsi m.
2. Serratus anterior m.
3. Angle of the 8th rib
4. Intercostal m.
5. Posterior intercostal a.
6. Pleura

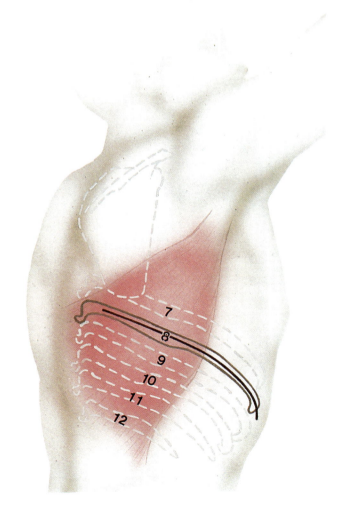

(Fig. 9-36) The skin and deep fascia are incised, the lateral edge of the latissimus dorsi [1] is identified, and the 7th to 9th digitations of the serratus anterior [2] are exposed.

1. Latissimus dorsi m.
2. Serratus anterior m.

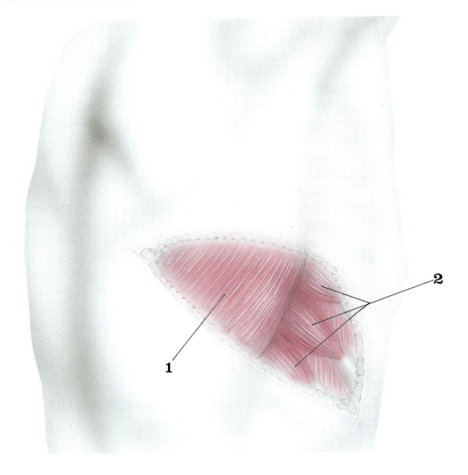

(Fig. 9-37) The latissimus dorsi [1] and serratus anterior [2] muscles are separated or detached from the ribs to expose the ribs and their intercostal spaces [4]. The latissimus dorsi muscle may be divided for further exposure.

1. Latissimus dorsi m.
2. Serratus anterior m.
4. Intercostal m.

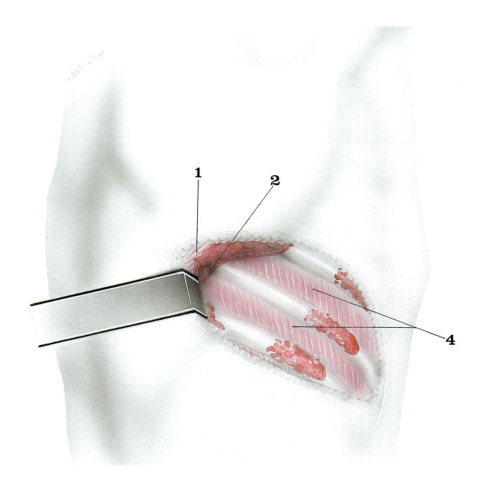

(Fig. 9-38) The erector spinae is separated and retracted to expose the angle of the rib [3] at which the neurovascular bundle [5] leaves the subcostal groove, to pass obliquely downward; the bundle can then be identified and isolated. The collateral branch can either be preserved or ligated.

The intercostal muscles [4] are divided layer by layer along the upper borders of the selected rib and the 9th rib below, avoiding incision damage to the pleura and to the intercostal neurovascular bundle. Simultaneously, the serratus posterior inferior muscle [7] can be divided in the course of dissection. Then, the pleura [6] is carefully dissected from the 8th rib.

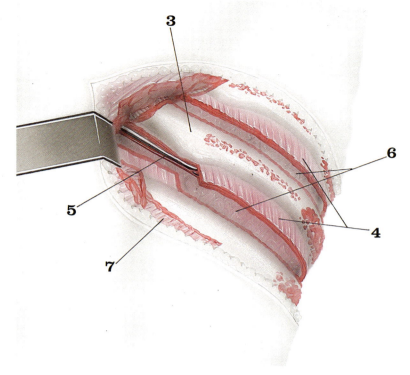

3. Angle of the 8th rib
4. Intercostal m.
5. Posterior intercostal a.
6. Pleura
7. Serratus anterior m.

(Fig. 9-39) According to the length and curvature required, the rib is divided at both ends, and the neurovascular bundle [5] on the distal end is ligated. The rib is thus isolated on the posterior intercostal neurovascular bundle. Further dissection to obtain a greater pedicle length can proceed over the tubercle of the rib, and the nutrient artery can be ligated.

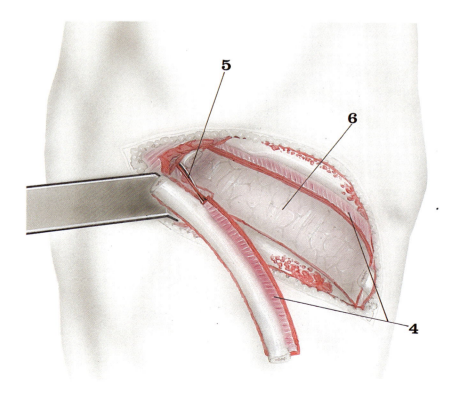

4. Intercostal m.
5. Posterior intercostal a.
6. Pleura

LATERAL INTERCOSTAL SKIN FLAP

(Fig. 9-40) The neurovascular pedicle selected is usually at T10 or T11. The flap is marked according to the following parameters. Its axis corresponds to the lateral cutaneous perforator of the posterior intercostal vessels of T10, for example. The posterior border of the flap should be at least 5.0 cm behind the posterior axillary line. Flap size ranges from 10 × 14 cm to 17 × 24 cm.

1. Latissimus dorsi m.
2. Lateral cutaneous perforator and n.
3. 10th rib
4. External oblique m.
5. Posteroinferior serratus m.
6. Anterior serratus m.
7. Intercostal m.
8. Pleura
9. Posterior intercostal a., v., and n.

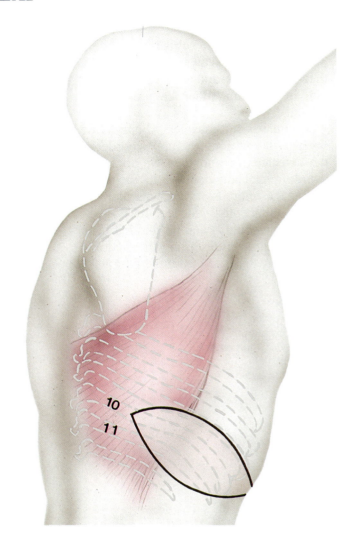

(Fig. 9-41) The posterior border of the flap is elevated with deep fascia to expose the lateral border of the latissimus dorsi [1]. Careful dissection should be undertaken anteriorly to identify the lateral cutaneous perforating bundles [2] of the 10th and 11th intercostal spaces that are just anterior to the edge of the latissimus dorsi [1]. The posterior branches of the bundles appear under the fascia of the flap at these points.

1. Latissimus dorsi m.
2. Lateral cutaneous perforator and n.

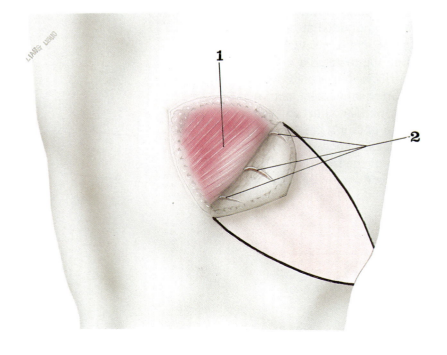

(**Fig. 9-42**) After a comparison of the 10th and 11th bundles, the larger is chosen. If the axis of the flap is to be changed, flap design is readjusted; the remaining bundles are ligated. Using the 10th bundle as an example: to trace the main bundle, the slip of the origin of the external oblique [4] below it is detached, and the latissimus dorsi [1] and serratus posteroinferior muscles [5] are incised and retracted to expose the 10th interspace.

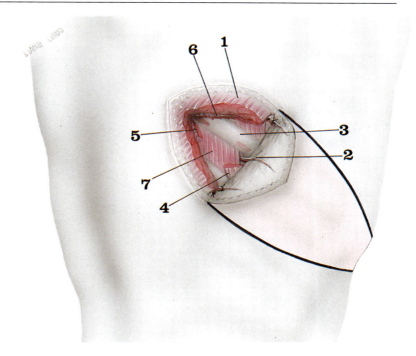

1. Latissimus dorsi m.
2. Lateral cutaneous perforator and n.
3. 10th rib
4. External oblique m.
5. Posteroinferior serratus m.
6. Anterior serratus m.
7. Intercostal m.

(**Fig. 9-43**) The external and internal intercostal muscles [7] are then cut from the lower border of the rib, identifying the junction of the lateral cutaneous perforator [2] with the posterior intercostal bundle [9].

The periosteum of the lower border of the rib is incised and reflected downward, and the periosteum on the roof of the subcostal groove is released subperiosteally, using an elevator. The intercostal bundle [9] is then delivered by pulling the incised edge of the periosteum downward.

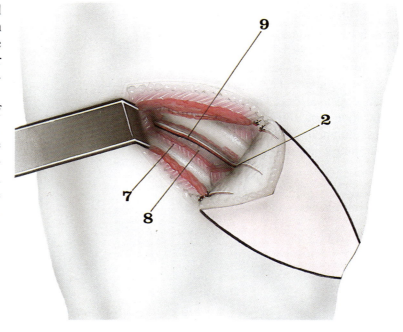

2. Lateral cutaneous perforator and n.
7. Intercostal m.
8. Pleura
9. Posterior intercostal a., v., and n.

(**Fig. 9-44**) The continuation of the posterior intercostal vessels [9] (after giving off the lateral cutaneous branch) is ligated. A desired length of pedicle can be dissected posteriorly; it is usually 8 to 15 cm in length. The lateral cutaneous nerve can be stripped from the main nerve. Remaining flap borders are incised down to and including the deep fascia, and the flap is quickly elevated.

2. Lateral cutaneous a., v., and n.
3. 10th rib
4. External oblique m.
7. Intercostal m.
8. Pleura
9. Posterior intercostal a., v., and n.

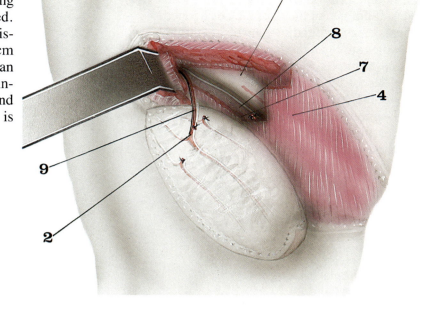

(**Fig. 9-45**) The surgeon is advised that caution is necessary in identifying the anterior branch of the lateral cutaneous perforator [2] *before* ligating the continuation of the posterior intercostal bundle [9]. This is because of anatomic variations at the incipient division of the lateral cutaneous branch deep in the intercostal space.

2. Lateral cutaneous a., v., and n.
8. Pleura
9. Posterior intercostal a., v., and n.

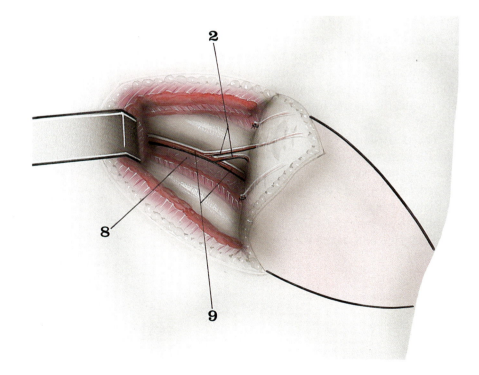

POSTERIOR COSTAL OSTEOCUTANEOUS FLAP

(**Fig. 9-46**) The skin flap is marked using the following parameters. The flap axis is the lateral cutaneous branch that emerges on the midaxillary line and is parallel to the selected rib. Assuming choice of the 9th rib, the posterior edge of the flap is located about 10 cm away from the midline of the back. Maximal flap size is about 20 × 12 cm.

1. Angle of the 9th rib
2. Posterior intercostal a., v., and n.
3. Intercostal m.
4. Latissimus dorsi m.
5. Pleura
6. Serratus anterior m.

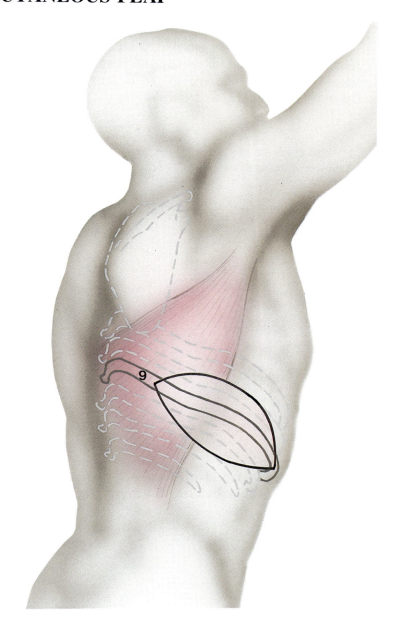

434 ATLAS OF MICROVASCULAR SURGERY

(**Fig. 9-47**) The posterior intercostal neurovascular bundle [2] is identified near the angle of the rib [1].

While deepening the incision, a subcutaneous vein is preserved for subsequent anastomosis. Skin should be fixed to the underlying intercostal muscle [3] to avoid shearing.

1. Angle of the 9th rib
2. Posterior intercostal a., v., and n.
3. Intercostal m.
4. Latissimus dorsi m.
5. Pleura
6. Serratus anterior m.

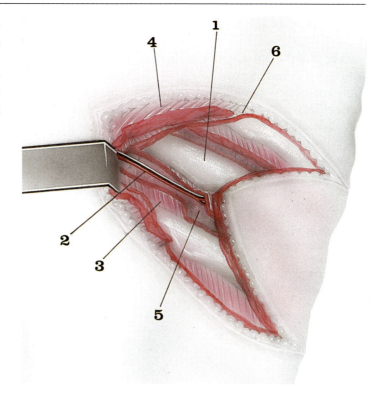

(**Fig. 9-48**) The costal osteocutaneous flap can be raised following principles similar to those of a free rib technique.

1. Angle of the 9th rib
2. Posterior intercostal a., v., and n.
3. Intercostal m.
4. Latissimus dorsi m.
5. Pleura
6. Serratus anterior m.

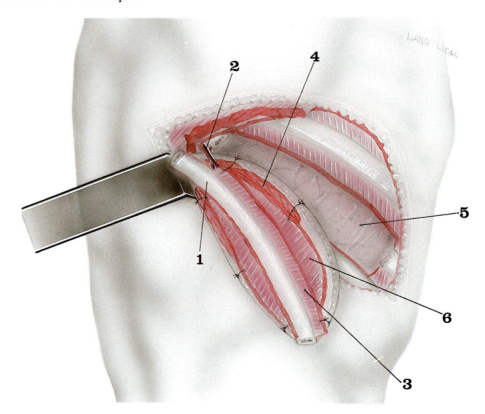

VASCULARIZED RIB GRAFT (Based on the Anterior Intercostal Artery)

(**Fig. 9-49**) The 5th and 6th ribs are choice donor sites for this procedure, because the transverse thoracic muscle separates the internal mammary vessels and its branches from the parietal pleura. An incision is placed directly over the selected rib. Using the 5th rib as an example, the incision would run from the anterior midline and as far laterally as necessary.

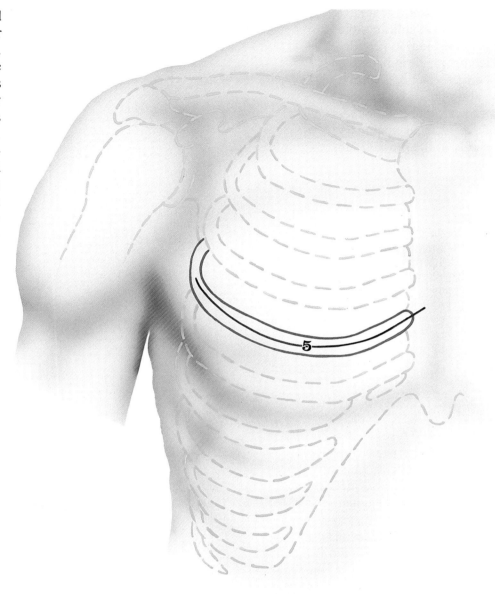

1. 5th rib
2. Pectoralis major m.
3. Pectoralis minor m.
4. Intercostal m.
5. Serratus anterior m.
6. Sternum
7. Internal mammary a. and v.
8. Anterior intercostal a., v., and n.
9. Transverse thoracic m.
10. Pleura

436 ATLAS OF MICROVASCULAR SURGERY

(Fig. 9-50) The 5th rib [1] and two interspaces [4] above and below it are exposed after splitting the pectoralis major [2], detaching the origin of the pectoralis minor [3], and ligating the direct cutaneous perforating branches of the internal mammary vessels in the 4th and 5th interspaces.

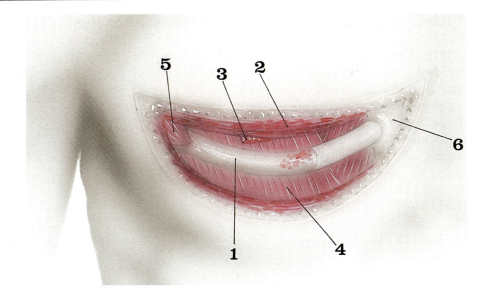

1. 5th rib
2. Pectoralis major m.
3. Pectoralis minor m.
4. Intercostal m.
5. Serratus anterior m.
6. Sternum

(Fig. 9-51) A segment of the costal cartilage is isolated and removed subpericondrially. Dissection proceeds, identifying and isolating the underlying internal mammary vessels [7] and the anterior intercostal vessels [8]. Attention should be paid to preservation of the pleura.

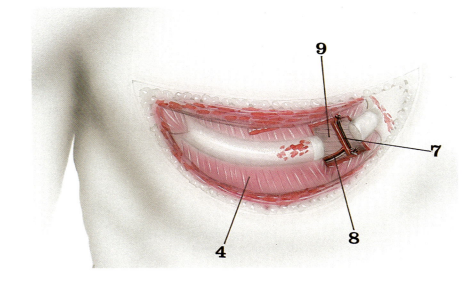

4. Intercostal m.
7. Internal mammary a. and v.
8. Anterior intercostal a., v., and n.
9. Transverse thoracic m.

(**Fig. 9-52**) After the vascular pedicle [8] is safely dissected, the intercostal muscles [4] of the 4th and 5th interspaces are incised below the 4th and above the 6th ribs, leaving as wide a muscle cuff as possible for the 5th rib, both superiorly and inferiorly.

4. Intercostal m.
7. Internal mammary a. and v.
8. Anterior intercostal a., v., and n.
9. Transverse thoracic m.
10. Pleura

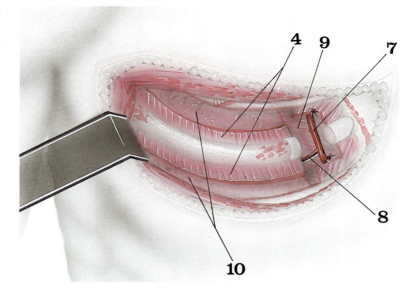

(**Fig. 9-53**) The 5th rib [1] is divided laterally as far as required, and the vascularized rib is elevated from the pleura [10]. The internal mammary vessels [7] inferior to the origin of the 5th anterior intercostal vessels are ligated. Then, the vascularized rib is based on the vessels superiorly. Pedicle length is about 6.0 cm.

1. 5th rib
4. Intercostal m.
7. Internal mammary a. and v.
8. Anterior intercostal a., v., and n.
9. Transverse thoracic m.
10. Pleura

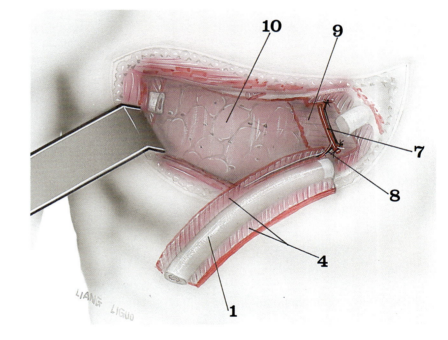

ANTERIOR COSTAL OSTEOCUTANEOUS FLAP

(**Fig. 9-54**) The axis of the flap is the intercostal space of the proposed rib (as an example, the 5th intercostal space). Flap size is up to about 10 × 30 cm, corresponding to the rib length required.

1. Internal mammary a.
2. Anterior intercostal a.
3. Direct cutaneous perforator
4. Pectoralis major m.
5. Sternum
6. Transverse thoracic m.
7. 5th rib
8. Pleura
9. Intercostal m.

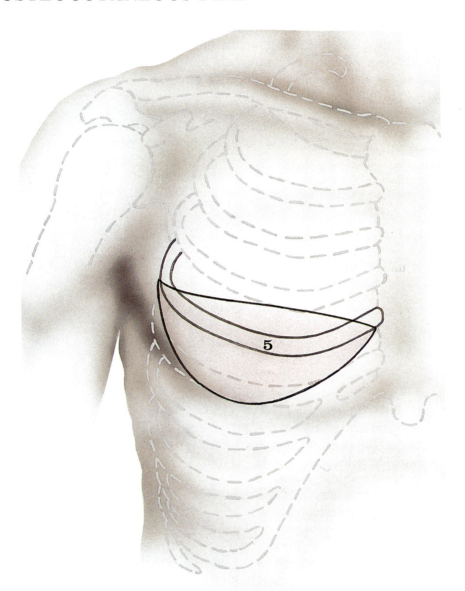

(**Fig. 9-55**) In the medial incision of the flap, the direct cutaneous perforator [3] from the internal mammary vessels [1] should be carefully identified and preserved, before dissecting the costal cartilage.

The skin should be kept intact and connected with the pectoralis [4] and intercostal muscles above and below the 5th rib during flap dissection. It is useful to anchor the skin to the underlying muscle to prevent shearing.

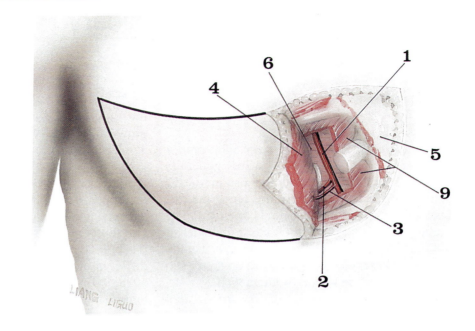

1. Internal mammary a.
2. Anterior intercostal a.
3. Direct cutaneous perforator
4. Pectoralis major m.
5. Sternum
6. Transverse thoracic m.
9. Intercostal m.

(**Fig. 9-56**) Following the technique of vascularized rib graft [7] based on the anterior intercostal artery [2], the anterior costal osteocutaneous flap is isolated on the internal mammary vessels [1].

1. Internal mammary a.
2. Anterior intercostal a.
3. Direct cutaneous perforator
4. Pectoralis major m.
6. Transverse thoracic m.
7. 5th rib
8. Pleura
9. Intercostal m.

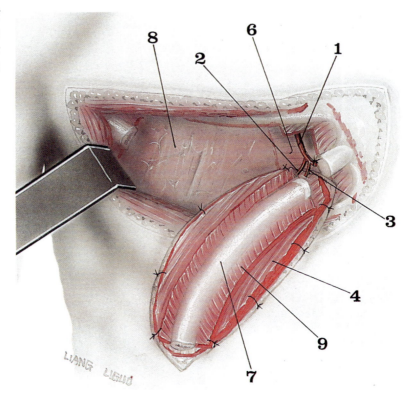

Lateral Thoracic Flap (Axillary Flap)

Arterial Anatomy (Fig. 9-57)

The anatomy for this area may be quite variable. There are perhaps three axial arteries to nourish this skin region.

The *cutaneous branch from the subscapular or thoracodorsal arteries* [4] arises generally within 2 to 5 cm beyond the origin of the subscapular artery and then runs along the free anterior border of the latissimus dorsi [6]. The cutaneous branch [4], which has a diameter of about 1.0 mm in 70% of cases, can usually supply a skin area of 10 × 20 cm on the posterior portion of the lateral thoracic wall.

The *cutaneous branch from the lateral thoracic artery* [3] usually serves as the terminal branch after giving off branches to the pectoralis muscles, and then runs along the lateral border of the pectoralis major [5]. In females, this terminal branch thickens as it goes to the breast. The cutaneous branch, present in 30% of cases, with a diameter of 1.5 mm, supplies a skin area of 8 × 15 cm in the anterior portion of this region.

The *accessory lateral thoracic artery* originates directly from the axillary or brachial artery [1] on its anterior aspect and goes from the center of the axillary fossa inferiorly along the middle axillary line; it then turns toward the nipple. The artery is present in 70% of cases and has a diameter of 1.4 mm; it supplies a skin area of 7 × 12 cm in the midportion of this region. It can also nourish the inner aspect of the upper arm.

Some authors believe that the accessory lateral thoracic artery is a variation of the cutaneous branch of the lateral thoracic artery, with a different takeoff (origin). They use a common term, "superficial lateral thoracic artery" for both vessels.

Venous Drainage

Usually, one or two venae comitantes accompany these arteries.

Innervation

The sensibility of this region is supplied segmentally by the intercostal nerves.

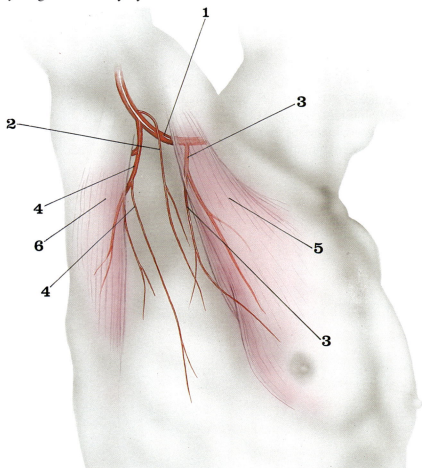

1. Axillary a.
2. Accessory lateral thoracic a.
3. Lateral thoracic a. and its cutaneous branch
4. Thoracodorsal a. and its cutaneous branch
5. Pectoralis major m.
6. Latissimus dorsi m.

COMMENT AND INSIGHTS

The color and texture of this flap are good matches for the head, neck, and hand. The donor scar is easy to conceal, and the donor defect can be closed directly. Axillary hair is available, if it is required in the transfer. A vascular pedicle can be created to a length of 10 cm. External diameters of the selected artery and vein are usually about 1.2 and 1.5 mm, respectively. The size of the flap can be approximately 10 × 20 cm.

One of the main disadvantages is the variable anatomy of the three axial arteries, requiring more extensive dissection. The dominant vessels should be determined and selected intraoperatively. For this reason, this flap is not widely used. It cannot be a sensory skin flap because its innervation is segmentally provided.

This flap is not recommended for routine use.

Harvesting Technique

(Fig. 9-58) The territory of the flap comprises: the upper border, pulsating path of the axillary artery; the posterior border, the lateral border of the latissimus dorsi; the anterior border, the lateral border of the pectoralis major; and the lower border, above the 8th rib. The flap location may be changed slightly back and forth, according to the arterial axis, with a sufficient diameter discovered during dissection.

The first incision is along the course of the axillary artery (the upper border of the flap).

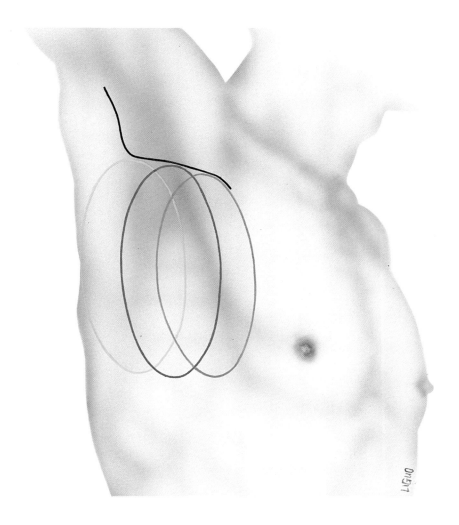

1. Axillary a. and v. and brachial plexus
2. Accessory lateral thoracic a. and v.
3. Lateral thoracic a. and v. and their cutaneous branches
4. Thoracodorsal a. and v. and their cutaneous branches
5. Pectoralis major m.
6. Latissimus dorsi m.
7. Serratus anterior m.

(**Fig. 9-59**) The accessory lateral thoracic artery [2] is first dissected because it courses through the most superficial layer. If its diameter is adequate, the vascular pedicle can be dissected to the axillary or brachial artery [1].

1. Axillary a. and v. and brachial plexus
2. Accessory lateral thoracic a. and v.
5. Pectoralis major m.
6. Latissimus dorsi m.

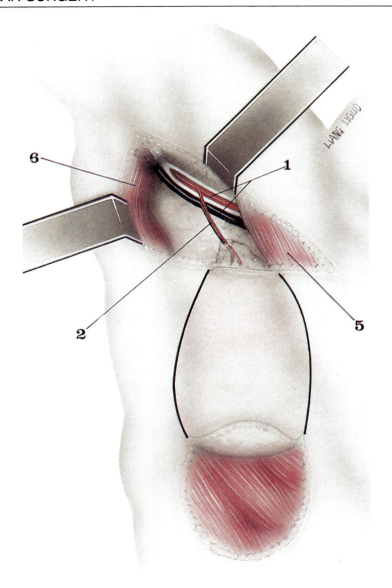

(**Fig. 9-60**) If the accessory lateral thoracic artery is absent or too small, the dissection is carried onto the anterior wall of the axillary fossa, along the lateral edge of the pectoralis major [5], to explore for the cutaneous branch of the lateral thoracic artery [3]. If the cutaneous branch is large enough, the lateral thoracic artery is dissected, and the skin flap is designed a little forward.

1. Axillary a. and v. and brachial plexus
3. Accessory lateral thoracic a. and v.
5. Pectoralis major m.
6. Latissimus dorsi m.

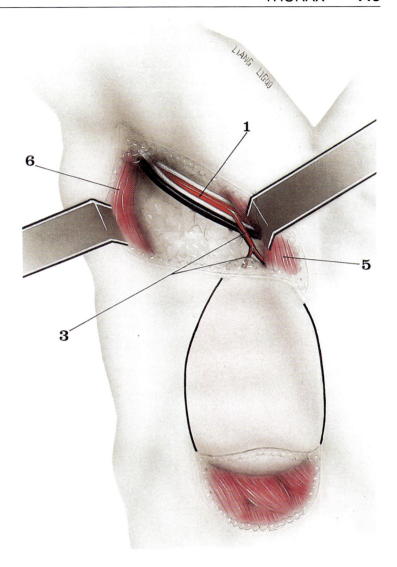

(Fig. 9-61) If both of these arteries are absent or too small, the dissection is turned to the posterior wall of the axillary fossa, along the anterolateral edge of the latissimus dorsi [6], to explore for the cutaneous branch of the thoracodorsal artery [4]. If this branch is sufficient, the thoracodorsal artery [4] is dissected out and the flap is designed somewhat back.

1. Axillary a. and v. and brachial plexus
4. Thoracodorsal a. and v. and their cutaneous branches
5. Pectoralis major m.
6. Latissimus dorsi m.

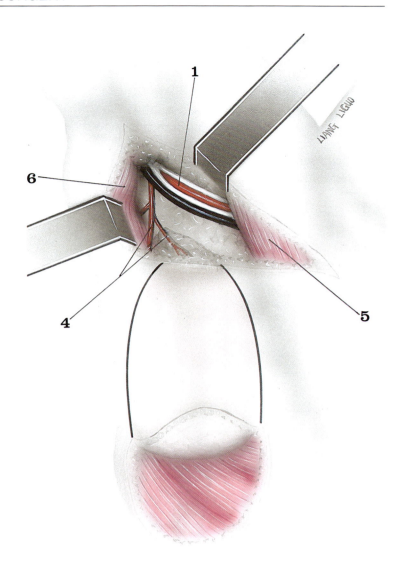

(Fig. 9-62) The lateral thoracic flap is elevated, based on the pedicle of the accessory lateral thoracic artery [2], as an example.

1. Axillary a. and v. and brachial plexus
2. Accessory lateral thoracic a. and v.
5. Pectoralis major m.
6. Latissimus dorsi m.
7. Serratus anterior m.

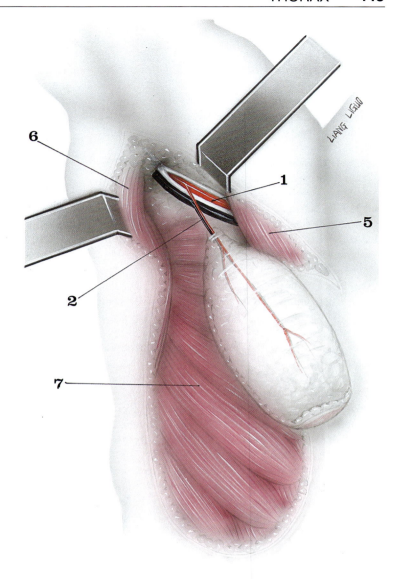

BIBLIOGRAPHY

Pectoralis Major Flap

Ariyan S: Further experiences with the pectoralis major myocutaneous flap for the immediate repair of defects from excisions of head and neck cancers. Plast Reconstr Surg 64:605, 1979.

Baek SM, Lawson W, Biller HF: An analysis of 133 pectoralis major myocutaneous flaps. Plast Reconstr Surg 69:460, 1982.

Bell MSG, Barron PT: The rib-pectoralis major osteomyocutaneous flap. Ann Plast Surg 6:347, 1981.

Clark JMP: Reconstruction of biceps brachii by pectoral muscle transplantation. Br J Surg 34:180, 1946.

Freeman JL, Walker EP, Wilson JSP, Shaw HJ: The vascular anatomy of the pectoralis major myocutaneous flap. Br J Plast Surg 34:3, 1981.

Green MF, Gibson JR, Bryson JR, Thomson E: A one-stage correction of mandibular defects using a split sternum pectoralis major osteomusculocutaneous transfer. Br J Plast Surg 34:11, 1981.

Holtmann B, Wray RC, Lowrey R, Weeks P: Restoration of elbow flexion. Hand 7:256, 1975.

Ikuta Y: Skeletal muscle transplantation in the severely injured upper extremity. In: Serafin D, Buncke HJ (eds): *Microsurgical Composite Tissue Transplantation*. St. Louis: CV Mosby, 1979, pp. 587–604.

Ikuta Y: Microneurovascular transfer of pectoralis major muscle and musculocutaneous flaps. In: Strauch B, Vasconez LO, Hall-Findlay E (eds): *Grabb's Encyclopedia of Flaps*, vol II. Boston: Little, Brown, 1990, pp. 1212–1214.

Lam KH, Wei WI, Siu KF: The pectoralis major costomyocutaneous flap for mandibular reconstruction. Plast Reconstr Surg 73:904, 1984.

Little JW III, McCulloch DT, Lyons JR: The lateral pectoral composite flap in one-stage reconstruction of the irradiated mandible. Plast Reconstr Surg 71:326, 1983.

Manktelow RT: Muscle transplantation. In: Serafin D, Buncke HJ (eds): *Microsurgical Composite Tissue Transplantation*. St. Louis: CV Mosby, 1979, pp. 369–390.

Manktelow RT, McKee NH: An anatomical study of the pectoralis major muscle as related to functioning free muscle transplantation. Plast Reconstr Surg 65:610, 1980.

Manktelow RT, McKee NH: Free muscle transplantation to provide active finger flexion. J Hand Surg 3:416, 1978.

Milroy BC, Korula P: Vascularized innervated transfer of the clavicular head of the pectoralis major muscle in established facial paralysis. Ann Plast Surg 230:75, 1988.

Morain WD, Colen LB, Hitchings JC: The segmental pectoralis major muscle flap: A function-preserving procedure. Plast Reconstr Surg 75:825, 1985.

Morain WD, Geurkink NA: Split pectoralis major myocutaneous flap. Ann Plast Surg 5:358, 1980.

Palmer JH, Batchelor AG: The functional pectoralis major musculocutaneous island flap in head and neck reconstruction. Plast Reconstr Surg 85:363, 1990.

Reid CD, Taylor GI, Waterhouse N: The clavicular head of pectoralis major musculocutaneous free flap. Br J Plast Surg 39:57, 1986.

Reid CD, Taylor GI: The vascular territory of the acromiothoracic axis. Br J Plast Surg 37:194, 1984.

Research Laboratory for Replantation of Severed Limbs, Shanghai Sixth People's Hospital: Free muscle transplantation by microsurgical neurovascular anastomoses: Report of a case. Chin Med J 2:47, 1976.

Sharzer LA, Kalisman M, Silver CE, Strauch B: The parasternal paddle: A modification of the pectoralis major myocutaneous flap. Plast Reconstr Surg 67:753, 1981.

Stepanov VS, Tatyanchenko VK: Surgical anatomy of the musculus pectoralis major. Arkhiv Anatomii, Gistologii i Embriologii (Leningrad) 79:98, 1980.

Tobin GR: Pectoralis major segmental anatomy and segmentally split pectoralis major flaps. Plast Reconstr Surg 75:814, 1985.

Wei WI, Lam KH, Wong J: The true pectoralis major myocutaneous island flap: An anatomical study. Br J Plast Surg 37:568, 1984.

Pectoralis Minor Muscle Flap

Harrison DH: The pectoralis minor vascularized muscle graft for the treatment of unilateral facial palsy. Plast Reconstr Surg 75:206, 1985.

Manstein CH, Manstein G, Somers RG, Barwick WJ: Use of pectoralis minor muscle in immediate reconstruction of the breast. Plast Reconstr Surg 76:566, 1985.

Terzis JK: Pectoralis minor: A unique muscle for correction of facial palsy. Plast Reconstr Surg 83:767, 1989.

Serratus Anterior Flap

Arnold PG, Pairolero PC, Waldorf JC: The serratus anterior muscle: Intrathoracic and extrathoracic utilization. Plast Reconstr Surg 73:240, 1984.

Bartlett SP, May JW Jr, Yaremchuk MJ: The latissimus dorsi muscle: A fresh cadaver study of the primary neurovascular pedicle. Plast Reconstr Surg 67:631, 1981.

Gordon L, Rosen J, Alpert BS, Buncke HJ: Free microvascular transfer of second toe ray and serratus anterior muscle for management of thumb loss at the carpometacarpal joint level. J Hand Surg 9A:642, 1984.

Grotting JC: Microneurovascular free transfer of the serratus anterior muscle. In: Strauch B, Vasconez LO, Hall-Findlay E (eds): *Grabb's Encyclopedia of Flaps*, vol I. Boston: Little, Brown, 1990, pp. 608–612.

Harii K, Yamada A, Ishihara K, Miki Y, Itoh M: A free transfer of both latissimus dorsi and serratus anterior flaps with thoracodorsal vessel anastomoses. Plast Reconstr Surg 70:620, 1982.

Moscona RA, Ullmann Y, Hirshowitz B: Free composite serratus anterior muscle-rib flap for reconstruction of severely damaged foot. Ann Plast Surg 20:167, 1988.

Richards MA, Poole MD, Godfrey AM: The serratus anterior/rib composite flap in mandibular reconstruction. Br J Plast Surg 38:466, 1985.

Takayanagi S, Ohtsuka M, Tsukie T: Use of the latissimus dorsi and the serratus anterior muscles as a combined flap. Ann Plast Surg 20:333, 1988.

Takayanagi S, Tsukie T: Free serratus anterior muscle and myocutaneous flaps. Ann Plast Surg 8:277, 1982.

Revascularized Costal Bone Graft and Intercostal Flap

Ariyan S, Finseth FJ: The anterior chest approach for obtaining free osteocutaneous rib grafts. Plast Reconstr Surg 62:676, 1978.

Badran HA, El-Helaly MS, Safe I: The lateral intercostal neurovascular free flap. Plast Reconstr Surg 73:17, 1984.

Buncke HJ, Furnas DW, Gordon L, Achauer BM: Free osteocutaneous flap from a rib to the tibia. Plast Reconstr Surg 59:799, 1977.

Daniel RK, Kerrigan CL, Gard DA: The great potential of the intercostal flap for torso reconstruction. Plast Reconstr Surg 61:653, 1978.

Harashina T, Nakajima H, Imai T: Reconstruction of mandibular defects with revascularized free rib grafts. Plast Reconstr Surg 62:514, 1978.

Little JW III: The intercostal neurovascular musculocutaneous rib flap. In: Strauch B, Vasconez LO, Hall-Findlay E (eds): *Grabb's Encyclopedia of Flaps*, vol III. Boston: Little, Brown, 1990, chap 318, pp. 1374–1378.

Little JW III, Fontana DJ, McCulloch DT: The upper-quadrant flap. Plast Reconstr Surg 68:175, 1981.

Serafin D, Riefkohl R, Thomas I, Georgiade NG: Vascularized rib-periosteal and osteocutaneous reconstruction of the maxilla and mandible: An assessment. Plast Reconstr Surg 66:718, 1980.

Serafin D, Villarreal-Rios A, Georgiade NG: A rib-containing free flap to reconstruct mandibular defects. Br J Plast Surg 30:263, 1977.

Lateral Thoracic Flap

Baudet J, Garbe JF, Guimberteau JC, Lemaire JM: Axillary flap. In: Serafin D, Buncke HJ (eds): *Microsurgical Composite Tissue Transplantation*. St. Louis: CV Mosby, 1979, pp. 317–335.

Baudet J, Guimberteau JC, Nascimento E: Successful clinical transfer of two free thoraco-dorsal axillary flaps. Plast Reconstr Surg 58:680, 1976.

Cabanie H, Garbe JF, Guimberteau JC: Les bases anatomiques du lambeau axillaire thoracodorsal en vue de son transfert par microchirurgie vasculaire. Anat Clin 2:65, 1979.

Cormack GC, Lamberty BGH: The anatomical vascular basis of the axillary fasciocutaneous pedicled flap. Br J Plast Surg 36:425, 1983.

Harii K, Torii S, Sekiguchi J: The free lateral thoracic flap. Plast Reconstr Surg 62:212, 1978.

Hu BC, Jian JB, Wang LB et al: Surgical anatomy of the free lateral thoracic flap: Providing a new arterial flap (in Chinese). Chin J Surg 19:479, 1981.

Roswell AR, Davies DM, Eisenberg D, Taylor GI: The anatomy of the subscapular-thoracodorsal arterial system: Study of 100 cadaver dissections. Br J Plast Surg 37:574, 1984.

Tolhurst DE, Haeseker B: Fasciocutaneous flaps in the axillary region. Br J Plast Surg 35:430, 1982.

10 ABDOMINAL WALL AND CAVITY

Rectus Abdominis Flap

Anatomy (Fig. 10-1)

The origins of the rectus abdominis muscle [8] are the symphysis pubis and pubic crest. Insertions are at the fifth, sixth, and seventh costal cartilages, interdigitating with the pectoralis major muscle. The rectus abdominis forms an important part of the anterior abdominal wall and flexes the vertebral column. It is a long strap muscle, thickly enclosed by the rectus sheath [6], except for the posterior part below the arcuate line [7] that is usually located midway between the umbilicus and symphysis pubis. The muscle has three tendinous intersections: one at the xiphoid, one at the umbilicus, and one in between. Average muscle length, width, and thickness are 30, 6, and 0.6 cm, respectively.

Blood Supply

The *superior epigastric artery* [3] comes from the internal mammary artery [4] at the level of the sixth intercostal space. It then runs down through the space between the costal and xiphoid origins of the diaphragm, before the lower fibers of the transversus thoracis and the upper fibers of the transversus abdominis. It pierces the sheath of the rectus abdominis lying behind the muscle, then enters it and supplies the muscle and its overlying skin.

The average length of the superior epigastric artery from its origin (the point of bifurcation with the musculophrenic artery [5]) to its entrance to the rectus is about 4.6 cm (range, 3.1 to 6.1 cm). The diameter at its origin is 2.1 mm (range, 1.2 to 3.8 mm), and the diameter at its entrance to the rectus is 1.9 mm (range, 1.2 to 2.6 mm).

The vessel generally has two venae comitantes, the diameter of which is 2.8 mm at the origin (range, 1.8 to 3.9 mm), and 1.3 mm at the muscular entrance (range, 1.1 to 2.6 mm).

The *inferior epigastric artery* [2] arises from the external iliac artery [1] immediately above the inguinal ligament. It then ascends obliquely and medially, penetrating the transversalis fascia, traveling in front of the arcuate line [7], and continuing upward between the rectus abdominis and the posterior wall of its sheath [6]. Generally, it divides into two or three large branches below the level of the umbilicus. These vessels pass upward in the muscle to communicate with the superior epigastric system [3] above the level of the umbilicus.

The average arterial length from its origin to its entrance to the rectus is 10.9 cm (range, 7.1 to 14.7 cm). Vessel diameters at the origin and entrance are, respectively, 2.7 mm (range, 1.6 to 3.5 mm) and 2.0 mm (range, 1.5 to 2.6 mm). The artery has two venae comitantes, the diameter of which is 3.0 mm (range, 1.7 to 3.8 mm) at the origin and 2.2 mm (range, 0.8 to 3.1 mm) at the entrance.

Segmental branches of the deep epigastric system pass upward and outward into the neurovascular plane of the lateral abdominal wall, anastomosing with the lower six intercostal arteries and deep circumflex iliac artery.

ABDOMINAL WALL AND CAVITY

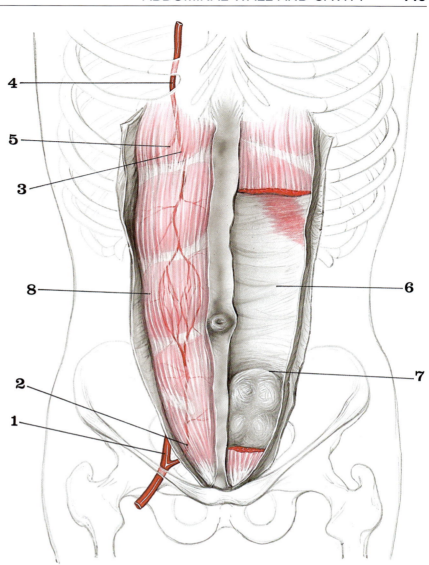

1. External iliac a.
2. Inferior epigastric a.
3. Superior epigastric a.
4. Internal mammary a.
5. Musculophrenic a.
6. Posterior sheath of rectus
7. Arcuate line
8. Rectus abdominis m.

Paraumbilical Perforators [1] (Fig. 10-2)

Many perforating arteries emerge through the anterior rectus sheath, but the highest concentration of major perforators (greater than 0.5 mm in diameter) is in the paraumbilical area. These vessels are terminal cutaneous branches of the inferior epigastric artery. They feed into a subcutaneous vascular network that radiates from the umbilicus like the spokes of a wheel: inferiorly, with the superficial inferior epigastric artery [2]; inferolaterally, with the superficial circumflex iliac artery [4]; and superiorly, with the superficial superior epigastric artery [3]. However, the dominant connections are superolaterally with the lateral cutaneous branches of the intercostal arteries [5]. They also connect with each other across the midline.

Innervation

The rectus abdominis is supplied by the ventral rami of the lower six or seven segmental thoracic spinal nerves [6].

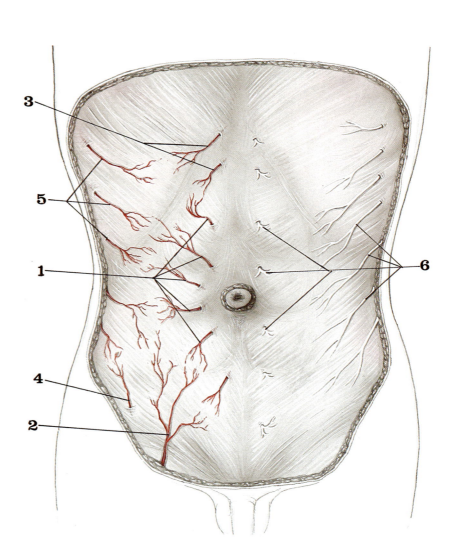

1. Paraumbilical perforator
2. Superficial inferior epigastric a.
3. Superficial superior epigastric a.
4. Superficial circumflex iliac a.
5. Lateral cutaneous branches of intercostal a.
6. Segmental thoracic spinal n.

COMMENT AND INSIGHTS

Use of the rectus abdominis muscle and musculocutaneous flap, based on the deep inferior epigastric vessels, has been a popular and acceptable procedure. The vascular pedicle is quite constant, reliable, and anatomically long, with large-sized vessels. Elevation of the flap and microvascular repair at a distant site are easily and rapidly accomplished.

Since the arterial system of the rectus abdominis has extensive circulatory connections with some of the circumferential arteries in the abdomen (e.g., intercostal arteries), the size and shape of the flap can be varied to suit any number of recipient site requirements. Abundant tissue is available. Subcutaneous tissue tends to be thicker, especially in obese patients; however, on the lateral thorax in a thoracoumbilical flap, it tends to be of moderate thickness.

The entire rectus abdominis muscle can survive on either superior or inferior pedicles. Nevertheless, the deep inferior epigastric artery has certain advantages over the superior epigastric artery: it is a larger vessel with a longer pedicle; the cutaneous vascular territory is greater; and it gives rise to the paraumbilical perforators, rather than merely connecting with them via a system of reduced caliber vessels within the rectus muscle. Taking these facts into account, the free transfer of the rectus abdominis is generally based on the inferior epigastric vessels. A flap based on the superior vessels can be used for more local transfer, e.g., in breast reconstruction.

The rectus muscle flap is generally used for wound coverage, rather than for functional reconstruction. The skin flap is not sensate because of multisegmental innervation.

Taking the rectus muscle and its anterior sheath can result in some weakness of the abdominal wall and may possibly cause abdominal herniation. For this reason, the resultant defect should be very carefully repaired, especially below the arcuate line.

RECTUS ABDOMINIS MUSCLE FLAP (Based on the Inferior Epigastric Vessels)

(**Fig. 10-3**) A paramedian incision is made; the lower part of an incision below the level midway between the umbilicus and symphysis pubis runs laterally down to the midpoint of the inguinal ligament.

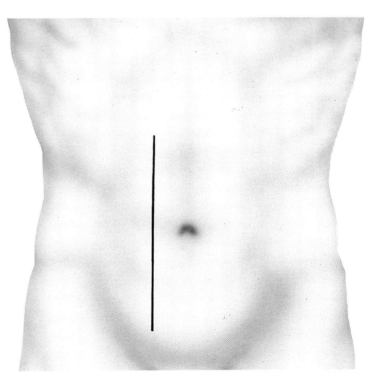

1. Rectus abdominis m.
2. Sheath of rectus
3. Inferior epigastric a.
4. Arcuate line

(Fig. 10-4) The skin, fascia, and anterior sheath [2] are incised, and the anterior surface of the rectus abdominis [1] is exposed.

1. Rectus abdominis m.
2. Sheath of rectus

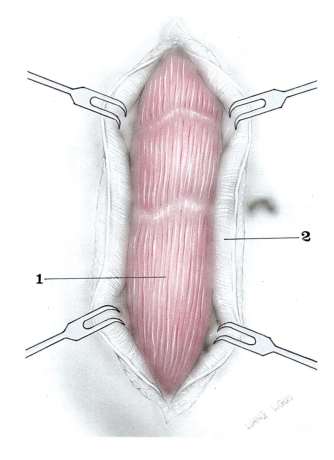

(Fig. 10-5) The inferior epigastric vascular bundle [3] is identified at the lateral border of the lower part of the muscle above the pubic tubercle. The origin on the symphysis pubis and pubic crest is detached.

1. Rectus abdominis m.
2. Sheath of rectus
3. Inferior epigastric a.
4. Arcuate line

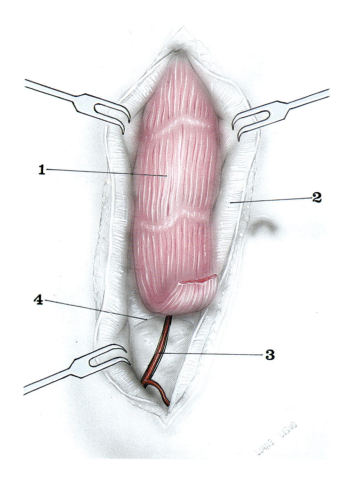

(Fig. 10-6) The rectus abdominis muscle [1] is separated from the posterior sheath. It can be divided at any tendinous intersection, even on its insertion, if necessary. After further dissection, the length of the vascular pedicle [3] can reach approximately 10 cm. The anterior sheath should be meticulously sutured after transfer of the muscle flap.

1. Rectus abdominis m.
2. Sheath of rectus
3. Inferior epigastric a.
4. Arcuate line

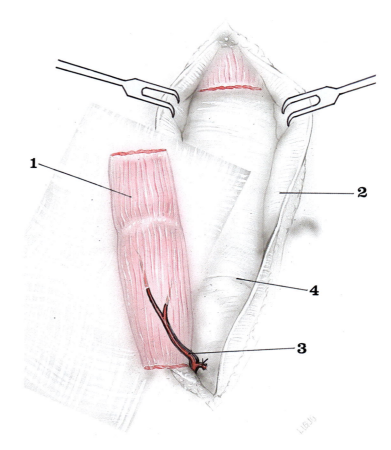

RECTUS ABDOMINIS MYOCUTANEOUS FLAP (Based on the Inferior Epigastric Vessels)

(Fig. 10-7) The base of the skin area of this flap is the rectus abdominis muscle, and the center of the base is the paraumbilical area within 3 to 5 cm of the umbilicus. Owing to the abundant interconnected circulation previously described, the flap on the base can be extended over the muscle area, even across the midline, to at least the lateral border of the opposite rectus muscle. The flap can be designed either transversely, obliquely, or vertically, on either the upper or lower abdomen.

Type A. Vertical rectus abdominis myocutaneous flap. The procedure is fairly similar to the muscle flap.

Type B. Lower transverse rectus abdominis myocutaneous flap (lower TRAM flap). The procedure will be described in detail later.

Type C. Middle transverse rectus abdominis myocutaneous flap (middle TRAM flap). The umbilicus is left in situ.

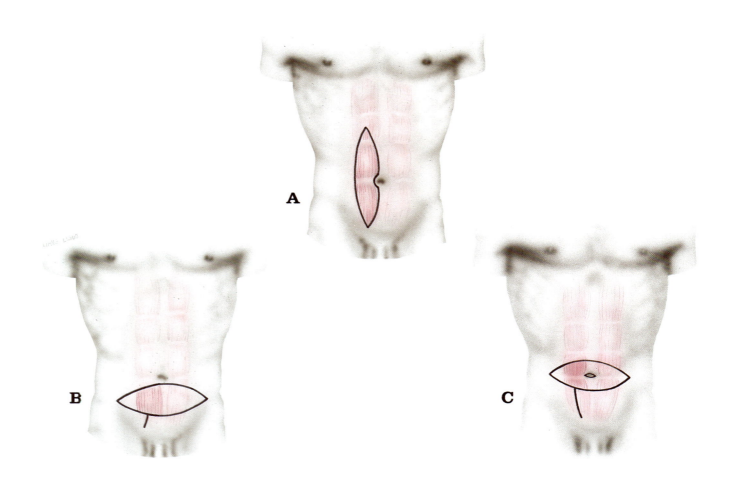

Type D. Thoracoumbilical flap (extended deep inferior epigastric flap). The procedure will be described in detail later.

Type E. Thoracoumbilical and vertical combined myocutaneous flap.

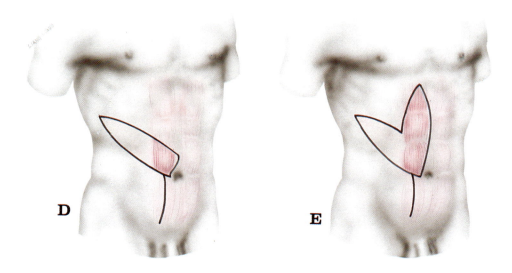

LOWER TRANSVERSE RECTUS ABDOMINIS MYOCUTANEOUS FLAP

For drawing the design of the lower TRAM flap, refer to type B of the rectus abdominis myocutaneous flaps (see Fig. 10-7).

The skin territory of the flap is defined below the umbilicus, above the inguinal ligament, and not extending to the anterosuperior iliac spines. Its maximum area may be 30 × 20 cm.

(Fig. 10-8) The skin flap is incised to the deep areolar fascia or sheath of the rectus [2]. Both lateral edges of the flap are raised, preserving the fascial layer on the undersurface of subcutaneous fat. Dissection proceeds medially to both borders of the carrier rectus muscle [1]. The anterior sheath [2] beneath the skin flap is incorporated into the flap, and several tacking stitches are applied at the edges, to prevent shearing of the musculocutaneous perforators.

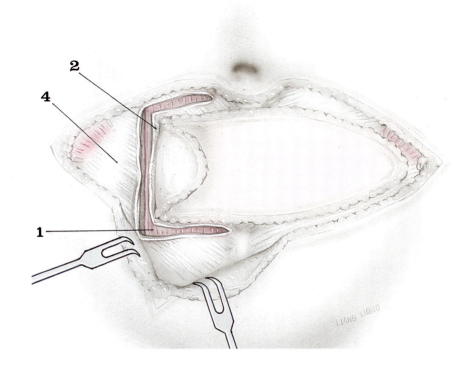

1. Rectus abdominis m.
2. Sheath of rectus
3. Inferior epigastric a.
4. External oblique m.
5. Synthetic mesh (Gor-Tex)

(Fig. 10-9) The rectus muscle [1] inferior to the skin flap is exposed, and the inferior epigastric vessels [3] are identified and dissected at the lateral border of the rectus above the pubic tubercle. The muscle is divided over the superior edge of the skin flap.

1. Rectus abdominis m.
2. Sheath of rectus
3. Inferior epigastric a.

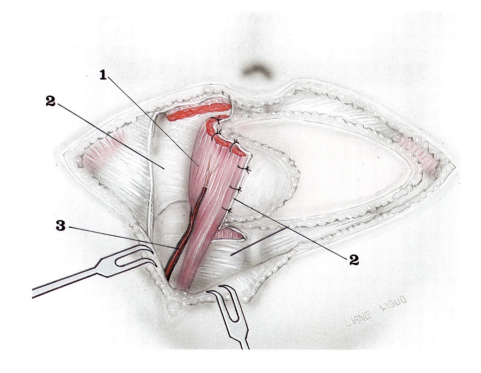

(**Fig. 10-10**) The muscle is divided along the lower border of the skin flap, with care to protect the inferior epigastric vessels. The flap is elevated after separating it from the posterior sheath [2].

1. Rectus abdominis m.
2. Sheath of rectus
3. Inferior epigastric a.

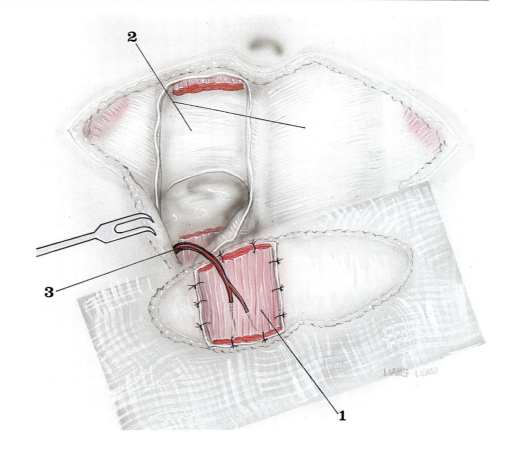

(**Fig. 10-11**) To prevent herniation at the donor site, the defect in the anterior sheath should be repaired with synthetic mesh [5] such as Gor-Tex, Mersilene, Prolene, Marlex, or nylon.

5. Synthetic mesh (Gore-Tex)

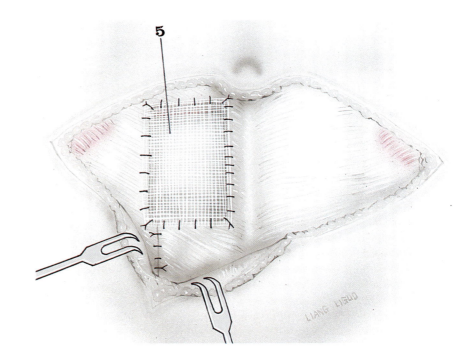

Note: The lower TRAM flap based on the superior epigastric vessels is commonly applied in breast reconstruction by local transfer.

MODIFIED LOWER TRAM FLAP

Because the major paraumbilical perforators are located in the medial two thirds of the rectus muscle, the lateral third of the rectus muscle and its anterior sheath can be saved in situ without damage of the circulation of the inferior TRAM flap. The defect can be closed directly, allowing for a more adequate closure.

(Fig. 10-12) Leaving the lateral third of the muscle and sheath in situ, the medial portion [1] is divided superiorly and then turned inferiorly to identify the vascular pedicle [3].

1. Rectus abdominis m.
2. Sheath of rectus
3. Inferior epigastric a.
4. External oblique m.

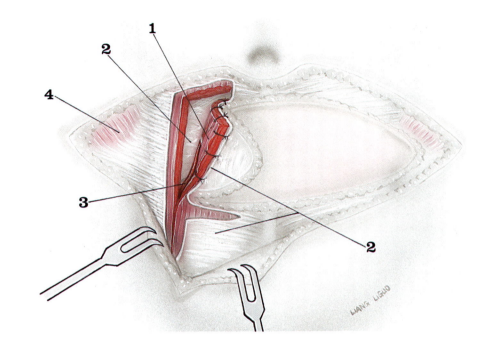

(Fig. 10-13) The pedicle of the inferior epigastric vessels [3] is isolated. The medial portion of the muscle [1] is divided at about 8 cm from the upper cut portion. The modified lower TRAM flap is raised.

1. Rectus abdominis m.
2. Sheath of rectus
3. Inferior epigastric a.

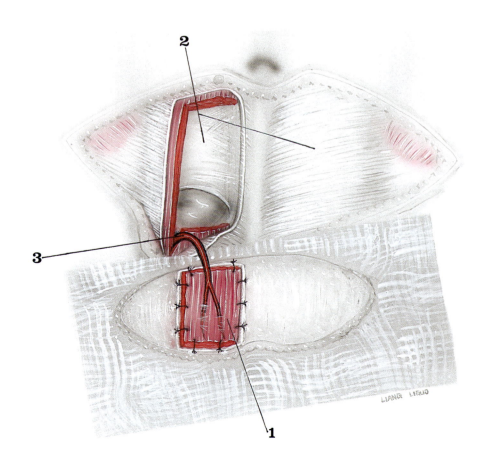

THORACOUMBILICAL FLAP

The extended deep inferior epigastric flap is designed on an axis between the umbilicus and the inferior angle of the scapula. Its medial edge is placed on or over the midline, running upward and laterally as far as the midaxillary line or even the posterior axillary line. Flap width ranges from 8 to 20 cm.

For drawing the design of the flap, see type D of the rectus abdominis myocutaneous flaps (Fig. 10-7).

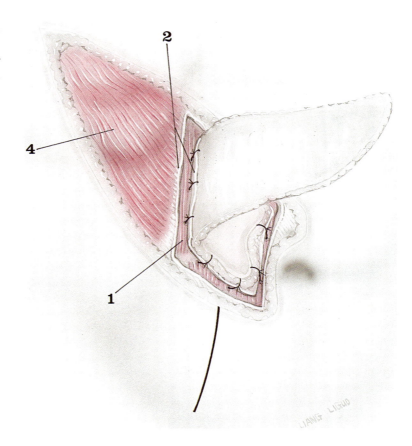

(Fig. 10-14) The lateral part of the flap is raised from the chest wall and external oblique muscle [4] up to the lateral edge of the rectus muscle [1]. The fascial areolar layer on the undersurface of the subcutaneous flap is preserved in the flap.

A disc of the anterior sheath [2] through which the paraumbilical perforators emerge is incised along the upper and lower borders of the skin flap and beside the midline and lateral edge of the rectus muscle, leaving 0.5 to 1.0 cm fringes on the medial and lateral borders for later repair. Care should be taken to keep this disc with both muscle and skin flap intact, and not to damage the perforators between them. It is advisable that several tacking stitches be made immediately after the disc of anterior sheath is created.

1. Rectus abdominis m.
2. Sheath of rectus
3. Inferior epigastric a.
4. External oblique m.

(Fig. 10-15) A paramedian incision on the lower part of the rectus is used to expose the muscle [1] and to identify the inferior epigastric vessels [3]. The rectus muscle [1] is divided along the upper border of the flap and dissected down from its posterior wall.

1. Rectus abdominis m.
2. Sheath of rectus
3. Inferior epigastric a.
4. External oblique m.

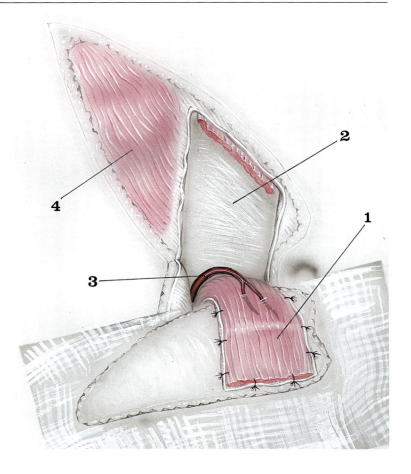

(**Fig. 10-16**) The muscle [1] can be retained in the vascular pedicle [3], with its origin detached from the pubis, or separated from the vascular stalk for a distance necessary to avoid bulkiness. The first method is simple, rapid, and safe. The defect of the anterior sheath superior to the arcuate line does not require repair.

1. Rectus abdominis m.
2. Sheath of rectus
3. Inferior epigastric a.
4. External oblique m.

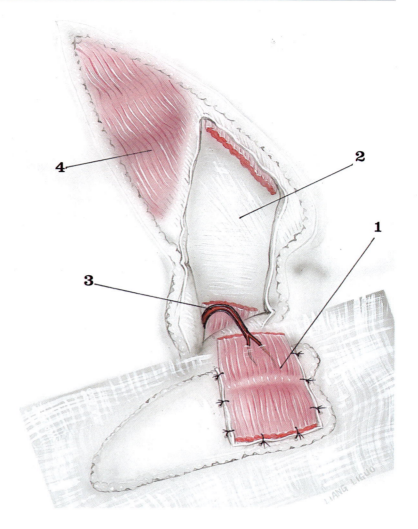

Greater Omentum Transfer

Anatomy (Fig. 10-17)

The largest peritoneal fold of the omentum is composed of four layers. It always contains some adipose tissue that is present in considerable quantity in obese patients. The two layers that descend from the stomach [1] and beginning of the duodenum pass downward in front of the small intestine for a variable distance. They then fold over and ascend as far as the anterosuperior aspect of the transverse colon. The function of the omentum is to limit the spread of infection in the peritoneal cavity.

Size

	Males		Females	
	Average (cm)	Range (cm)	Average (cm)	Range (cm)
Length	25	14–36	24	14–34
Width	35	23–46	33	20–46

Blood Supply

The *right and left gastroepiploic arteries* [6,5] are the terminal branches of the gastroduodenal and splenic arteries [3,4], respectively. They course along the greater curvature of the stomach [1] and anastomose with each other, forming the *gastroepiploic arterial arch* [7] that lies about a fingerbreadth from the greater curvature between its anterior two layers.

From the gastroepiploic arterial arch [7], several short branches arise upward to the greater curvature of the stomach, and the three major *omental arteries* (*right* [9], *middle* [10], and *left* [11]) go downward to the greater omentum. The middle omental artery [10] at its terminal portion branches into right and left terminal segments that anastomose with the corresponding branches of the right and left omental arteries [9,11] to form the arterial network of the great omentum. On the right side, there is an accessory omental artery [8] that branches from the right gastroepiploic artery and does not join the arterial network.

The right gastroepiploic artery is the dominant vessel.

Diameter (mm)

	Right Gastroepiploic		Left Gastroepiploic	
	Artery	Vein	Artery	Vein
Average	2.8	3.2	1.8	2.4
Range	1.5–4.5	1.5–4.5	1.0–3.0	1.0–4.5

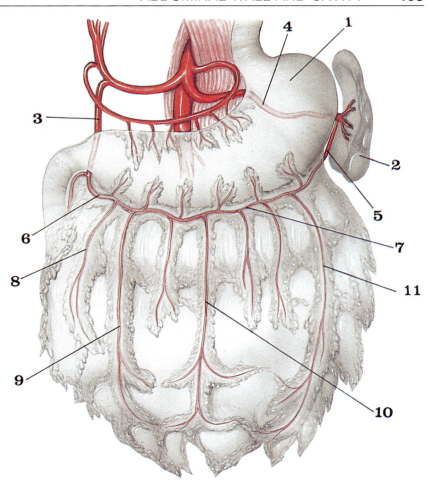

1. Stomach
2. Spleen
3. Gastroduodenal a.
4. Splenic a.
5. Left gastroepiploic a.
6. Right gastroepiploic a.
7. Gastroepiploic arterial arch
8. Accessory omental a.
9. Right omental a.
10. Middle omental a.
11. Left omental a.

COMMENT AND INSIGHTS

The greater omentum has an abundant blood supply and lymphatic circulation. It therefore can eliminate or limit infection and, when used as a donor, can improve circulation at the recipient site, as in the treatment of radionecrotic lesion. A large amount of soft tissue is available and sizeable defects can be reconstructed. A single procedure using a split-thickness skin graft to cover the transfer is also possible. In addition, the omental transfer is especially useful in filling depressed areas such as occur in hemifacial microsomia. With a clear and constant anatomy, harvesting is easy and an excellent vascular pedicle allows facile transfer with microsurgical techniques. Postoperative atrophy of the transplanted omentum is not a usual expectation.

The compound flap of stomach and omentum provides a vascularized tube with a plenitude of soft tissue, especially useful in reconstructing pharyngoesophageal defects with heavily irradiated surrounding tissue. Removal of the gastric flap may reduce the stomach to a diameter of 2.5 cm, but without functional consequences. Still, the acid secretion of the gastric flap may irritate the lower esophagus.

Despite its advantages, use of the omentum may not be a first choice. Laparotomy can lead to complications such as peritonitis, adhesion, or even volvulus. On occasion, the omentum may not incorporate with recipient soft tissue; several pull-out bolster sutures are advisable in augmentation procedures, to prevent gravitational pull from moving the transfer. Other contraindications are a history of abdominal disease or previous abdominal surgery.

FREE OMENTUM TRANSFER

(Fig. 10-18) An upper middle abdominal incision is made.

1. Transverse colon
2. Stomach
3. Small intestine
4. Right gastroepiploic a.
5. Left gastroepiploic a.
6. Accessory omental a.
7. Right omental a.
8. Middle omental a.
9. Left omental a.

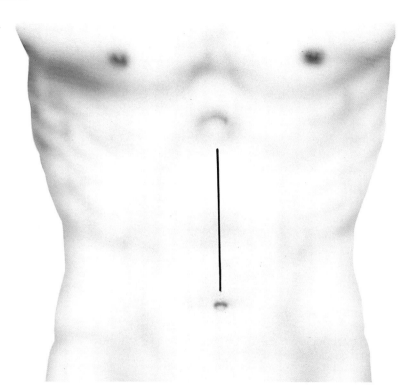

(Fig. 10-19) The greater omentum is delivered from the abdominal cavity, and the stomach [2] and right and left gastroepiploic vessels [4,5] are identified.

2. Stomach
4. Right gastroepiploic a.
5. Left gastroepiploic a.
6. Accessory omental a.
7. Right omental a.
8. Middle omental a.
9. Left omental a.

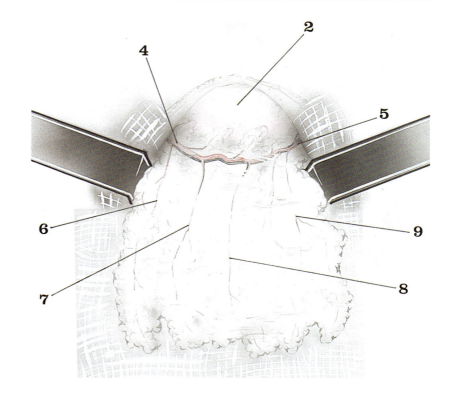

(Fig. 10-20) All the short branches from the gastroepiploic arterial arch to the greater curvature of the stomach [2] are ligated and divided. The omentum is separated from the transverse colon [1] in an avascular plane.

1. Transverse colon
2. Stomach
3. Small intestine
4. Right gastroepiploic a.
5. Left gastroepiploic a.
6. Accessory omental a.
7. Right omental a.
8. Middle omental a.
9. Left omental a.

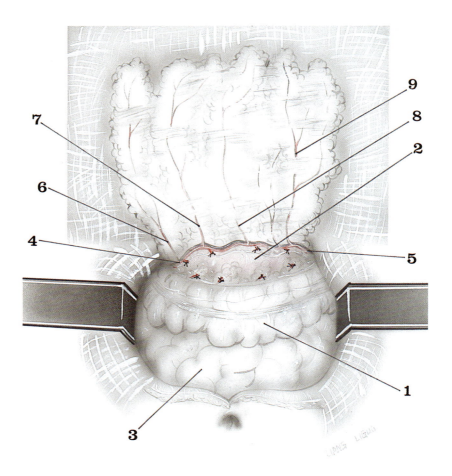

(Fig. 10-21) The left gastroepiploic vessels [5] are ligated, and an omental flap is isolated on the right gastroepiploic vessels [4] with a pedicle length of 9 to 12 cm.

1. Transverse colon
2. Stomach
3. Small intestine
4. Right gastroepiploic a.
5. Left gastroepiploic a.

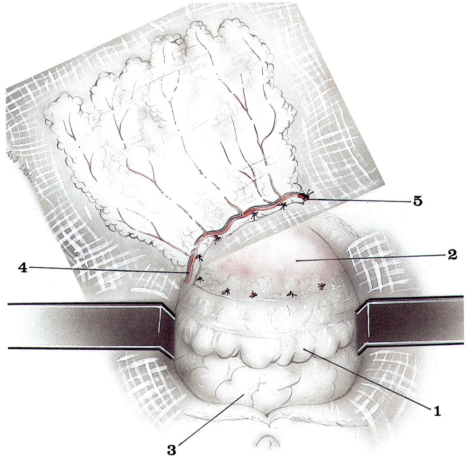

EXTENDING GREATER OMENTUM

(Fig. 10-22) If it is necessary to cover a long defect at the recipient site, or for local transfer, omental length can be extended using the following technique.

The gastroepiploic arterial arch [5] is ligated and divided between the origins of the right and middle omental arteries [6,7]. The middle omental artery [7] is ligated and divided at a point before it gives off the right and left terminal branches.

1. Stomach
2. Right gastroepiploic a.
3. Accessory omental a.
4. Left gastroepiploic a.
5. Gastroepiploic arterial arch
6. Right omental a.
7. Middle omental a.
8. Left omental a.

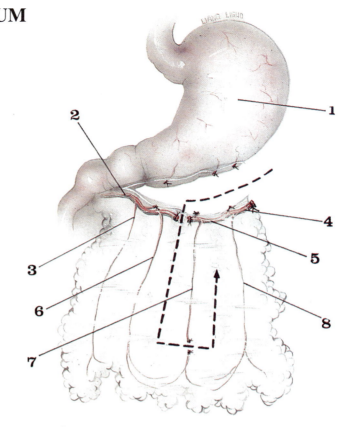

(Fig. 10-23) Referring to the arrow line in Figure 10-22, omental length can be increased without damage to the blood supply.

2. Right gastroepiploic a.
4. Left gastroepiploic a.
5. Gastroepiploic arterial arch
7. Middle omental a.
8. Left omental a.

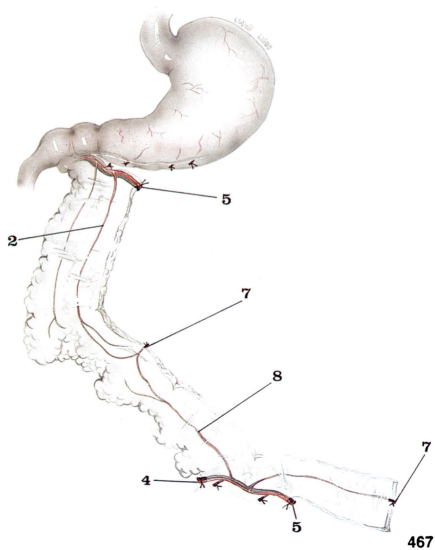

COMPOSITE FLAP OF STOMACH AND OMENTUM

(Fig. 10-24) The greater omentum [7] is separated from the transverse colon [1] and mesocolon, and the left gastroepiploic vessel [5] is ligated. The posterior wall of the stomach [3] is exposed.

1. Colon
2. Small intestine
3. Stomach
4. Right gastroepiploic a.
5. Left gastroepiploic a.
6. Lesser sac
7. Greater omentum
8. Omental a.
9. Gastroepiploic arterial arch

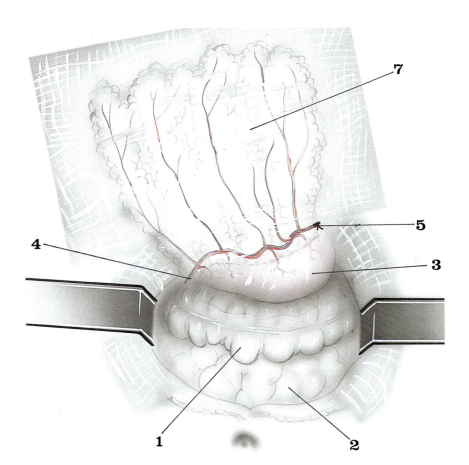

ABDOMINAL WALL AND CAVITY 469

(Fig. 10-25) The above procedure is diagrammed in cross-section.

1. Colon
3. Stomach
6. Lesser sac
7. Greater omentum
8. Omental a.
9. Gastroepiploic arterial arch

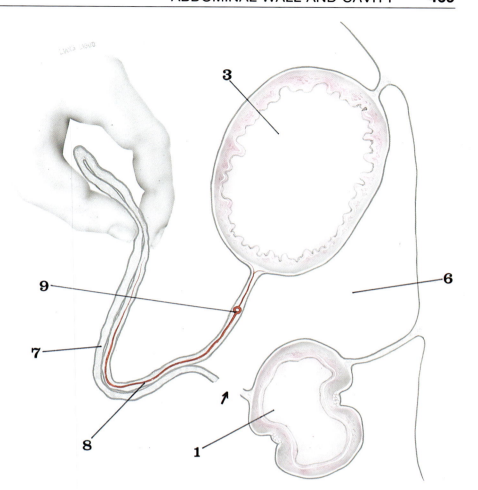

(Fig. 10-26) The right gastroepiploic vessel [4] is isolated, and the stomach [3] clamped on the body and fundus, parallel to the greater curvature. The distance between the edge of the curvature and the clamp is 4 cm. The largest available dimensions of the stomach flap are about 13 cm in length and 8 cm in width.

3. Stomach
4. Right gastroepiploic a.
7. Greater omentum
9. Gastroepiploic arterial arch

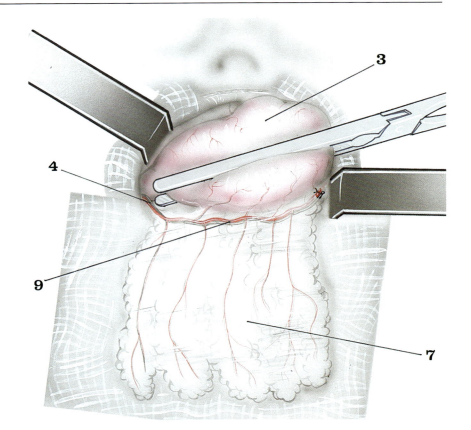

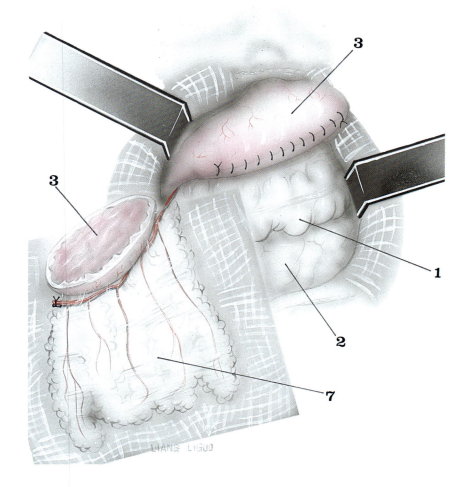

(Fig. 10-27) The gastric flap [3] is excised in continuity with the greater omentum [7], preserving the short gastric vessels that supply the flap at this level. The stomach is closed in two layers with deep interrupted extramucosal sutures and running superficial sutures.

1. Colon
2. Small intestine
3. Stomach
7. Greater omentum

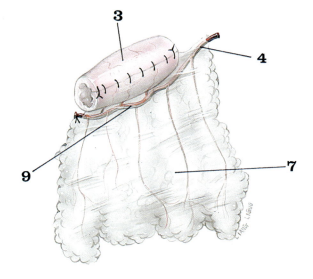

(Fig. 10-28) The flap is immersed in a chilled heparinized solution and is stitched into a tube before transfer to the recipient site.

3. Stomach
4. Right gastroepiploic a.
7. Greater omentum
9. Gastroepiploic arterial arch

Free Jejunum Transfer

Anatomy (Fig. 10-29)

The duodenal jejunal flexure is located to the left of the aorta at the level of the upper border of the second lumbar vertebra. It is fixed by a fibromuscular band, termed the "ligament of Treitz," that arises from the right crus of the diaphragm, close to the right side of the esophagus. The jejunum comprises the first two fifths of the 7 m length from the duodenal jejunal flexure to the ileocecal valve. Jejunal diameter is about 4 cm.

The mesentery is fan-shaped and its vertebral root is about 15 cm long. It is attached to the posterior abdominal wall along a line running from the left side of the second lumbar vertebral body to the right sacroiliac joint. The average width from the vertebral to the intestinal border is about 20 cm, but widest in the middle.

Blood Supply

There are an average of five jejunal branches [7] from the superior mesenteric artery [6], with a total of about 12 to 15 branches to the jejunum and ileum [2]. They run almost parallel to one another between the mesenteric layers, each vessel dividing into two, that unite with adjacent branches to form a series of arcades [8]. From the terminal arcade, numerous vasa recta [9] pass to the mesenteric border of the jejunum. Usually, the upper portion of the jejunum contains a single arcade giving off long vasa recta; the lower portion contains two to three arcades giving off shorter vasa recta; and the terminal ileum contains four arcades giving off much shorter vasa recta.

The first intestinal branch is usually not selected as a vascular pedicle for the following reasons. As a variation, it frequently has a common stem with the inferior pancreatic duodenal artery. The pedicle length is short and its origin much too high and deep. Also, the length of the intestinal segment it supplies is short and sometimes lacks an arcade.

The second, third, and fourth intestinal branches are preferred choices, and the most common choice is the second.

Measurement of Intestinal Branches of Superior Mesenteric Vessels

		Intestinal branches			
		#1	*#2*	*#3*	*#4*
Average diameter (mm)	Artery	3.5	3.8	4.0	4.3
	Vein	5.0	5.0	5.0	5.0
Length of pedicle		25 cm	36 cm	4.5 cm	4.2 mm
Average no. arcades		1.5	2.4	2.7	3.2
Length of intestinal segment supplied (cm)		37	53	60	100

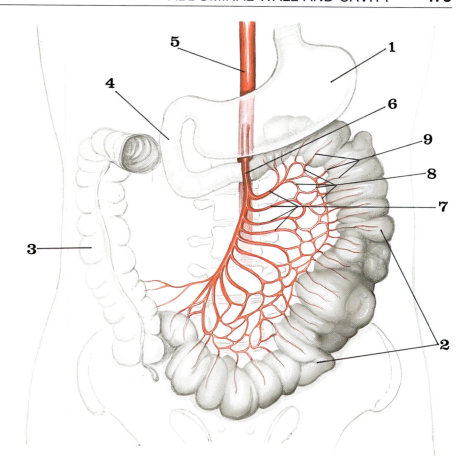

1. Stomach
2. Small intestine (jejunum and ileum)
3. Colon
4. Duodenum
5. Aorta
6. Superior mesenteric a.
7. Jejunal branch
8. Arterial arcade
9. Vasa recta

COMMENT AND INSIGHTS

The main application of free jejunum transfer remains the reconstruction of defects following extensive excision of the hypopharynx and cervical esophagus, as well as the replacement of oral mucosa. The removal of a jejunal segment does not affect digestive or absorbent functions.

Earlier reports endorsed the application of free ileum, colon, or gastric antrum for reconstruction of conduits in the hypopharynx and esophagus. However, these procedures have lost favor because the removal of ileum may result in a malabsorption syndrome. In addition, the dimensions of the colon and gastric antrum are too large to match the esophagus, and there is also a higher risk in colon surgery.

With the use of the free jejunum transfer, complications following laparotomy may include peritonitis or adhesions, among other sequelae. Contamination should be stringently avoided throughout the procedure. Needless to emphasize, the clinician should be well experienced in all aspects of abdominal surgery.

474 ATLAS OF MICROVASCULAR SURGERY

Harvesting Technique

(**Fig. 10-30**) Depending on the surgeon's preference, an upper midline incision is made, or a paramedian or transverse incision may be used.

1. Jejunum
2. Duodenal jejunal flexure
3. First jejunal branch
4. Second jejunal branch
5. Third jejunal branch

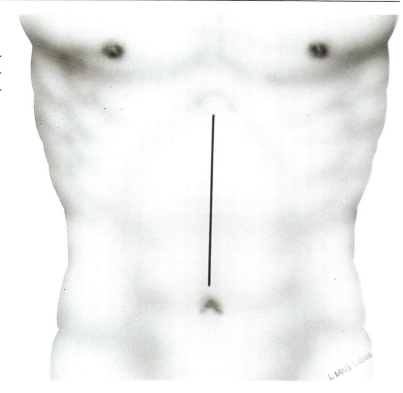

(**Fig. 10-31**) The abdomen is entered, the upper part of the small intestine is delivered, and the duodenal jejunal flexure [2] is identified. The intestinal branches [3,4,5] of the superior mesenteric vessels are carefully inspected, and the second intestinal branch [4], with its arcades and vasa recta, is identified and evaluated.

1. Jejunum
2. Duodenal jejunal flexure
3. First jejunal branch
4. Second jejunal branch
5. Third jejunal branch

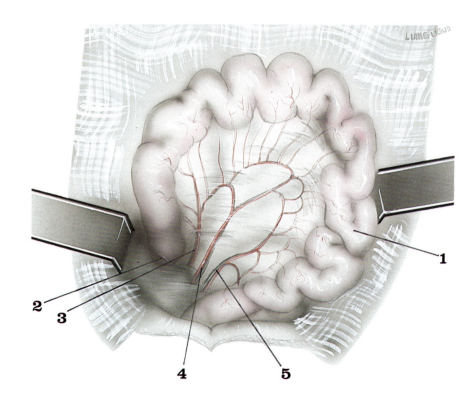

(Fig. 10-32) Depending on the main distribution of the second intestinal branch [4] and recipient site requirements, 10 to 20 cm or more of jejunum [1] can be harvested. The jejunum is emptied manually.

1. Jejunum
2. Duodenal jejunal flexure
3. First jejunal branch
4. Second jejunal branch
5. Third jejunal branch

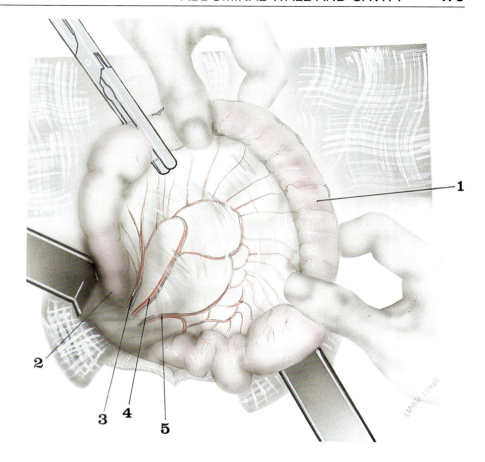

(Fig. 10-33) Intestinal clamps are applied to both sides of the jejunal segment [1] and it is divided. The mesentery is separated between the vasa recta and between the first, second, and third intestinal branches [3,4,5]. The arcades beyond the jejunal segment are ligated. The vascular pedicle can be dissected up to its origin at the superior mesenteric artery.

1. Jejunum
2. Duodenal jejunal flexure
3. First jejunal branch
4. Second jejunal branch
5. Third jejunal branch

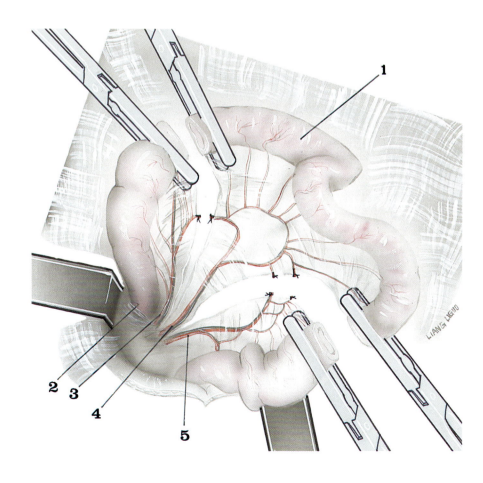

(Fig. 10-34) The free jejunal segment [1] is then bathed in saline slush solution for 5 to 10 minutes before transfer to the recipient site. Intestinal continuity is restored with an end-to-end jejunal anastomosis.

1. Jejunum
4. Second jejunal branch

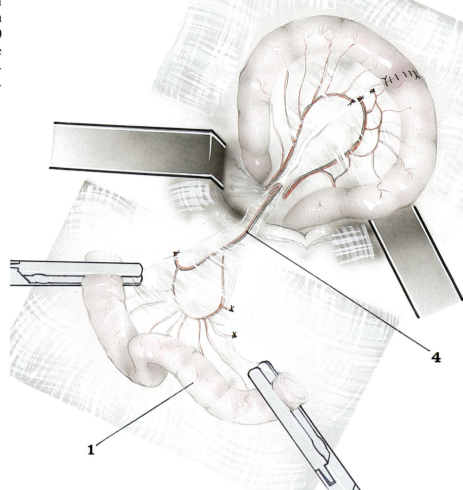

Note. The proximal end of the jejunal segment should be marked to ensure isoperistaltic anastomosis at the recipient site and to avoid regurgitation. Also, only the antimesenteric border can be incised for enlarging the proximal stoma of the jejunal segment, in order to reconstruct a pharyngeal defect or to create a free intestinal patch to replace intraoral lining.

RECIPIENT SITE EXPOSURES

Inferior Epigastric Artery

(Fig. 10-35) A paramedian incision below the umbilical level is made, extending inferomedially to the pubic symphysis.

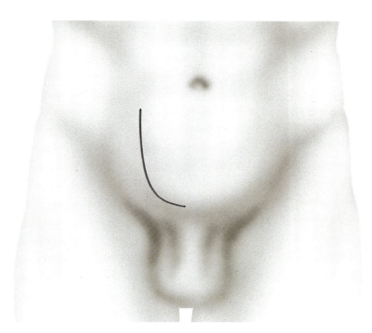

1. Oblique abdominis (aponeurosis and muscle)
2. Rectus sheath
3. Spermatic cord
4. Rectus abdominis m.
5. Inferior epigastric a. and v.
6. Arcuate line
7. External iliac a. and v.

(Fig. 10-36) The anterior sheath [2] of the rectus abdominis and aponeurosis of the oblique abdominis [1] are identified. Care should be taken not to injure the spermatic cord [3] in the lower part of the incision.

1. Oblique abdominis (aponeurosis and muscle)
2. Rectus sheath
3. Spermatic cord

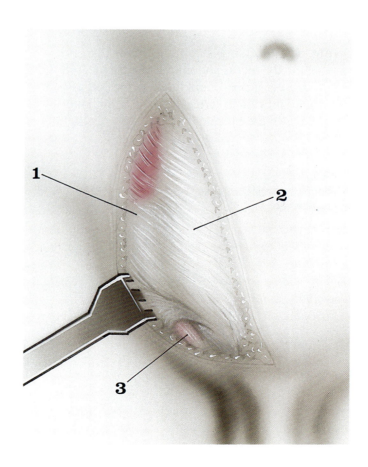

(Fig. 10-37) The anterior wall of the rectus sheath [2] is divided longitudinally near its lateral border, and the rectus abdominis [4] and its lateral edge are then exposed.

1. Oblique abdominis (aponeurosis and muscle)
2. Rectus sheath
4. Rectus abdominis m.

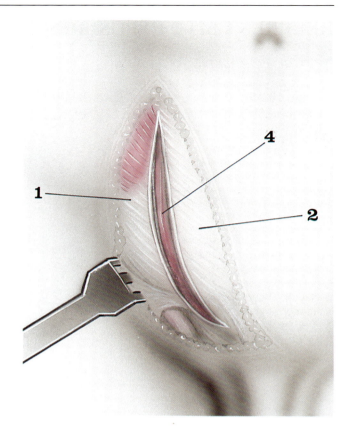

(Fig. 10-38) Using sharp and blunt dissection behind the rectus abdominis muscle [4], its lateral edge is flipped, and the inferior epigastric artery and vein [5] are visualized behind the lower edge of the muscle.

4. Rectus abdominis m.
5. Inferior epigastric a. and v.
6. Arcuate line

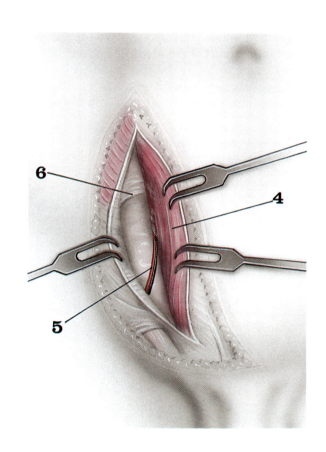

(Fig. 10-39) The inferior epigastric vessels [5] are dissected to their origin from the external iliac vessels [7].

4. Rectus abdominis m.
5. Inferior epigastric a. and v.
7. External iliac a. and v.

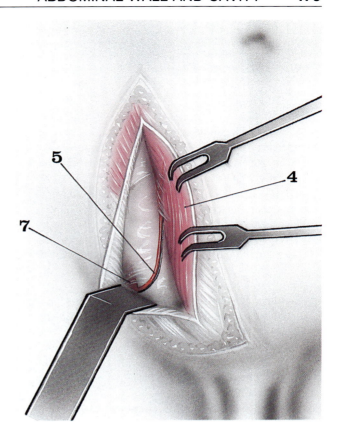

BIBLIOGRAPHY

Rectus Abdominis Flap

Arnez SM, Bajec J, Bardsley AF, et al: Experience with 50 free TRAM flap breast reconstructions. Plast Reconstr Surg 87:470, 1991.

Boyd JB, Taylor GI, Corlett R: The vascular territories of the superior epigastric and the deep inferior epigastric systems. Plast Reconstr Surg 73:1, 1984.

Brown RG, Vasconez LO, Jurkiewicz MJ: Transverse abdominal flaps and the deep epigastric arcade. Plast Reconstr Surg 55:416, 1975.

Bunkis J, Walton RL, Mathes SJ, Krizek TJ, Vasconez LO: Experience with the transverse lower rectus abdominis operation for breast reconstruction. Plast Reconstr Surg 72:819, 1983.

De la Plaza R, Arroyo JM, Vasconez LO: Upper transverse rectus abdominis flap: The flag flap. Ann Plast Surg 12:411, 1984.

Drever JM, Hodson-Walker N: Closure of the donor defect for breast reconstruction with rectus abdominis myocutaneous flaps. Plast Reconstr Surg 76:558, 1985.

Ebihara H, Maruyama Y: Free abdominal flaps: Variations in design and application to soft tissue defects of the head. J Reconstr Microsurg 5:193, 1989.

Friedman RJ, Argenta LC, Anderson R: Deep inferior epigastric free flap for breast reconstruction after radical mastectomy: Case report. Plast Reconstr Surg 76:455, 1985.

Gandolfo EA: Breast reconstruction with a lower abdominal myocutaneous flap. Br J Plast Surg 25:452, 1982.

Gottlieb ME, Chandrasekhar B, Terz JJ, Sherman R: Clinical applications of the extended deep inferior epigastric flap. Plast Reconstr Surg 78:782, 1986.

Holmstrom H: The free abdominoplasty flap and its use in breast reconstruction: An experimental study and clinical case report. Scand J Plast Reconstr Surg 13:423, 1979.

Jones NF, Sekhar LN, Schramm VL: Free rectus abdominis muscle flap reconstruction of the middle and posterior cranial base. Plast Reconstr Surg 78:471, 1986.

Logan SE, Mathes SJ: The use of a rectus abdominis myocutaneous flap to reconstruct a groin defect. Br J Plast Surg 37:351, 1984.

Mathes SJ, Bostwick J III: A rectus abdominis myocutaneous flap to reconstruct abdominal wall defects. Br J Plast Surg 30:282, 1977.

Mixter RC, Wood WA, Dibbell DG Sr: Retroperitoneal transposition of rectus abdominis myocutaneous flaps to the perineum and back: Case report. Plast Reconstr Surg 85:437, 1990.

Miyamoto Y, Harada K, Kodama Y, Takahashi H, Okano S: Cranial coverage involving scalp, bone and dura using free inferior epigastric flap. Br J Plast Surg 39:483, 1986.

Pennington DG, Pelly AD: The rectus abdominis myocutaneous free flap. Br J Plast Surg 33:277, 1980.

Stevenson TR, Hester TR, Duus EC, Dingman RO: The superficial inferior epigastric artery flap for coverage of hand and forearm defects. Ann Plast Surg 12:333, 1984.

Tai Y, Hasegawa H: A transverse abdominal flap for reconstruction after radical operations for recurrent breast cancer. Plast Reconstr Surg 53:52, 1974.

Taylor GI, Corlett R, Boyd JB: The extended deep inferior epigastric flap: A clinical technique. Plast Reconstr Surg 72:751, 1983.

Taylor GI, Corlett RJ, Boyd JB: The versatile deep inferior epigastric (inferior rectus abdominis) flap. Br J Plast Surg 37:330, 1984.

Greater Omentum Transfer

Alday ES, Goldsmith HS: Surgical technique for omental lengthening based on arterial anatomy. Surg Gynecol Obstet 135:103, 1972.

Arnold PG, Irons GB: The greater omentum: Extensions in transposition and free transfer. Plast Reconstr Surg 67:169, 1981.

Baudet J, Panconi B, Vidal L: Microvascular free transfer of a compound flap of stomach and omentum. In: Strauch B, Vasconez LO, Hall-Findlay E (eds): *Grabb's Encyclopedia of Flaps*, vol I. Boston: Little, Brown, 1990, pp. 752–756.

Das SK: The size of the human omentum and methods of lengthening it for transplantation. Br J Plast Surg 29:170, 1976.

Das SK, Lesavoy MA: Omental flap for cheek, neck, and intraoral reconstruction. In: Strauch B, Vasconez LO, Hall-Findlay E (eds): *Grabb's Encyclopedia of Flaps*, vol I. Boston: Little, Brown, 1990, pp. 539–540.

Ikuta Y: Omental transplantation. In: Serafin D, Buncke HJ (eds): *Microsurgical Composite Tissue Transplantation*. St. Louis: CV Mosby, 1979, pp. 361–368.

Ikuta Y: Autotransplant of omentum to cover large denudation of the scalp. Plast Reconstr Surg 55:490, 1975.

Ikuta Y: Microvascular free transfer of omentum. In: Strauch B, Vasconez LO, Hall-Findlay E (eds): *Grabb's Encyclopedia of Flaps*, vol I. Boston: Little, Brown, 1990, pp. 37–39.

McLean DH, Buncke HJ Jr: Autotransplant of omentum to a large scalp defect, with microsurgical revascularization. Plast Reconstr Surg 49:268, 1972.

Ohtsuka H, Shioya N: The fate of free omental transfers. Br J Plast Surg 38:478, 1985.

Samson R, Pasternak BM: Current status of surgery of the omentum. Surg Gynecol Obstet 149:437, 1979.

Spear SL, Oldham RJ: A lengthened omental pedicle in facial reconstruction. Plast Reconstr Surg 77:828, 1986.

Free Jejunum Transfer

Acland RD, Flynn MB: Free intestinal transplantation for esophageal reconstruction. In: Serafin D, Buncke HJ (eds): *Microsurgical Composite Tissue Transplantation*. St. Louis: CV Mosby, 1979, pp. 357–360.

Buckspan GS, Newton ED, Franklin JD, Lynch JB: Split jejunal free-tissue transfer in oropharyngoesophageal reconstruction. Plast Reconstr Surg 77:717, 1986.

Harashina T, Inoue T, Andoh T, Sugimoto C, Fujino T: Reconstruction of cervical oesophagus with free double-folded intestinal graft. Br J Plast Surg 38:483, 1985.

Harashina T, Kakegawa T, Imai T, Suguro Y: Secondary reconstruction of oesophagus with free revascularised ileal transfer. Br J Plast Surg 34:17, 1981.

Hester TR, McConnel FMS, Nahai F, Jurkiewicz MJ, Brown RG: Reconstruction of cervical esophagus, hypopharynx and oral cavity using free jejunal transfer. Am J Surg 140:487, 1980.

Jones BM, Gustavson EH: Free jejunal transfer for reconstruction of the cervical oesophagus in children: A report of two cases. Br J Plast Surg 36:162, 1983.

Jurkiewicz MJ: Vascularized intestinal graft for reconstruction of the cervical esophagus and pharynx. Plast Reconstr Surg 36:509, 1965.

Katsaros J, Tan E: Free bowel transfer for pharyngo-oesophageal reconstruction: An experimental and clinical study. Br J Plast Surg 35:268, 1982.

Nahai F, Stahl RS, Hester TR, Clairmont AA: Advanced applications of revascularized free jejunal flaps for difficult wounds of the head and neck. Plast Reconstr Surg 74:778, 1984.

Peters CR, McKee DM, Berry BE: Pharyngoesophageal reconstruction with revascularized jejunal transplants. Am J Surg 121:675, 1971.

Roberts RE, Douglass FM: Replacement of the cervical esophagus and hypopharynx by a revascularized free jejunal autograft. N Engl J Med 264:342, 1961.

Robinson DW, MacLeod A: Microvascular free jejunum transfer. Br J Plast Surg 35:258, 1982.

Schusterman MA, Shestak K, deVries EJ, et al: Reconstruction of the cervical esophagus: Free jejunal transfer versus gastric pull-up. Plast Reconstr Surg 85:16, 1990.

Stahl RS, Jurkiewicz MJ: Microvascular free transfer of intestine. In: Strauch B, Vasconez LO, Hall-Findlay E (eds): *Grabb's Encyclopedia of Flaps*, vol I. Boston: Little, Brown, 1990, pp. 746–751.

11 BACK

Latissimus Dorsi Flap

Anatomic Outline of the Latissimus Dorsi Muscle (**Fig. 11-1**)

Origin

The origin of the muscle is the spinous processes of T7-12, L1-5, and sacrum; the posterior part of the iliac crest; and the external surface of the four inferior ribs.

Insertion

In the axilla, the muscle spirals 180° around the teres major and inserts on the intertubercular groove in front of the proximal humerus.

Function

Functions of the muscle include extension, adduction, rotation of the arm medially, and drawing the shoulder downward and backward.

Shape

The muscle is flat, broad, and triangular. Its length is 38 cm, its width is 20 cm, and its thickness is 0.8 cm.

Blood Supply

The dominant blood supply to the muscle is the thoracodorsal artery [3], the continuation of the subscapular artery [2], which arises from the third portion of the axillary artery [1]. At about 3 cm from its origin, the subscapular artery divides into the circumflex scapular artery [4] that courses posteriorly through the triangular space, and the thoracodorsal artery [3] that continues inferiorly to supply the latissimus dorsi [7] as a dominant vessel.

The entrance of the thoracodorsal artery [3] to the muscle is located, on average, 8.7 cm (range, 6.0 to 11.5 cm) distal to the origin of the subscapular artery, and about 2.6 cm (range, 1 to 4 cm) medial to the lateral border of the muscle. After its entrance, the thoracodorsal artery immediately divides into the lateral and medial branches [5,6]. The lateral branch [5] is usually the larger; it courses parallel to the lateral border of the muscle, keeping approximately 2.1 cm medial to the border. Within the distal part of the muscle, the lateral branch gives off one or more branches that parallel the medial branch. The medial branch [6] courses parallel to the upper border of the muscle, remaining approximately 3.5 cm below and parallel to the upper border, at a 45° angle to the lateral branch.

Before its entrance to the muscle, the thoracodorsal artery gives off one or two branches to the serratus anterior muscle.

There is only a single vena comitans accompanying the thoracodorsal artery.

The latissimus dorsi is also supplied segmentally by a minor pedicle from the intercostal and lumbar arteries that enter the deep surface of the posterior part of the muscle.

Innervation

The thoracodorsal nerve arises from the posterior cord of the brachial plexus and travels lateroinferiorly behind the axillary artery and vein. It usually is located 3 cm medial to the origin of the subscapular artery in the axilla. It then runs to join the vasculature within 3 to 4 cm. The nerve divides into lateral and medial branches 1.3 cm proximal to the neurovascular hilum. Each branch runs with its vascular counterpart.

Measurement of Diameters

Artery		Vein		Nerve
Subscapular	Thoracodorsal	Subscapular	Thoracodorsal	Thoracodorsal
3–4 mm	1.5–3.0 mm	3.5–4.5 mm	2.5–4.5 mm	1.5–2.1 mm

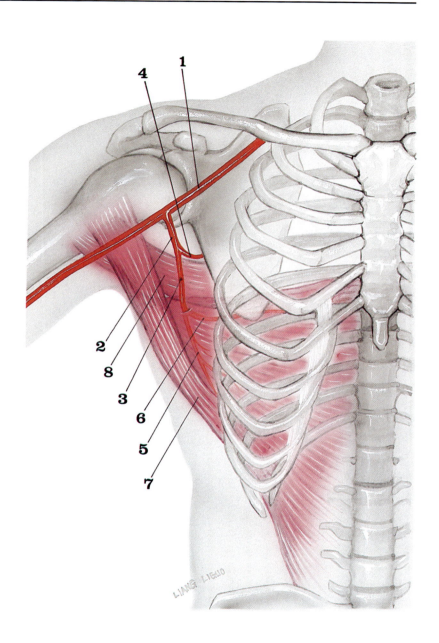

1. Axillary a.
2. Subscapular a.
3. Thoracodorsal a.
4. Circumflex scapular a.
5. Lateral branch
6. Medial branch
7. Latissimus dorsi m.
8. Teres major m.

Variations in Branching of the Thoracodorsal Neurovascular Bundle (Fig. 11-2)

Type A. Typical branching pattern (86% of cases)

Type B. No identifiable medial branch, but the lateral branch gives off several smaller vessels coursing from lateral to medial (14% of cases).

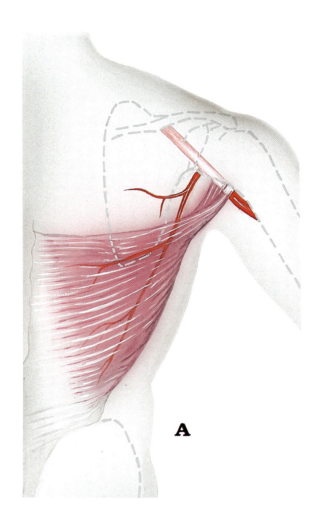

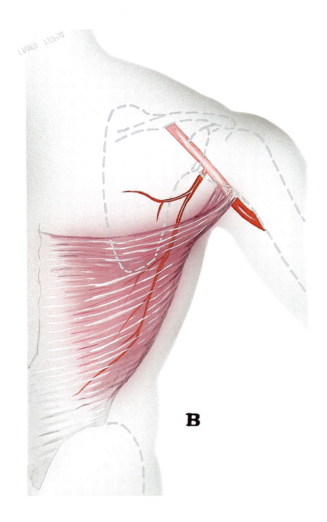

Variations of the Subscapular Artery and Vein (Fig. 11-3)

Type A. Typical origin and branching of the subscapular artery and vein [3,4] (62% of cases)

Type B. The circumflex scapular artery [7] arises directly from the axillary artery (4% of cases)

Type C. The circumflex scapular vein [8] arises directly from the axillary vein (12% of cases)

Type D. Double circumflex veins [8] (14% of cases)

Type E. Double circumflex arteries [7] (8% of cases)

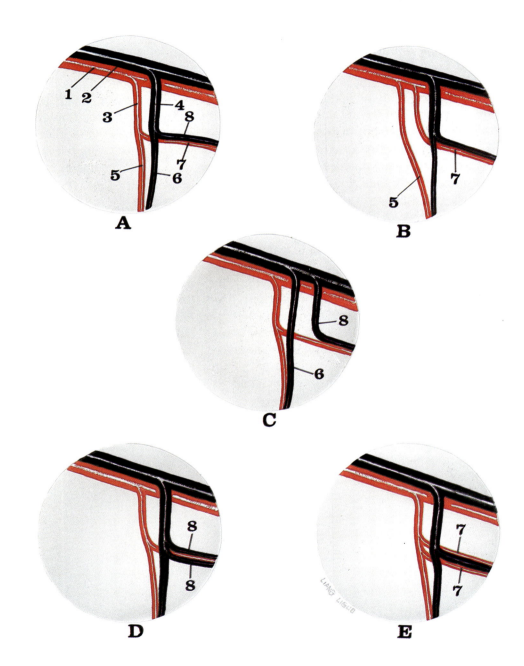

1. Axillary a.
2. Axillary v.
3. Subscapular a.
4. Subscapular v.
5. Thoracodorsal a.
6. Thoracodorsal v.
7. Circumflex scapular a.
8. Circumflex scapular v.

COMMENT AND INSIGHTS

The latissimus dorsi muscle flap is one of the most widely applicable and reliable free tissue flaps, with a long pedicle and large diameter of the dominant vessels. Because its neurovascular anatomy is quite constant, the flap can be easily isolated. This is a large flap and it provides a large amount of soft tissue.

Clinically, there is no notable residual functional problem from loss of the latissimus dorsi (because of the compensatory action of the teres major and pectoralis major), but the procedure should be used prudently for the patient on crutches. The flap can also be used for functional muscle repair and for treatment of chronic osteomyelitis.

During dissection of the neurovascular pedicle in the axillary fossa, extreme abduction of the arm should be avoided. Failure to attend to this warning may cause the posterior bow of the clavicle to impinge on the upper trunk of the brachial plexus against the cervical spine, resulting in transient weakness and sensory changes in the ipsilateral upper extremity.

The bilobed split latissimus flap provides two flaps that can be used simultaneously. The lateral or medial split flap can be transferred as a smaller muscle or myocutaneous flap, preserving the function of the latissimus dorsi to a certain extent, with the intact half of the muscle.

The rib-latissimus dorsi osteomyocutaneous flap can be applied in reconstruction of a compound bony defect of the extremities; however, for bony defects of the tibia or femur, the flap should include two ribs. It can be used also as an island transfer in reconstructions of mandibular defects.

(For a description of the properties of rib, refer to Chapter 9 on free costal bone graft.)

The flap can also be combined with the serratus anterior, scapular, or parascapular flap, or with vascularized scapular bone, using one vascular pedicle of the subscapular vessels. However, the flap is too bulky to be used in such sites as the hand. In addition, the skin of the myocutaneous flap does not have sensibility, and this flap is not recommended for use on the weight-bearing parts of the heel and sole.

There are methods of mitigating the bulkiness of the flap: the lateral or medial split latissimus dorsi flap produces less bulk; the muscle flap with skin graft is much thinner than the myocutaneous flap; and, in addition, the volume of muscle in a noninnervated muscle flap will atrophy about 25 to 50%. Furthermore, the muscle flap can also be thinned of one third of its thickness by resection of the superficial layer, since the thoracodorsal neurovascular bundle and its branches consistently remain on the deep surface of the muscle for their entire course.

LATISSIMUS DORSI MUSCLE FLAP

(Fig. 11-4) The patient is placed on his side, with the donor side upward and the shoulder joint abducted. An incision is made from the posterior axillary fold, running posteroinferiorly toward the loin, 3 to 5 cm posterior to the lateral margin of the muscle. The length of the incision accords with the size of the muscle flap required. At times, a small skin island is designed, remaining on the muscle as a monitor for the integrity of the circulation.

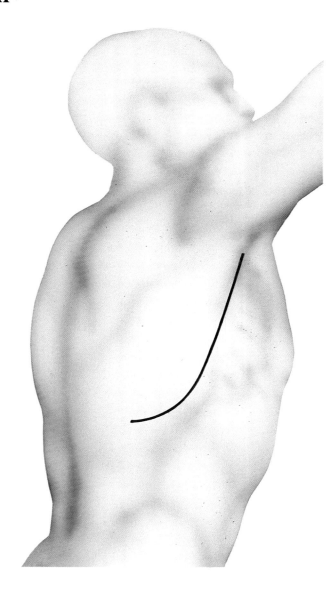

1. Latissimus dorsi m.
2. Serratus anterior m.
3. Teres major m.
4. Rhomboid major m.
5. Infraspinatus m.
6. Axillary a. and v.
7. Subscapular a. and v.
8. Thoracodorsal a., v., and n.
9. Circumflex scapular a. and v.
10. Branch to serratus anterior
11. Serratus posterior inferior m.
12. Intercostalis externus m.
13. Pectoralis major m.

(Fig. 11-5) The skin and subcutaneous layers are incised. Anterior and posterior flaps are raised with undermining, to expose the superficial surface of the latissimus dorsi muscle [1]. Then, the lateral and superior borders of the muscle are identified.

1. Latissimus dorsi m.
2. Serratus anterior m.
3. Teres major m.
4. Rhomboid major m.

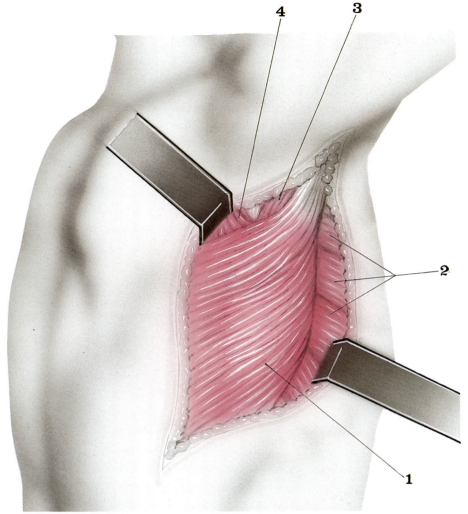

(**Fig. 11-6**) At its lateral border, dissection proceeds between the latissimus dorsi [1] and serratus anterior [2] muscles. The middle portion of the latissimus dorsi is separated from the chest wall.

1. Latissimus dorsi m.
2. Serratus anterior m.
10. Branch to serratus anterior

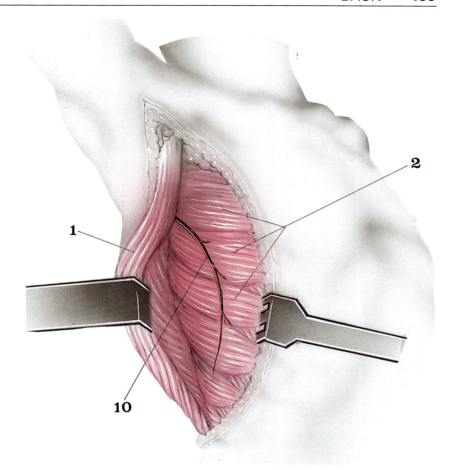

(Fig. 11-7) In the axillary dissection, the thoracodorsal neurovascular pedicle [8] is identified under the latissimus dorsi [1], approximately 2 to 3 cm medial to the lateral border of the muscle. Its entrance to the muscle can be defined about 9 cm below the apex of the axilla.

One or two branches [10] to the serratus anterior are ligated, and the thoracodorsal neurovascular pedicle [8] is then isolated and marked with a vascular loop. The proximal part of the muscle is isolated and retracted with a Penrose drain. After identification of the circumflex scapular artery [9], the pedicle can be dissected up to the origins of the subscapular vessels [7].

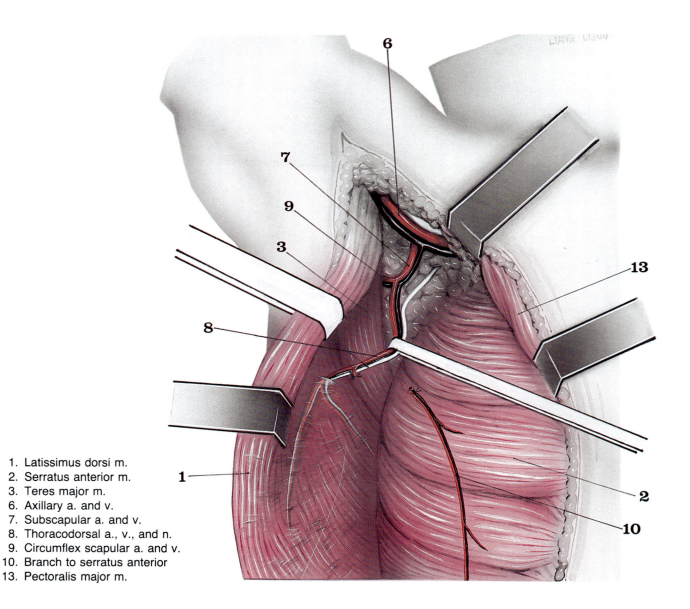

1. Latissimus dorsi m.
2. Serratus anterior m.
3. Teres major m.
6. Axillary a. and v.
7. Subscapular a. and v.
8. Thoracodorsal a., v., and n.
9. Circumflex scapular a. and v.
10. Branch to serratus anterior
13. Pectoralis major m.

(Fig. 11-8) After dissecting between the muscle and the chest wall toward the back midline and the iliac crest, and ligating the branches from the intercostal and lumbar arteries, the distal portion of the muscle is divided at a level depending on the amount of tissue required at the recipient site. As the muscle flap is elevated from the chest wall proximally, some perforating branches from the chest wall to the deep surface are encountered and ligated.

2. Serratus anterior m.
3. Teres major m.
4. Rhomboid major m.
5. Infraspinatus m.
11. Serratus posterior inferior m.
12. Intercostalis externus m.

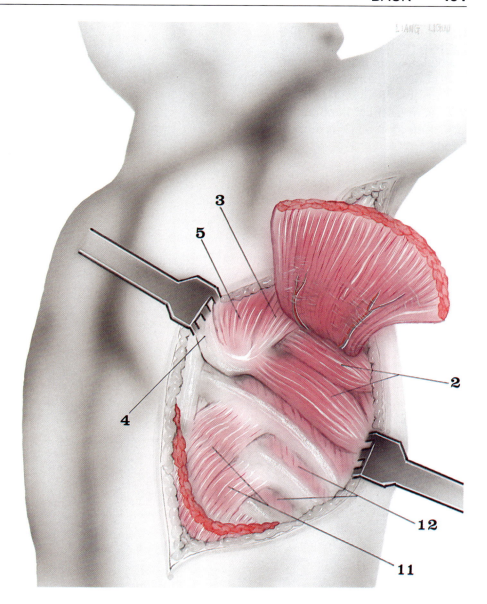

(Fig. 11-9) The proximal portion of the muscle [1] is divided near its insertion, with protection of the neurovascular pedicle [8]. Tethered only by the neurovascular bundle, the latissimus dorsi [1] is almost freed.

1. Latissimus dorsi m.
6. Axillary a. and v.
7. Subscapular a. and v.
8. Thoracodorsal a., v., and n.

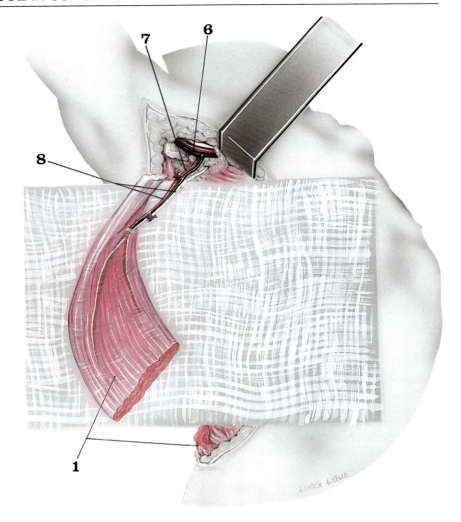

LATISSIMUS DORSI MYOCUTANEOUS FLAP

(Fig. 11-10) The lateral and upper borders of the muscle should be identified by palpation. A skin paddle of the required size is outlined at the proper location on the muscle. Generally, the myocutaneous perforators from the latissimus dorsi are more numerous over the proximal two thirds of the muscle.

If the skin paddle is larger than 10 cm in width, donor site closure may require a split-thickness skin graft. The maximum dimensions are approximately 40 × 20 cm.

1. Latissimus dorsi m.
2. Serratus anterior m.
3. Thoracodorsal a., v., and n.
4. Axillary a. and v.
5. Subscapular a.
6. Teres major m.

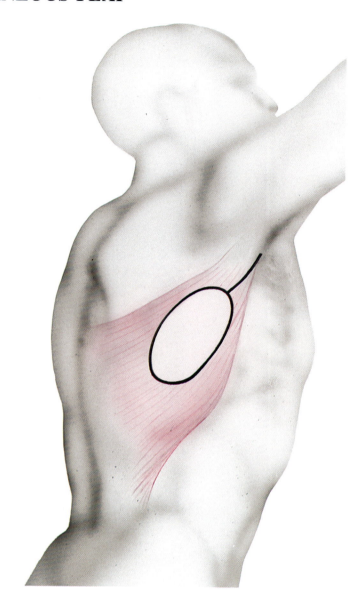

(Fig. 11-11) A circumferential incision of the skin flap is carried out and extended proximally to the axillary fossa. The anterior and posterior skin over the rest of the latissimus dorsi [1] is raised to expose the lateral and upper borders of the latissimus dorsi muscle. The skin margin of the flap is sutured to the muscle fascia with several tacking sutures, to avoid shearing injury to the myocutaneous perforators.

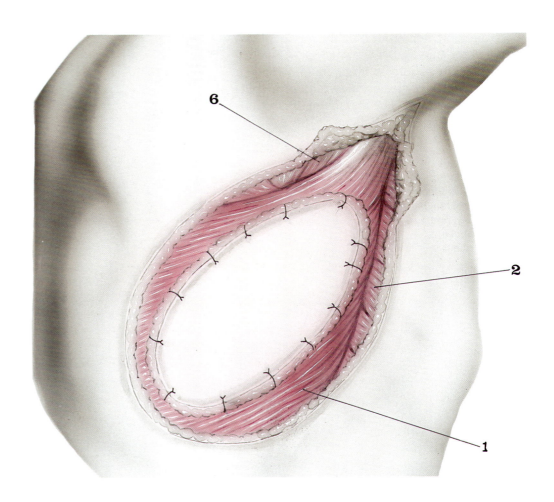

1. Latissimus dorsi m.
2. Serratus anterior m.
6. Teres major m.

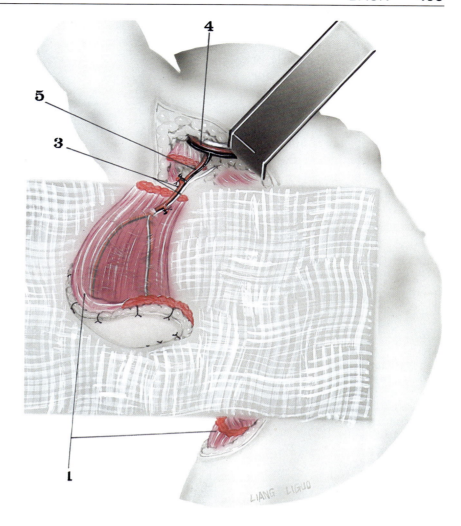

(**Fig. 11-12**) The latissimus dorsi [1] with its skin paddle is elevated, and its neurovascular pedicle [3] dissected, as described in the section on muscle flap harvesting.

1. Latissimus dorsi m.
3. Thoracodorsal a., v., and n.
4. Axillary a. and v.
5. Subscapular a.

BILOBED SPLIT LATISSIMUS DORSI FLAP

(**Fig. 11-13**) The muscle or myocutaneous flap based on the thoracodorsal neurovascular pedicle [3] is raised as has already been described. On the deep surface, the entrance of the neurovascular pedicle is identified and the lateral and medial neurovascular branches [4,5] are traced from it. The neurovascular pattern may be defined by transillumination and with the use of a stimulator. It can be marked with several needles passed through the flap.

1. Latissimus dorsi m.
2. Teres major m.
3. Thoracodorsal a. and v.
4. Lateral branch
5. Medial branch
6. Axillary a. and v.
7. Thoracodorsal n.
8. Serratus anterior m.

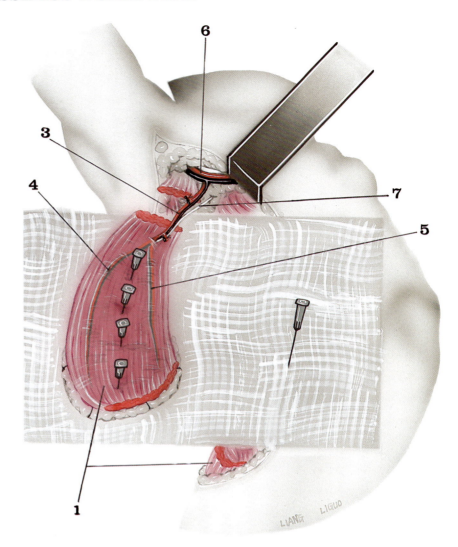

(**Fig. 11-14**) The skin paddle is incised and the muscle is split along the previously marked neurovascular pattern.

4. Lateral branch
5. Medial branch

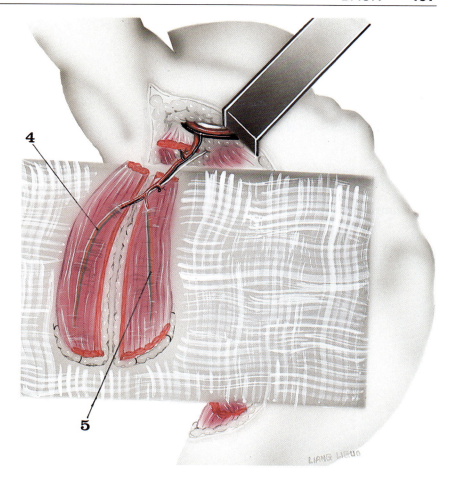

LATERAL SPLIT LATISSIMUS DORSI FLAP

(**Fig. 11-15**) An incision is made from the posterior axillary fold, running along the lateral border of the latissimus dorsi muscle. (If a myocutaneous flap is required, the skin paddle is designed on the lateral part of the muscle.)

1. Latissimus dorsi m.
2. Teres major m.
3. Thoracodorsal a. and v.
4. Lateral branch
5. Medial branch
6. Axillary a. and v.
7. Thoracodorsal n.
8. Serratus anterior m.

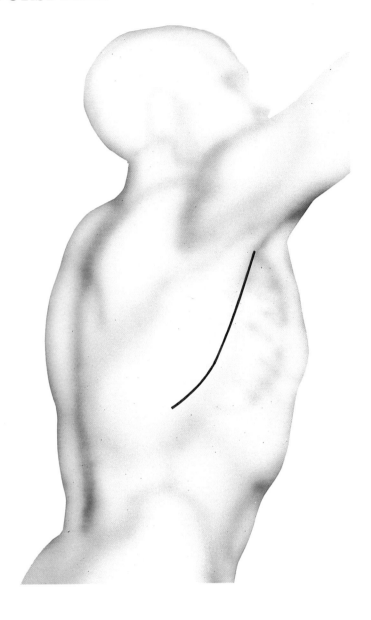

(**Fig. 11-16**) The muscle is elevated to expose the thoracodorsal neurovascular bundle [3], and its entrance and lateral branches [4] are then identified.

1. Latissimus dorsi m.
2. Teres major m.
3. Thoracodorsal a. and v.
4. Lateral branch
5. Medial branch
6. Axillary a. and v.
7. Thoracodorsal n.
8. Serratus anterior m.

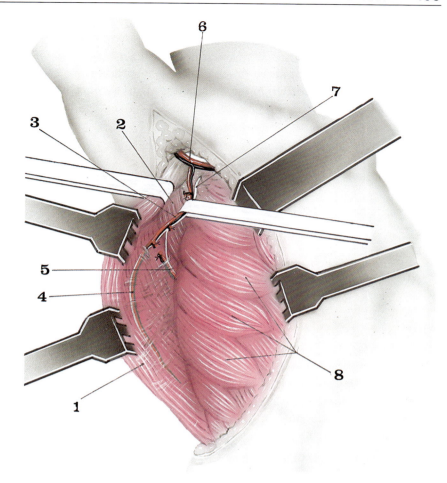

(**Fig. 11-17**) Taking care that the lateral branch [4] is included, the lateral part of the muscle is split, and the medial vascular branch [5] is ligated. The lateral nerve branch is separated from the medial branch in the thoracodorsal nerve [7] and divided to be as long as possible, leaving the medial nerve branch intact. The lateral split latissimus dorsi flap, based on the thoracodorsal-lateral branch neurovascular bundle, is isolated.

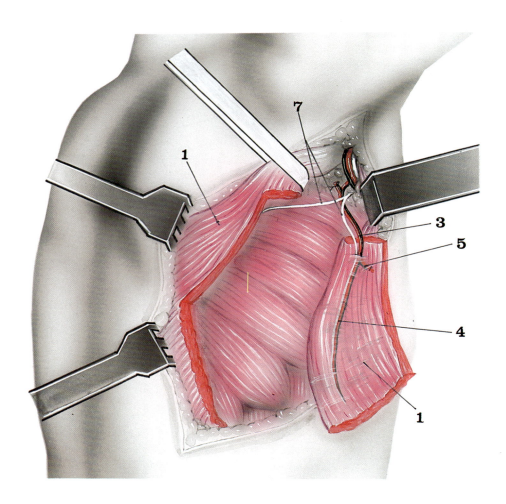

1. Latissimus dorsi m.
3. Thoracodorsal a. and v.
4. Lateral branch
5. Medial branch
7. Thoracodorsal n.

RIB-LATISSIMUS DORSI OSTEOMYOCUTANEOUS FLAP

(**Fig. 11-18**) The latissimus dorsi muscle covers the lower ribs from the back midline to the posterior axillary line. There are vascular communications between the thoracodorsal artery and the periosteal vessels of the ribs. The ninth or tenth ribs may be selected to be combined in the flap. A bony length of about 12 cm is available.

1. Latissimus dorsi m.
2. Intercostalis m.
3. 9th rib
4. Pleura
5. Thoracodorsal a., v., and n.

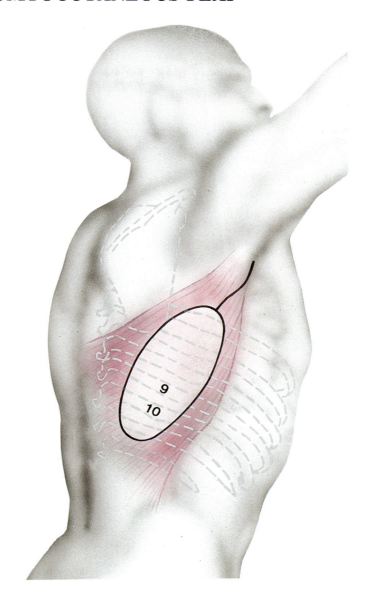

(Fig. 11-19) Flap elevation is begun distally and must stop at the intercostal space inferior to the selected ribs. Then, the intercostal muscles [2] are incised in the intercostal space, and the rib is divided at both ends. The rib [3] is separated from the pleura [4]. The component is then flipped proximally, keeping it intact with the muscle flap.

1. Latissimus dorsi m.
2. Intercostalis m.
3. 9th rib
4. Pleura

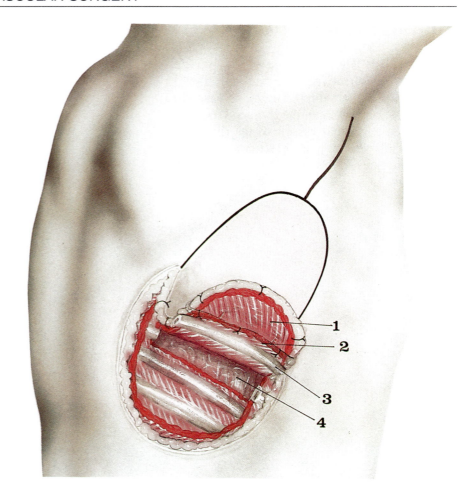

(**Fig. 11-20**) Intercostal muscles proximal to the selected ribs are incised, and the osteomyocutaneous flap is isolated on the thoracodorsal neurovascular pedicle [5], as was already described.

1. Latissimus dorsi m.
3. 9th rib
5. Thoracodorsal a., v., and n.

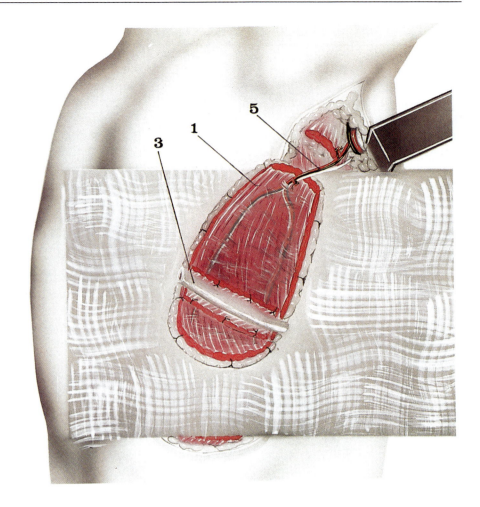

(Refer to Chapter 9 for additional details on harvesting a vascularized rib.)

Scapular and Parascapular Flaps

Anatomy (Fig. 11-21)

The *circumflex scapular artery* [7] arises from the subscapular artery [6] approximately 3 to 4 cm from its origin at the axillary artery [5]. (For variations in its origin, see section on the latissimus dorsi.) The artery [7] passes posteriorly through the triangular space bordered by the teres minor [4] above, the teres major [3] below, and the long head of the triceps [2] laterally, and in this space it usually gives off the following branches:

1. The infrascapular branch [9] enters the subscapular fossa deep to the subscapularis.
2. One or two muscular branches run to the teres major and teres minor.
3. The *descending branch* [10] goes back as its continuation and emerges posteriorly from the triangular space; it then divides into two main cutaneous branches, [11,1], right at the edge of the lateral border of the scapula.
4. The *cutaneous scapular branch* [11] runs horizontally over the posterior aspect of the scapula.
5. The *cutaneous parascapular branch* [1] proceeds to the inferior angle of the scapula.
6. Before dividing into the two main cutaneous branches, the circumflex scapular artery [7] gives off several small branches that penetrate the lateral border of the scapula.

Both the circumflex scapular and the cutaneous arteries are accompanied by two veins, one of which usually has a larger diameter than the other (2.5 to 4 mm). These are responsible for the venous drainage of the area.

Measurements of Arteriovenous Scapular System

		Diameter (mm)	Length (cm)
Subscapular	Artery	3–4	3–4
	Vein	3.5–4.5	
Circumflex scapular	Artery	2.5–3.5	3–4
	Vein	2.5–4.0	
Descending	Artery	1.5–2.0	4–6
	Vein	2.0–2.5	
Cutaneous scapular	Artery	0.8–1.5	
	Vein	1.0–2.0	
Cutaneous parascapular	Artery	0.8–1.5	
	Vein	1.0–2.0	

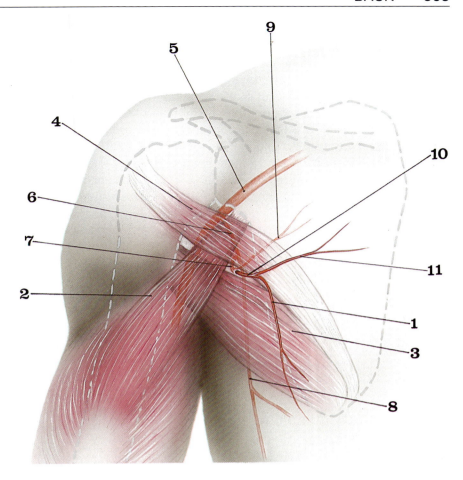

1. Cutaneous parascapular branch
2. Long head of triceps m.
3. Teres major m.
4. Teres minor m.
5. Axillary a.
6. Subscapular a.
7. Circumflex scapular a.
8. Thoracodorsal a.
9. Subscapular branch
10. Descending branch
11. Cutaneous scapular branch

COMMENT AND INSIGHTS

Clinically, this scapular area supplied by the circumflex scapular artery, has become one of the most frequently used donor sites in reconstructive microsurgery because of consistent vascular anatomy, easily accessible vascular pedicle, desirable vessel diameter and length, and flap safety and reliability.

There is a moderate amount of subcutaneous tissue and generally hairless skin. Flap size can reach 10 × 25 cm in the scapular flap and 15 × 30 cm in the parascapular flap. There is, however, no large single nerve that can be used to innervate these flaps.

The lateral border of the scapula can provide vascularized bone, especially useful for face and hand reconstruction.

Generally, the donor site defect can be closed directly, with acceptable scarring and little postoperative morbidity.

Based on the subscapular arterial system, scapular or parascapular osteocutaneous flaps can be combined with the latissimus dorsi and serratus anterior or their myocutaneous flaps.

SCAPULAR FLAP

(Fig. 11-22) The location of the triangular space is marked using the following method. The distance from the midpoint of the scapular spine can be derived from the formula: $D_1 = (D-1)/2$, where D is the distance between the midpoint of the spine and the tip of the scapula. The location of the triangular space can be confirmed with bidigital palpation.

The flap is outlined according to the following parameters. Its axis corresponds to the cutaneous scapular artery that runs from the marked triangular space medially and parallel to the scapular spine. Flap design may vary, although an elliptical shape is preferred for easy closure, with the lateral end of the ellipse positioned just over the triangular space. The medial end can extend all the way to the midline of the back; the superior limit is the spine of the scapula and the inferior limit is the tip of the scapula. A flap can be harvested larger than 10 cm in width and 20 cm in length.

The patient can be positioned in either lateral decubitus, prone, or three quarter position, depending on whether the recipient site is posterior or anterior.

There are two options for exposing the emergence of the cutaneous branches.

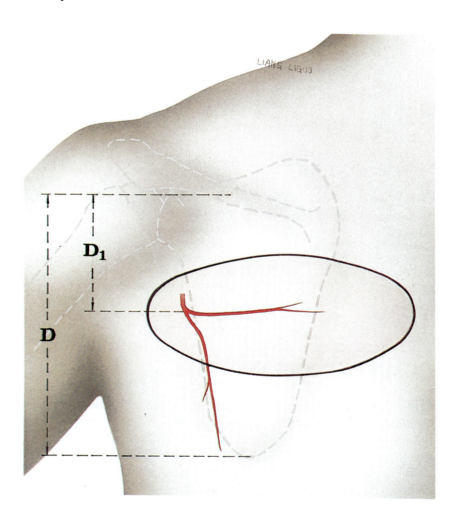

1. Deltoid m.
2. Teres major m.
3. Teres minor m.
4. Long head of triceps m.
5. Descending branch of circumflex scapular a.
6. Infraspinatus m.
7. Trapezius m.
8. Rhomboideus major m.
9. Latissimus dorsi m.
10. Axillary a.
11. Subscapular a.
12. Circumflex scapular a.
13. Thoracodorsal a. and n.
14. Subscapularis m.

Lateral Exposure of Vascular Emergence (Fig. 11-23)

The first incision is started on the upper lateral portion of the ellipse described previously. The posterior margin of the deltoid [1] is identified and the muscle is retracted superiorly, revealing the teres minor [3]. Dissection proceeds along the surface of the teres minor; a fibrofatty tissue through which the cutaneous branches [5] of the circumflex scapular vessels course can be exposed.

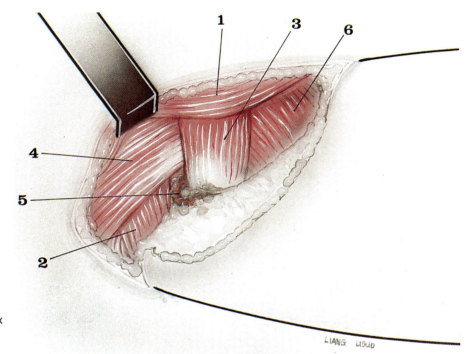

1. Deltoid m.
2. Teres major m.
3. Teres minor m.
4. Long head of triceps m.
5. Descending branch of circumflex scapular a.
6. Infraspinatus m.

Medial Exposure of Vascular Emergence (Fig. 11-24)

Elevation of the flap begins medially in an avascular plane, just above the superficial fascia of the infraspinatus [6] and teres major [2] muscles. Once the triangular space is reached near the lateral border of the scapula, the vessels can be seen emerging in a fibrofatty tissue between the teres minor and major muscles.

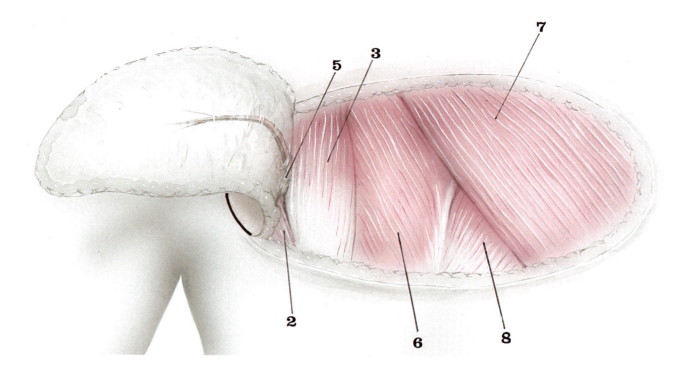

2. Teres major m.
3. Teres minor m.
5. Descending branch of circumflex scapular a.
6. Infraspinatus m.
7. Trapezius m.
8. Rhomboideus major m.

(Fig. 11-25) The vascular pedicle [5] and triangular space should be further identified while raising the remainder of the flap. It is not necessary to dissect the vessels in the fibrofatty tissue; the optimal way to isolate the pedicle is to stay close to the muscular walls, freeing the fibrofatty tissue toward the center of the space.

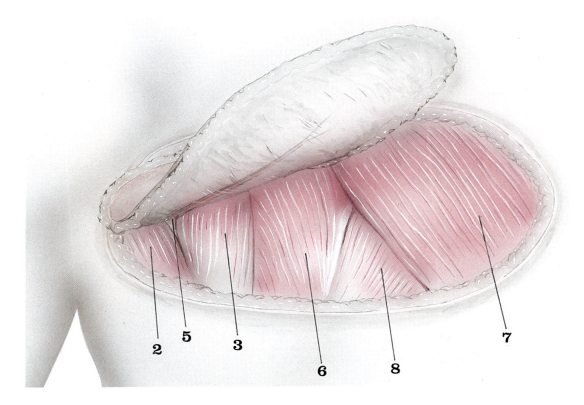

2. Teres major m.
3. Teres minor m.
5. Descending branch of circumflex scapular a.
6. Infraspinatus m.
7. Trapezius m.
8. Rhomboideus major m.

(**Fig. 11-26**) For further dissection, the long head of the triceps and the teres major and minor [2,3] should be retracted in their respective directions to gain better exposure. The branches to the teres major and minor, infraspinatus and infrascapular branches, are ligated successively. In this manner, a vascular pedicle length of 6 to 9 cm can be obtained.

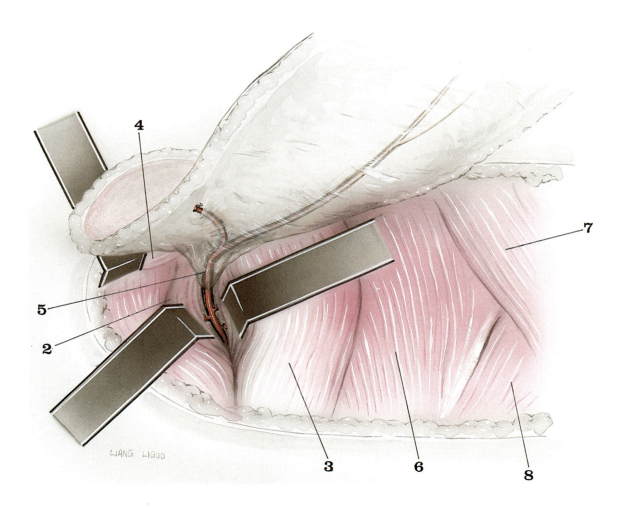

2. Teres major m.
3. Teres minor m.
4. Long head of triceps m.
5. Descending branch of circumflex scapular a.
6. Infraspinatus m.
7. Trapezius m.
8. Rhomboideus major m.

(**Fig. 11-27**) When a longer pedicle or further and better exposure are necessary, a 5 cm incision is made in the midaxilla. The subscapular artery [11] is identified and a tunnel is bluntly dissected under the teres minor to connect the triangular and axillary spaces. Once the thoracodorsal vessels [13] are ligated, a maximum pedicle length can reach 11 to 14 cm.

2. Teres major m.
9. Latissimus dorsi m.
10. Axillary a.
11. Subscapular a.
12. Circumflex scapular a.
13. Thoracodorsal a. and n.
14. Subscapularis m.

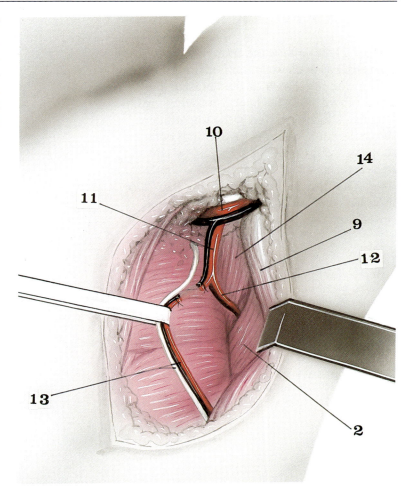

(Note that in 4% of cases the circumflex scapular artery originates independently from the axillary artery.)

PARASCAPULAR FLAP

(Fig. 11-28) Once the triangular space is located, as in the scapular flap described before, the main axis of the parascapular flap is drawn along the lateral border of the scapula. The upper edge of the flap is at or above the level of emergence of the cutaneous vessels; the lower edge can be situated as far as 25 to 30 cm from the upper edge. The maximum width of this flap is about 15 cm and the donor site can be closed directly.

1. Teres major m.
2. Teres minor m.
3. Latissimus dorsi m.
4. Infraspinatus m.
5. Long head of triceps
6. Descending branch of circumflex scapular a.
7. Cutaneous parascapular branch
8. Cutaneous scapular branch

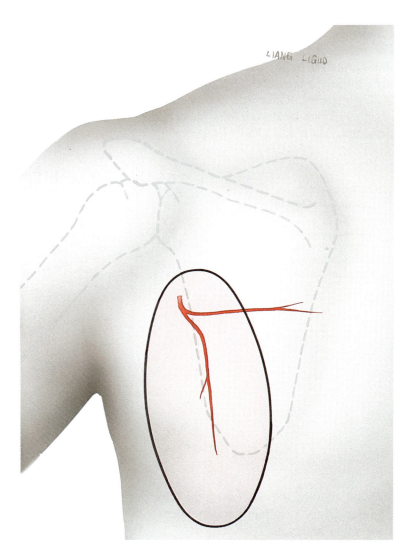

(Fig. 11-29) Procedures for raising the flap, dissection, and isolation of the vascular pedicle [6] are similar to the scapular flap.

1. Teres major m.
2. Teres minor m.
3. Latissimus dorsi m.
4. Infraspinatus m.
5. Long head of triceps
6. Descending branch of circumflex scapular a.
7. Cutaneous parascapular branch
8. Cutaneous scapular branch

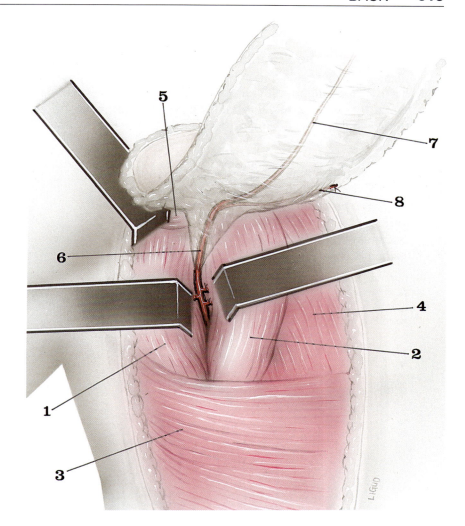

SCAPULAR OSTEOCUTANEOUS FLAP

Measurements of the Scapula

The length of the lateral scapular border (from the glenoid fossa to the inferior angle) ranges from 10 to 14 cm and the thickness of the lateral border is between 0.7 and 1.2 cm. The midportion of the scapula is quite thin, approximately 0.2 cm, making it ideal for palatal or orbital floor reconstruction.

(Fig. 11-30) The skin flap can be designed and elevated following the procedures and techniques for either scapular or parascapular flap (or both), as described before.

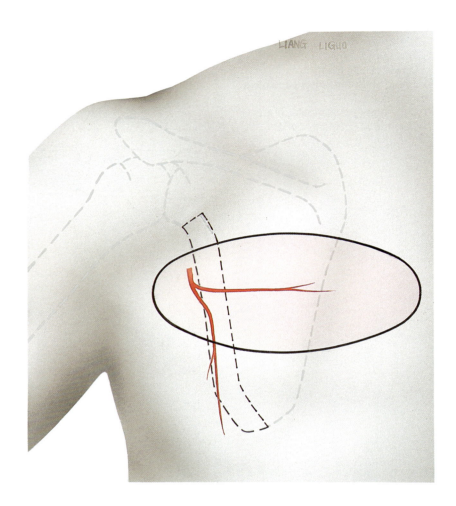

1. Teres major m.
2. Teres minor m.
3. Latissimus dorsi m.
4. Infraspinatus m.
5. Trapezius m.
6. Rhomboideus major m.
7. Descending branch of circumflex scapular a.
8. Scapula bone
9. Nutrient branch to scapula
10. Subscapular m.
11. Serratus anterior m.

(Fig. 11-31) The emergence of the vascular bundle [7] in the fibrofatty tissue is identified, with care taken not to divide the small, easily observed branches [9] to the bone over the lateral scapular border [8]. The circumflex scapular artery is dissected in its lateral aspect, preserving these bone branches in its medial aspect.

An incision is made directly through the muscles [4] overlying the scapula [8] and, using a periosteal elevator, the periosteum is stripped sufficiently to perform osteotomies.

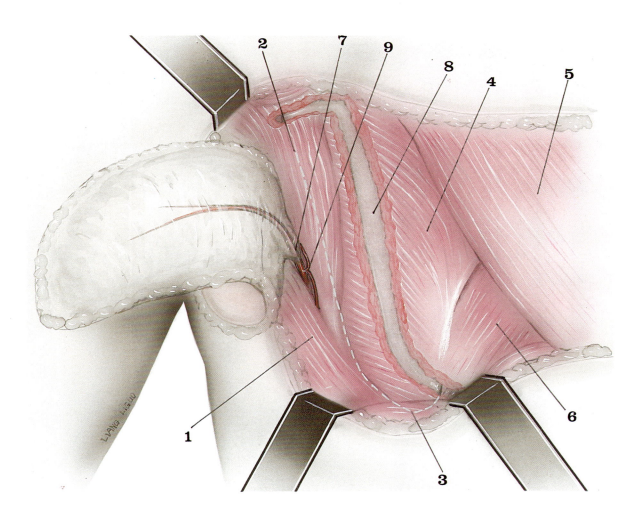

1. Teres major m.
2. Teres minor m.
3. Latissimus dorsi m.
4. Infraspinatus m.
5. Trapezius m.
6. Rhomboideus major m.
7. Descending branch of circumflex scapular a.
8. Scapula bone
9. Nutrient branch to scapula

(Fig. 11-32) The bone [8] is divided vertically with an oscillating saw along the transition between the thick lateral border and thin blade and transversely just below the glenoid fossa.

The muscular origins of the serratus anterior [11], subscapularis [10], and teres major and minor [2] are detached sharply from the remnants of the lateral border and inferior angle of the scapula [8], leaving a 0.5 cm muscular sleeve. The vascular pedicle [7] is further dissected to its proximal limits either at the junction of the thoracodorsal artery or to the axillary artery, if necessary.

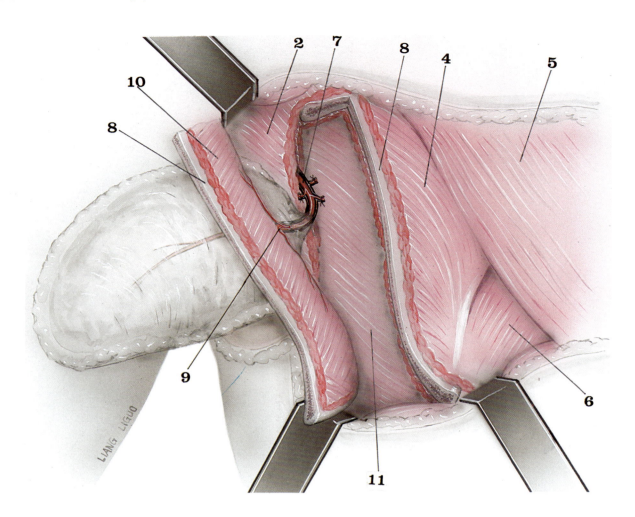

2. Teres minor m.
4. Infraspinatus m.
5. Trapezius m.
6. Rhomboideus major m.
7. Descending branch of circumflex scapular a.
8. Scapula bone
9. Nutrient branch to scapula
10. Subscapular m.
11. Serratus anterior m.

Note for Donor Closure. All muscle origins at the donor site are reattached to the scapula through drill holes while closing the donor site.

SCAPULAR AND PARASCAPULAR COMBINED FLAP

(**Fig. 11-33**) After determining the emergence point of the circumflex scapular artery, both scapular and parascapular flaps are designed according to the courses of the cutaneous scapular and parascapular arteries as axes of both flaps. Thus, an inverted L-shaped flap (Pacman flap)—a scapular and parascapular combined flap—is formed to meet the requirements of shape and size for the recipient site.

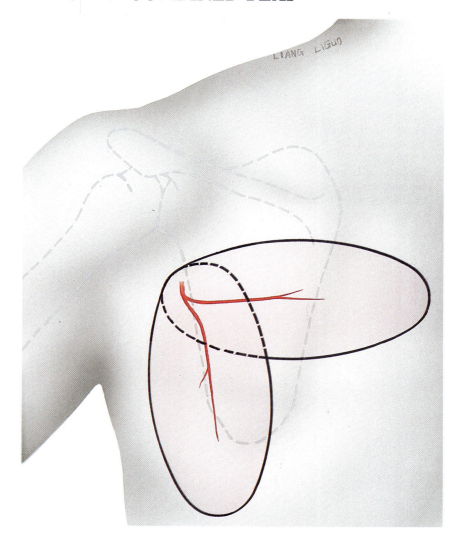

1. Teres major m.
2. Teres minor m.
3. Latissimus dorsi m.
4. Infraspinatus m.
5. Trapezius m.
6. Descending branch of circumflex scapular a.
7. Cutaneous scapular branch
8. Cutaneous parascapular branch

(Fig. 11-34) The flap is raised following the procedure described for the scapular flap.

1. Teres major m.
2. Teres minor m.
3. Latissimus dorsi m.
4. Infraspinatus m.
5. Trapezius m.
6. Descending branch of circumflex scapular a.
7. Cutaneous scapular branch
8. Cutaneous parascapular branch

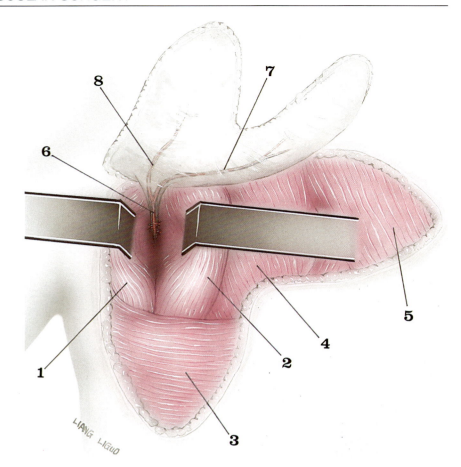

SCAPULAR AND LATISSIMUS DORSI COMBINED FLAP

(Fig. 11-35) The scapular flap is initially designed as described previously. From its lateral border, an incision is made to the axillary fossa and another incision runs downward from the inferior border of the flap.

1. Latissimus dorsi m.
2. Teres major m.
3. Teres minor m.
4. Trapezius m.
5. Rhomboideus major m.
6. Circumflex scapular a.
7. Thoracodorsal a. and n.
8. Subscapular a.
9. Serratus anterior m.

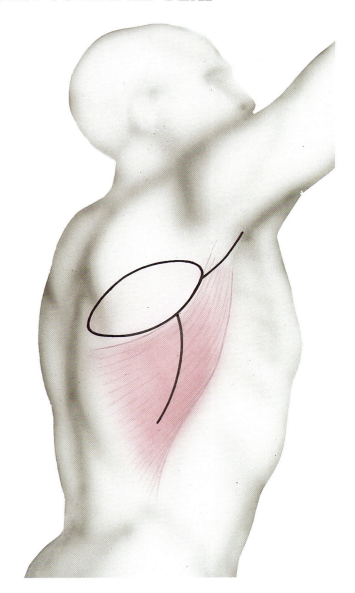

(Fig. 11-36) First, the circumflex scapular artery [6] is identified in the triangular space. The scapular flap is raised. Then the lateral and inferior flaps are turned laterally and inferiorly, respectively. The outer surface and the anterior border of the latissimus dorsi [1] are exposed.

1. Latissimus dorsi m.
2. Teres major m.
3. Teres minor m.
4. Trapezius m.
5. Rhomboideus major m.
6. Circumflex scapular a.

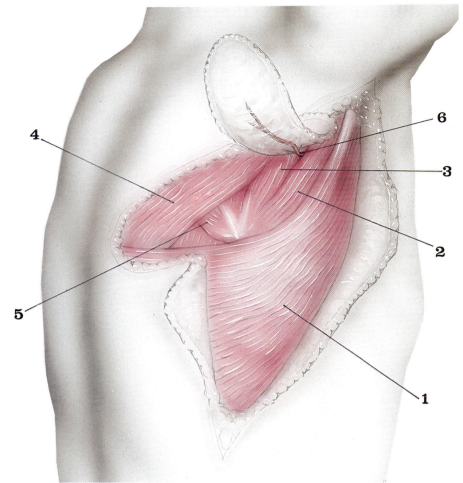

(Fig. 11-37) The latissimus dorsi muscle flap [1] is isolated (see section on latissimus dorsi) with care to keep the bifurcation of the circumflex scapular [6] and thoracodorsal arteries [7] intact. The teres major muscle [2] is identified and the circumflex scapular artery is dissected under the muscle.

1. Latissimus dorsi m.
2. Teres major m.
3. Teres minor m.
4. Trapezius m.
5. Rhomboideus major m.
6. Circumflex scapular a.
7. Thoracodorsal a. and n.
8. Subscapular a.
9. Serratus anterior m.

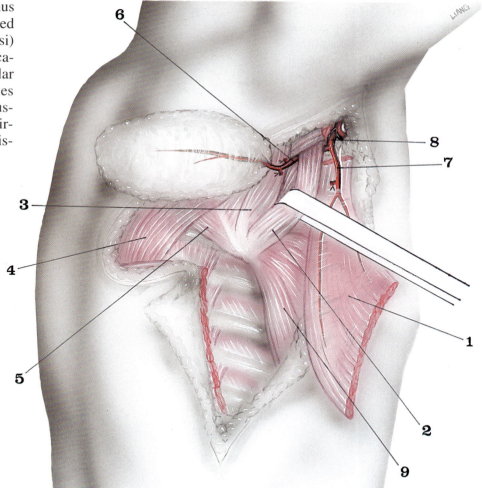

(Fig. 11-38) If the scapular flap is not very large, it can be passed through to the axillary fossa under the teres major muscle [2]. If necessary, the teres major muscle [2] can be divided so that the scapular flap is delivered safely.

1. Latissimus dorsi m.
2. Teres major m.
3. Teres minor m.
4. Trapezius m.
5. Rhomboideus major m.
6. Circumflex scapular a.
7. Thoracodorsal a. and n.
8. Subscapular a.
9. Serratus anterior m.

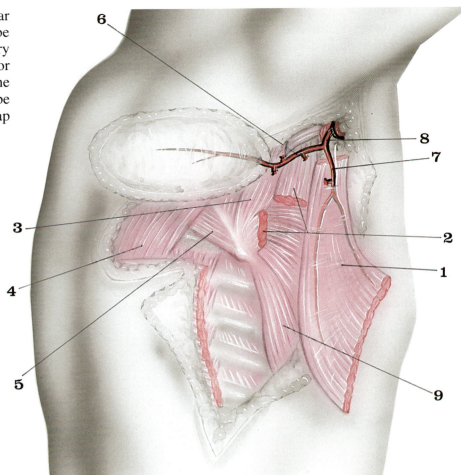

BIBLIOGRAPHY

Latissimus Dorsi Flap

Anderl H, Kerschbaumer S: Early correction of the thoracic deformity of Poland's syndrome in children with the latissimus dorsi muscle flap: Long term follow-up of two cases. Br J Plast Surg 39:167, 1986.

Barton RM: Microneurovascular transfer of the latissimus dorsi muscle and musculocutaneous flaps to the forearm. In: Strauch B, Vasconez LO, Hall-Findlay E (eds): *Grabb's Encyclopedia of Flaps*, vol II. Boston: Little, Brown, 1990, pp 1205–1206.

Barton RM, Vasconez LO: Microvascular free transfer of a latissimus dorsi muscle and musculocutaneous flap. In: Strauch B, Vasconez LO, Hall-Findlay E (eds): *Grabb's Encyclopedia of Flaps*, vol III. Boston: Little, Brown, 1990, pp 1773–1777.

Bostwick J III, Nahai F, Wallace JG, Vasconez LO: Sixty latissimus dorsi flaps. Plast Reconstr Surg 63:31, 1979.

Cohen BE: Shoulder defect correction with the island latissimus dorsi flap. Plast Reconstr Surg 74:650, 1984.

Dellon AL, Mackinnon SE: Segmentally innervated latissimus dorsi muscle: Microsurgical transfer for facial reanimation. J Reconstr Microsurg 2:7, 1985.

Fisher J, Bostwick J III, Powell RW: Latissimus dorsi blood supply after thoracodorsal vessel division: The serratus collateral. Plast Reconstr Surg 72:502, 1983.

Freedlander E: Brachial plexus cord compression by the tendon of a pedicled latissimus dorsi flap. Br J Plast Surg 39:514, 1986.

Gordon L, Buncke HJ, Alpert BS: Free latissimus dorsi muscle flap with split-thickness skin graft cover: A report of 16 cases. Plast Reconstr Surg 70:173, 1982.

Hirasé H, Kojima T, Kinoshita Y, et al: Composite reconstruction for chest wall and scalp using multiple ribs: Latissimus dorsi osteomyocutaneous flaps as pedicled and free flaps. Plast Reconstr Surg 87:555, 1991.

Laitung JK, Peck F: Shoulder function following the loss of the latissimus dorsi muscle. Br J Plast Surg 38:375, 1985.

Logan AM, Black MJM: Injury to the brachial plexus

resulting from shoulder positioning during latissimus dorsi flap pedicle dissection. Br J Plast Surg 38:380, 1985.

Maruyama Y, Onishi K, Iwahira Y, et al.: Free compound rib-latissimus dorsi osteomusculocutaneous flap in reconstruction of the leg. J Reconstr Microsurg 3:13, 1986.

Maruyama Y, Urita Y, Ohnishi K: Rib-latissimus dorsi osteomyocutaneous flap in reconstruction of a mandibular defect. Br J Plast Surg 38:234, 1985.

Maxwell GP, Manson PN, Hoopes JE: Experience with thirteen latissimus dorsi myocutaneous free flaps. Plast Reconstr Surg 64:1, 1979.

Maxwell GP, McGibbon BM, Hoopes JE: Vascular considerations in the use of a latissimus dorsi myocutaneous flap after a mastectomy with an axillary dissection. Plast Reconstr Surg 64:771, 1979.

Maxwell GP, Stueber K, Hoopes JE: A free latissimus dorsi myocutaneous flap. Plast Reconstr Surg 62:462, 1978.

May JW Jr, Gallico GG III, Jupiter J, Savage RC: Free latissimus dorsi muscle flap with skin graft for treatment of traumatic chronic bony wounds. Plast Reconstr Surg 73:641, 1984.

McCraw JB, Penix JO, Baker JW: Repair of major defects of the chest wall and spine with the latissimus dorsi myocutaneous flap. Plast Reconstr Surg 62:197, 1978.

Noever G, Brueser P, Koehler L: Reconstruction of heel and sole defects by free flaps. Plast Reconstr Surg 78:345, 1986.

Olivari N: Use of thirty latissimus dorsi flaps. Plast Reconstr Surg 64:654, 1979.

Quillen CG, Shearin JC Jr, Georgiade NG: Use of the latissimus dorsi myocutaneous island flap for reconstruction in the head and neck area. Plast Reconstr Surg 62:113, 1978.

Rosen HM: Double island latissimus dorsi muscle-skin flap for through-and-through defects of the forefoot. Plast Reconstr Surg 76:461, 1985.

Rowsell AR, Davies DM, Eisenberg N, Taylor GI: The anatomy of the subscapular-thoracodorsal arterial system: Study of 100 cadaver dissections. Br J Plast Surg 37:574, 1984.

Rowsell AR, Eisenberg N, Davies DM, Taylor GI: The anatomy of the thoracodorsal artery within the latissimus dorsi muscle. Br J Plast Surg 39:206, 1986.

Rowsell AR, Godfrey AM, Richards: The thinned latissimus dorsi free flap: A case report. Br J Plast Surg 39:210, 1986.

Salibian AH, Tesoro VR, Wood DL: Staged transfer of a free microvascular latissimus dorsi myocutaneous flap using saphenous vein grafts. Plast Reconstr Surg 71:543, 1983.

Serafin D, Goodkind DJ: Microsurgical free transfer of a latissimus dorsi musculocutaneous flap. In: Strauch B, Vasconez LO, Hall-Findlay E (eds): *Grabb's Encyclopedia of Flaps*, vol III. Boston: Little, Brown, 1990, pp. 1314–1318.

Stevenson T, Rohrich RJ, Pollack RA, Dingman RO, Bostwick J III: More experience with the "reverse" latissimus dorsi musculocutaneous flap: Precise location of blood supply. Plast Reconstr Surg 74:237, 1984.

Tobin GR, Moberg AW, DuBou RH, Weiner LJ, Bland KI: The split latissimus dorsi myocutaneous flap. Ann Plast Surg 7:272, 1981.

Tobin GR, Schusterman M, Peterson GH, et al.: The intramuscular neurovascular anatomy of the latissimus dorsi muscle: The basis for splitting the flap. Plast Reconstr Surg 67:637, 1981.

Watson JS, Craig RDP, Orton CI: The free latissimus dorsi myocutaneous flap. Plast Reconstr Surg 64:299, 1979.

Scapular and Parascapular Flaps

Barwick WJ, Goodkind DJ, Serafin D: The free scapular flap. Plast Reconstr Surg 69:779, 1982.

Chiu DT, Sherman JE, Edgerton MT: Coverage of the calvarium with a free parascapular flap. Ann Plast Surg 12:60, 1984.

Fonseca dos Santos L, Gilbert A: The free scapular flap. In Strauch B, Vasconez LO, Hall-Findlay E (eds): *Grabb's Encyclopedia of Flaps*, vol. 3. Boston: Little, Brown, 1990, pp. 412 ff.

Fonseca dos Santos L: The vascular anatomy and dissection of the free scapular flap. Plast Reconstr Surg 73:599, 1984.

Gahhos FN, Tross RB, Salomon JC: Scapular free-flap dissection made easier. Plast Reconstr Surg 75:115, 1985.

Gilbert A, Teot L: The free scapular flap. Plast Reconstr Surg 69:601, 1982.

Hamilton SGL, Morrison WA: The scapular free flap. Br J Plast Surg 35:2, 1982.

Kim PS, Gottlieb JR, Harris GD, et al: The dorsal thoracic fascia: Anatomic significance with clinical applications in reconstructive microsurgery. Plast Reconstr Surg 779:72, 1987.

Kim PS, Lewis VL Jr: Use of a pedicled parascapular flap for anterior shoulder and arm reconstruction. Plast Reconstr Surg 76:942, 1985.

Koshima I, Soeda S: Repair of a wide defect of the lower leg with the combined scapular and parascapular flap. Br J Plast Surg 38:518, 1985.

Mayou BJ, Whitby D, Jones BM: The scapular flap—An anatomical and clinical study. Br J Plast Surg 35:8, 1982.

Nassif TM, Vidal L, Bovet JL, Baudet J: The parascapular flap: A new cutaneous microsurgical free flap. Plast Reconstr Surg 69:591, 1982.

Rautio J, Asko-Seljavaara S, Laasonen L, Harma M: Suitability of the scapular flap for reconstructions of the foot. Plast Reconstr Surg 85:922, 1990.

Serra JM, Muirragui A, Tadjalli H: The circumflex scapular flap for reconstruction of mandibulofacial atrophy. J Reconstr Microsurg 1:263, 1985.

Swartz WM, Banis JC, Newton ED, et al.: The osteocutaneous scapular flap for mandibular and maxillary reconstruction. Plast Reconstr Surg 77:530, 1986.

Urbaniak JR, Koman LA, Goldner RD, et al.: The vascularized cutaneous scapular flap. Plast Reconstr Surg 69:772, 1982.

Yanai A, Nagata S, Hirabayashi S, Nakamura N: Inverted-U parascapular flap for the treatment of axillary burn scar contracture. Plast Reconstr Surg 76:126, 1985.

Yang LM, Shi WY, Zhong SZ, et al: Clinical application and anatomical studies of the parascapular flap. Med J PLA of China 8:326, 1983.

Part Four
HEAD AND NECK

12 HEAD AND NECK

Temporoparietal Flap

Arterial Anatomy (Fig. 12-1)

The *superficial temporal artery* [1], a terminal branch of the external carotid artery, lies between the deep and superficial lobes of the parotid gland at its origin and is covered there by the facial nerve. As it emerges from between the lobes, it lies lateral to the temporomandibular joint and gives off the *middle temporal* [2] and *transverse facial arteries* [3]. At the zygomatic arch, it blends into the superficial temporal fascia. In 80% of cases, it bifurcates above the zygomatic arch into anterior and posterior branches [4,5]. The internal caliber at this level ranges from 1.8 to 2.7 mm. Its length ranges from 2.5 to 5.0 cm, averaging 3.4 cm.

The *middle temporal artery* [2] arises from the superficial temporal artery [1] at or just below and superficial to the zygomatic arch. Immediately above the zygomatic arch, it enters the deep temporal fascia and arborizes within it. The middle temporal vein accompanies the artery throughout its course.

The *superficial temporal vein*, measuring between 2.1 and 3.3 mm in diameter, usually lies anterior to the artery and within 0.8 cm of it. However, the vein can be as distant as 3 cm away from the artery. Near the origin of the artery, the superficial temporal vein joins the maxillary vein to form the retromandibular vein, which drains into the external jugular vein.

The *auriculotemporal nerve*, a sensory branch of the trigeminal nerve, lies posterior to the superficial temporal vessels and above the superficial temporal fascia; it proceeds to innervate the temporal scalp.

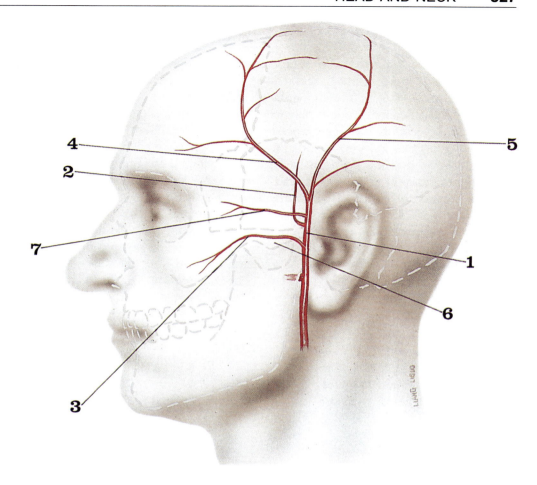

1. Superficial temporal a.
2. Middle temporal a.
3. Transverse facial a.
4. Anterior branch
5. Posterior branch
6. Zygomatic arch
7. Zygomatico-orbital a.

COMMENT AND INSIGHTS

The temporoparietal fascia free flap is a thin, highly vascularized unit having a consistently reliable pedicle. Its versatility stems from its nonbulky, supple property. It can drape over cartilage stripped of perichondrium and maintain the definition of the underlying framework in ear and nasal reconstruction. Likewise, it can contour into bony concavities as part of the treatment of chronic osteomyelitis. Temporoparietal fascial free flaps have proven especially useful in hand reconstruction, in simultaneously restoring a gliding apparatus for tendons denuded of paratenon and providing an elastic vascularized surface in wound closure. The scalp donor site scar is relatively inconspicuous. The operation accommodates a two-team approach.

Drawbacks of this flap include alopecia at the donor site and tedious elevation of the scalp flaps. Alopecia is usually transient and resolves in several months. It may be prevented by deepening the dissection and not exposing the hair follicles when raising the scalp flaps. Redundant wound margins may also be excised.

An osteofascial flap consisting of outer table of frontoparietal calvarium may be transferred by the superficial temporal pedicle. Because it is vascularized and contains membranous bone, this flap is appropriate for bony reconstructions in unfavorable recipient sites, e.g., scarred, irradiated beds, hypoplastic zygomaticomaxillary complex reconstructions in Treacher-Collins syndrome, or clinically infected hand defects requiring grafting to the metacarpals.

TEMPOROPARIETAL FASCIA FLAP

The *superficial temporal fascia* (temporoparietal fascia) is a thin, highly vascular layer of connective tissue that is a component of the superficial musculoaponeurotic system (SMAS). It is continuous with the galea aponeurotica superiorly, the occipitalis posteriorly, the frontalis anteriorly, and the deep investing fascia overlying the parotid gland and the muscles of facial expression inferiorly. It lies immediately beneath the hair follicles of the temporoparietal scalp and is progressively more adherent to the subdermal fibrofatty layer in which they lie, as it proceeds from the level of the zygomatic arch cephalad toward the vertex of the skull. The subdermal layer of the scalp is also attached to the superficial temporal fascia by numerous small vessels. The superficial temporal fascia overlies the deep temporal fascia and is separated from it by a loose, areolar plane. The superficial temporal fascia is 1.4 to 3.8 mm thick in the preauricular region of children, and 2.2 to 4.2 mm thick in adults. Its expansion is upward of 14 × 17 cm. Near the lateral orbital rim in the frontozygomatic area, the frontal branches of the facial nerve lie deep to an attenuated portion of the superficial temporal fascia, thus increasing its vulnerability during dissection.

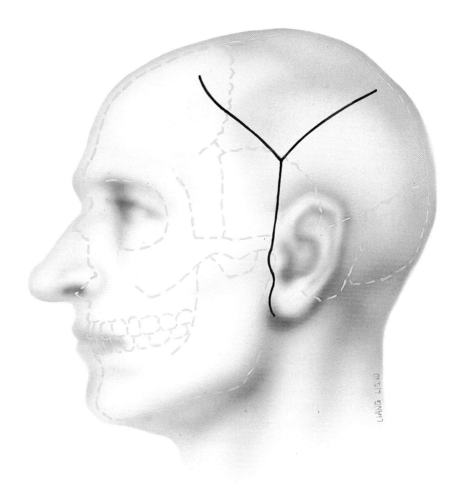

(Fig. 12-2) The pulse of the superficial temporal artery is appreciated in the preauricular area by palpation and Doppler probe. A rhytidectomy incision is outlined to extend vertically and to bifurcate in lofty "Y" fashion two thirds of the distance to the apex of the skull at the upper temporal fossa.

1. Superficial temporal a. and v.
2. Superficial temporal fascia
3. Frontal branch of facial n.
4. Auriculotemporal n.
5. Deep temporal fascia
6. Parotid gland

(Fig. 12-3) The superficial temporal vessels [1] are identified pretragally. Elevation of the scalp flaps begins inferiorly where the plane between the dermis and superficial temporal fascia [2] is more easily identified. As dissection proceeds cephalad, separation becomes increasingly difficult, because the fibrous septae and piercing vessels within the subcutaneous fat connecting the superficial temporal artery to the overlying scalp are quite dense. This plane is painstakingly developed so that it is deep enough to avoid exposure of the hair follicles, yet superficial enough not to injure the superficial temporal fascia [2]. Hemostasis is maintained by liberal use of the bipolar cautery. When dissecting in the frontozygomatic region, a nerve stimulator may help in localizing the frontal branch of the facial nerve [3]. The auriculotemporal nerve [4] is invariably incorporated within the fascial flap.

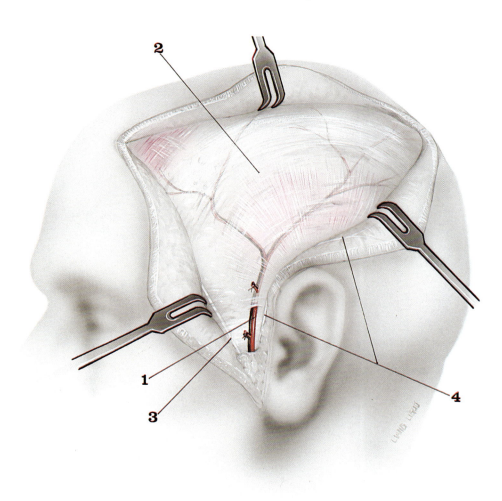

1. Superficial temporal a. and v.
2. Superficial temporal fascia
3. Frontal branch of facial n.
4. Auriculotemporal n.

(**Fig. 12-4**) After the scalp flaps are completely reflected, a template outlining the required geometry of the flap is applied to the superficial temporal fascia [2] and marked. The superficial temporal fascia is incised and readily elevated along with its pedicle in retrograde fashion. This is expedited by the loose, areolar plane that separates the superficial and deep temporal fasciae [2,5].

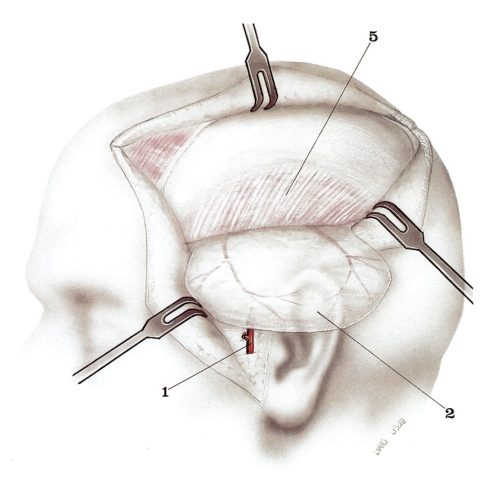

1. Superficial temporal a. and v.
2. Superficial temporal fascia
5. Deep temporal fascia

(Fig. 12-5) The superficial temporoparietal fascia flap [2] is completely raised from the deep fascia. In order to avoid damage to the branches of the facial nerve, further dissection of the vascular pedicle [1] in the parotid gland [6] is not recommended.

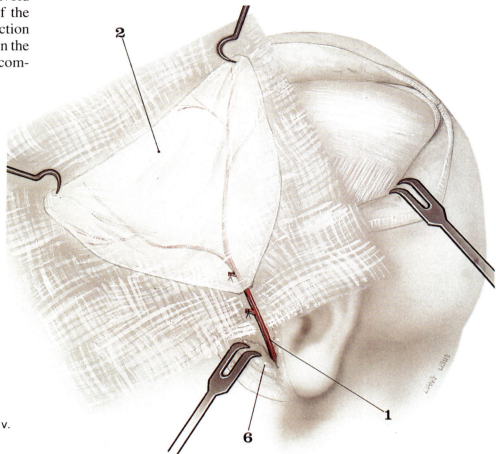

1. Superficial temporal a. and v.
2. Superficial temporal fascia
6. Parotid gland

BILOBED TEMPORAL FASCIA FLAP

When more tissue is required, a bilobed flap consisting of the superficial and deep temporal fascial leaves may be developed on the superficial temporal arterial pedicle.

The *deep temporal fascia* is a dense, semicircular fascial sheath that invests the temporal muscle. At each margin, this fascial layer ends by attaching to the periosteum of the frontal, temporal, and parietal bones, and the upper edge of the zygomatic arch. It measures approximately 7 cm in both dimensions. The deep temporal fascia is supplied by the middle temporal artery.

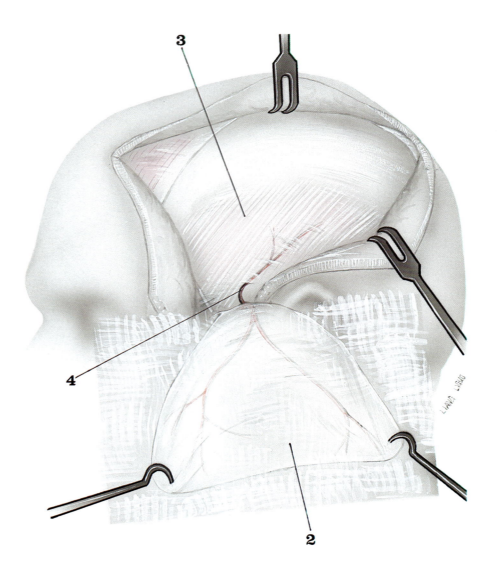

(Fig. 12-6) The superficial fascial flap [2] is raised as described in the section on the superficial temporal fascial flap.

1. Superficial temporal a. and v.
2. Superficial temporal fascia
3. Deep temporal fascia
4. Middle temporal a. and v.
5. Temporalis m.

(**Fig. 12-7**) The deep temporal fascia [3] is lifted off the underlying temporalis muscle [5] and sharply separated below from its zygomatic attachment. The middle temporal vessel [4] originating from the superficial temporal artery [1] and supplying the deep temporal fascia [3] is preserved. The double-leaf arrangement is particularly suited to tendon reconstruction in simultaneously providing vascularized coverage and an envelope of gliding surfaces.

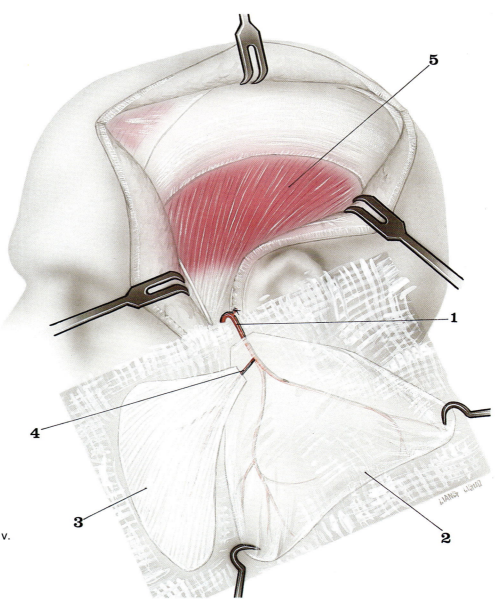

1. Superficial temporal a. and v.
2. Superficial temporal fascia
3. Deep temporal fascia
4. Middle temporal a. and v.
5. Temporalis m.

TEMPOROCALVARIAL OSTEOFASCIAL FLAP

As has already been mentioned, the SMAS is continuous with the galea through the temporoparietal fascia. The superficial temporal, occipital, and supratrochlear vessels form a rich, anastomotic network located just above the galea. As part of this complex, the superficial temporal artery, approximately 1 to 2 cm beyond the temporal line (a ridge that begins at the zygomatic process of the frontal bone coursing upward and backward across the frontal and parietal bones and ending at the supramastoid crest, representing the cephalic-most portion of the temporalis muscle), sends perforators down through the galea and periosteum. In the frontoparietal region, these perforators, in turn, anastomose through the diploë with branches of the middle meningeal artery, the dominant blood supply to the calvarium.

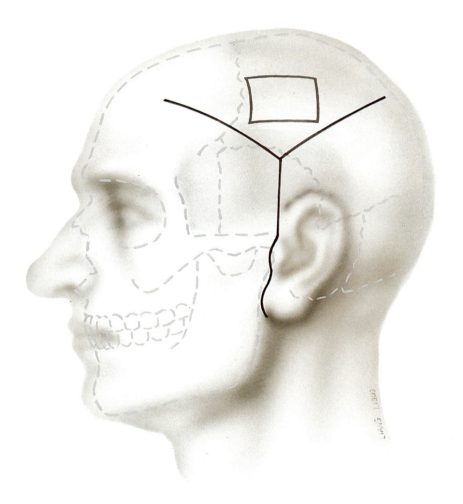

(Fig. 12-8) The skin incision and proposed outer table of calvarial bone are illustrated. The bone is outlined above the temporal line [6].

1. Frontoparietal bone
2. Superficial temporal a. and v.
3. Outer table of calvarial bone
4. Inner table of calvarial bone
5. Superficial temporal fascia
6. Temporal line

(Fig. 12-9) In harvesting the partial-thickness vascularized bone flap, care must be taken to incorporate all layers—galea bearing the overlying superficial temporal vascular network [2], periosteum, and outer table of calvarium [3]—as a composite. This is accomplished by suturing the galea and periosteal layers and drilling holes at the periphery of the bone, to prevent shearing at the deep surface of the galea. On its superficial surface where the galea is densely adherent to the scalp, dissection necessarily proceeds tediously, exposing the hair follicles of the dermis and preserving the superficial temporal vascular network covering the superficial surface of the galea. To augment the circulation in a partial-thickness bone flap, or when full-thickness calvarium is favored, the deep temporal fascia continuous with the periosteum above the temporal line is elevated along with the superficial temporal fascia [5], as part of the composite flap, thereby adding contributions from the middle temporal arteries. Moreover, the deep temporal fascia and its middle temporal arterial system are sufficient to carry the outer table of calvarium [3].

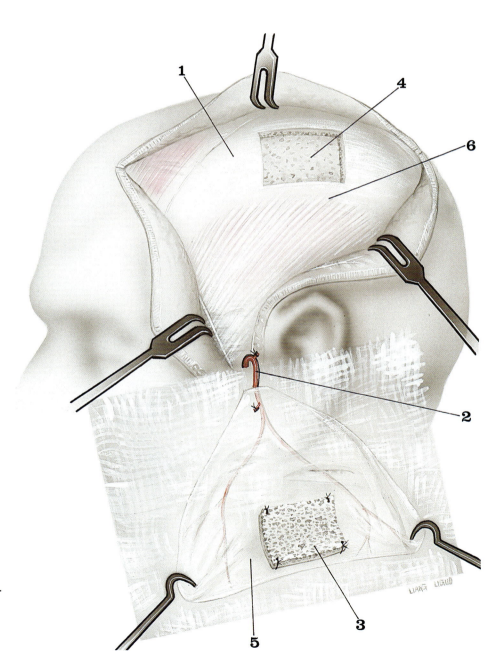

1. Frontoparietal bone
2. Superficial temporal a. and v.
3. Outer table of calvarial bone
4. Inner table of calvarial bone
5. Superficial temporal fascia
6. Temporal line

FREE SCALP SKIN FLAP

(**Fig. 12-10**) The superficial temporal arterial pedicle may be used to carry overlying scalp in correcting male-pattern baldness and temporal alopecia cicatrices (bald scars) in burn and trauma patients. Hair-bearing scalp flaps as small as 2.5 × 12 cm and as large as 6 × 35 cm have been successfully transferred.

1. Superficial temporal a. and v.
2. Hair-bearing scalp flap
3. Periosteum of calvarial bone
4. Deep temporal fascia

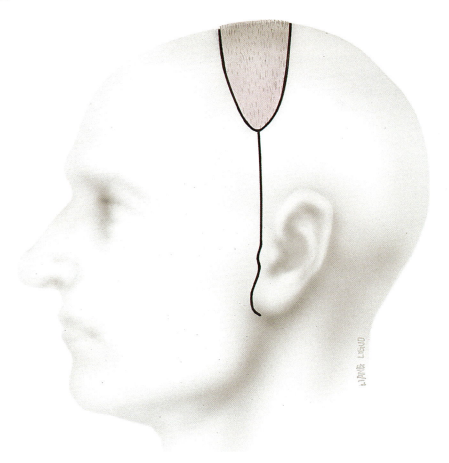

(**Fig. 12-11**) A top view of the flap design.

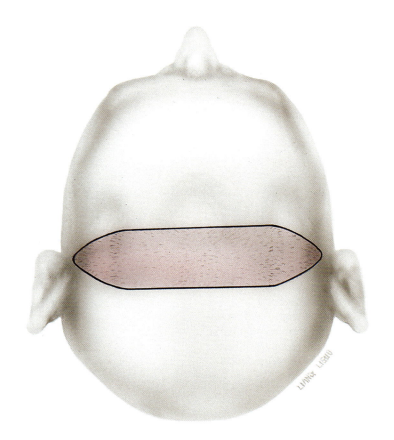

(Fig. 12-12) This composite flap consists of the scalp and underlying superficial temporal fascia bearing the superficial temporal arterial network [1]. The recipient vessels are usually the contralateral superficial temporal artery and vein. The transplanted scalp bears hair of normal density that grows in a natural anterior direction. The hair stream covers the inconspicuous scar. Donor defects up to 4 cm wide may be closed primarily.

1. Superficial temporal a. and v.
2. Hair-bearing scalp flap
3. Periosteum of calvarial bone
4. Deep temporal fascia

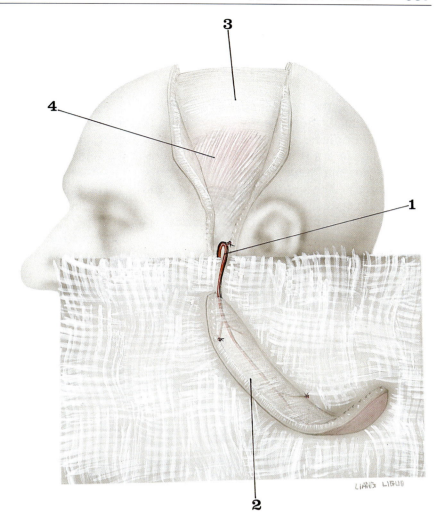

Superficial Cervical Flap

Arterial Anatomy (Fig. 12-13)

In most cases, the *superficial cervical artery* [5] arises directly from the thyrocervical trunk [2], which originates from the first portion of the subclavian artery [1] and almost immediately divides into three branches (the inferior thyroid artery [3], suprascapular artery [4], and superficial cervical artery [5] itself).

At its inception, the superficial cervical artery lies in front of the scalenus anterior, phrenic nerve, and brachial plexus, and behind the sternocleidomastoid and internal jugular vein. It runs laterally to cross the posterior cervical triangle. After passing over the brachial plexus and behind the inferior belly of the omohyoid, it divides into ascending and descending branches.

The *ascending branch* [6] runs superficially, giving off several small branches to the skin area of the posterior cervical triangle and ascending along the anterior border of the trapezius, where it anastomoses with the descending branch of the occipital artery. The *descending branch* [7] of the superficial cervical artery goes, along with the spinal accessory nerve, to the undersurface of the trapezius as its main blood supply.

The superficial cervical artery measures 1.0 to 1.5 mm in diameter at its origin.

Innervation of the Posterior Cervical Triangle

The *anterior, middle, and posterior supraclavicular nerves* emerge from the cervical plexus deep to the posterior margin of the sternocleidomastoid muscle. They course inferiorly across the triangle and branch out to the overlying skin. The middle trunk innervates the majority of this skin territory.

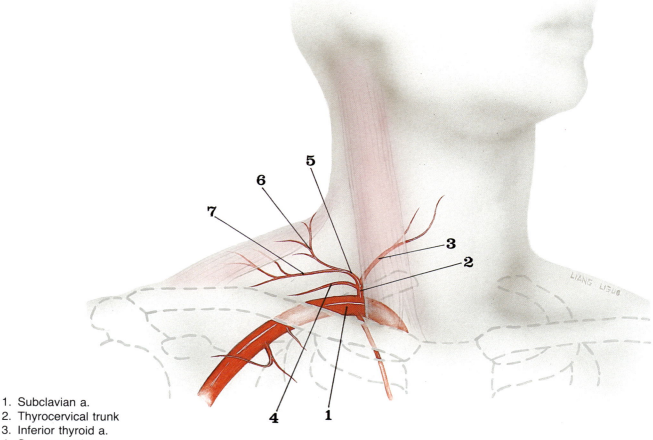

1. Subclavian a.
2. Thyrocervical trunk
3. Inferior thyroid a.
4. Suprascapular a.
5. Superficial cervical a.
6. Ascending branch
7. Descending branch

Variations in the Superficial Cervical Artery (Fig. 12-14)

Type A. In the majority of cases, the superficial cervical artery independently arises from the thyrocervical trunk [4], whereas the transverse cervical artery [2] originates from the second or third portion of the subclavian artery [5], to supply the muscles near the scapula.

Type B. In a minority of cases, the superficial cervical artery [1] arises from the transverse cervical artery [2], which originates from the thyrocervical trunk [4] and runs posteriorly to the scapular area.

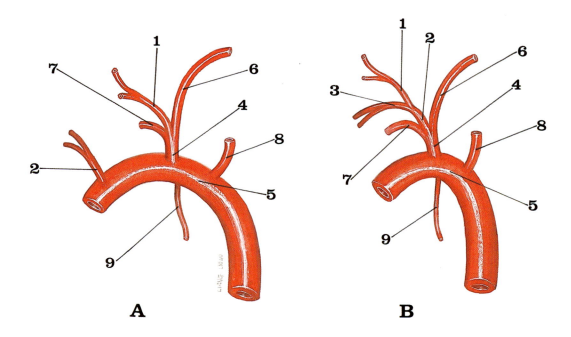

1. Superficial cervical a.
2. Transverse cervical c.
3. Deep branch of transverse cervical a.
4. Thyrocervical trunk
5. Subclavian a.
6. Inferior thyroid a.
7. Suprascapular a.
8. Vertebral a.
9. Internal mammary a.

COMMENT AND INSIGHTS

The superficial cervical free flap is fairly thin and its origin in the neck provides favorable thickness and color match in resurfacing facial defects. As an innervated flap, it is useful in offering both stable coverage and restoring sensibility in hand, heel, ankle, and transmetatarsal amputation site reconstruction.

Disadvantages of this flap are mainly related to its anatomy. Pedicle components do not course together in "comitante" fashion. Instead, the artery, vein, and nerve enter the flap at different points, making dissection tedious and restricting the flap orientation at the recipient site. The proximal dissection at the thyrocervical trunk is fairly deep, necessitating working in a hole. Moreover, the arterial diameter is smaller when compared with that of other thin, cutaneous, free flaps, e.g., the radial forearm free flap.

Donor site morbidity includes potential injury to the great auricular and spinal accessory nerves. Donor site closure may result in a widened scar of skin graft in a fairly conspicuous location.

Harvesting Technique

(**Fig. 12-15**) The flap is outlined in the posterior triangle of the neck, which is defined by the posterior margin of the sternocleidomastoid anteriorly, the anterior margin of the trapezius posteriorly, and the middle third of the clavicle inferiorly, centered along the axis of the superficial cervical artery that is marked from the sternoclavicular joint to the midpoint of the lateral margin of the trapezius (between the acromion and the external occipital protuberance). Depending on skin laxity, flaps as large as 8 × 15 cm can be transferred without having to skin graft the donor site.

1. Superficial cervical a.
2. Omohyoid m.
3. Sternocleidomastoid m.
4. Clavicle bone
5. Trapezius m.
6. Spinal accessory n.
7. External jugular v.
8. Supraclavicular n.
9. Thyrocervical trunk

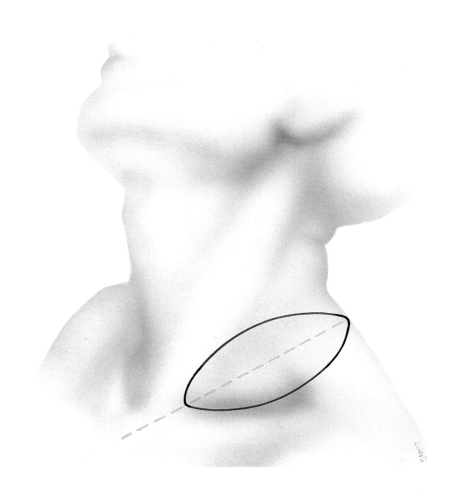

(Fig. 12-16) The anterior skin incision of the flap is made first, so as to identify the superficial cervical artery [1], and is carried through platysma and deep fascia. The omohyoid [2] is divided and the entrance of the superficial cervical artery to the flap is identified. The artery is traced to its origin at the thyrocervical trunk in the supraclavicular triangle, bordered by the posterior belly of the omohyoid [2] superiorly, clavicle [4] inferiorly, and clavicular insertion of the sternocleidomastoid muscle [3] medially.

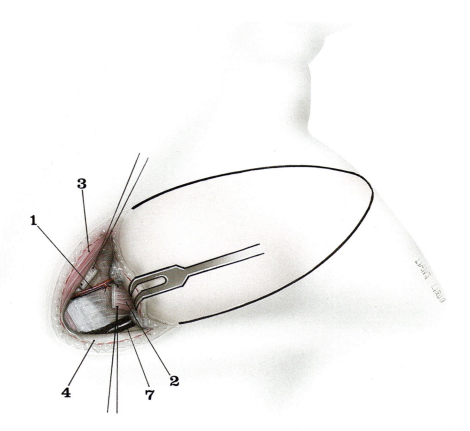

1. Superficial cervical a.
2. Omohyoid m.
3. Sternocleidomastoid m.
4. Clavicle bone
7. External jugular v.

(Fig. 12-17) The dorsal margin of the flap is incised and elevated proximally so as to incorporate the superficial cervical arteriovenous pedicle [1]. The plane of dissection is beneath the supraclavicular fat pad through which course the artery, vein, and nerves. Care must be taken at this point to avoid injury to the spinal accessory nerve [6] when dividing the artery as it enters the trapezius muscle [5].

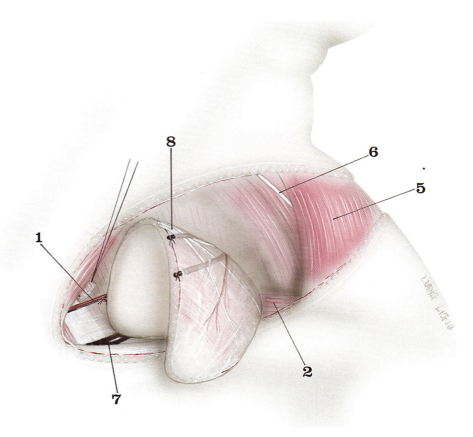

1. Superficial cervical a.
2. Omohyoid m.
5. Trapezius m.
6. Spinal accessory n.
7. External jugular v.
8. Supraclavicular n.

(Fig. 12-18) The venae comitantes of the superficial and other venous tributaries within the flap are followed to the external jugular vein [7] that is used as the pedicle. When taken as a sensory flap, the supraclavicular nerves [8] may be identified by tracing the great auricular nerve downward as it courses over the sternocleidomastoid muscle. As it dives behind the midposterior border of the muscle, the supraclavicular nerves are encountered arising from the cervical plexus.

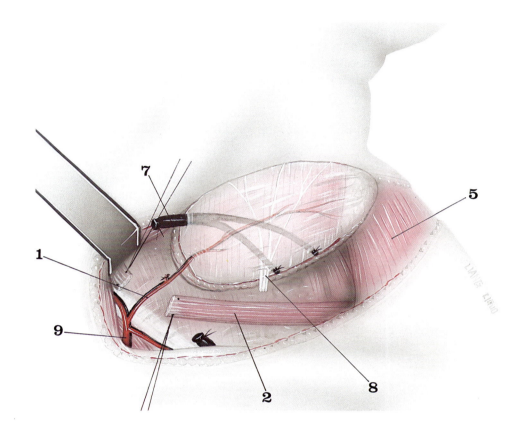

1. Superficial cervical a.
2. Omohyoid m.
5. Trapezius m.
7. External jugular v.
8. Supraclavicular n.
9. Thyrocervical trunk

Submental Flap

Anatomy (Fig. 12-19)

The *facial artery* [2] arises from the external carotid artery [1], a little above the level of the greater cornu of the hyoid bone. It runs upward behind the stylohyoid [7] and the posterior belly of the digastric [8] to enter the groove between the submandibular gland [4] and the medial pterygoid muscle, where it gives off three or four branches to the gland. It then goes forward to reach the lower border of the mandible. At the anterior edge of the masseter [6], it turns upward around the mandible toward the medial palpebral commissure.

The *submental artery* [5] is given off from the facial artery [2] immediately after the facial artery leaves the submandibular gland [4] and before it turns upward. It goes forward between the mylohyoid [9] and platysma in the submental region toward the chin. At the chin, it turns upward over the base of the mandible, where it divides into superficial and deep branches. In its course, the submental artery gives off some branches to the platysma and overlying skin. The diameter of this artery usually exceeds 1 mm and it is accompanied by its venae comitantes. The submental artery supplies a skin area of the ipsilateral mental and submental region.

Venous Drainage

After crossing over the mandible, the facial vein receives the submental vein, and then runs obliquely backward *separately* from the facial artery, superficial to the submandibular gland, digastric, and stylohyoid muscles. It communicates with the external jugular vein before draining to the internal jugular vein at the level of the hyoid bone. The submental venae comitantes travel with the artery and join the facial vein proximally.

Innervation

The sensibility of the submental area is supplied by several terminal branches of the transverse cutaneous nerve of the neck, which derives from the cervical plexus.

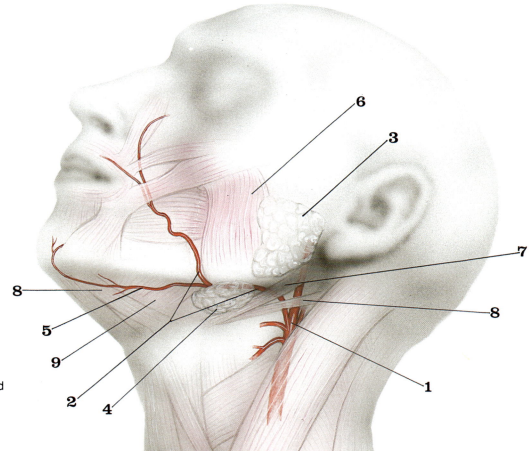

1. External carotid a.
2. Facial a.
3. Parotid gland
4. Submandibular gland
5. Submental a.
6. Masseter m.
7. Stylohyoid m.
8. Digastric m.
9. Mylohyoid m.

COMMENT AND INSIGHTS

This is a newly developed flap. According to preliminary reports of flap anatomy and clinical application, this flap would be useful in reconstructive surgery of the head and neck, especially with ipsilateral pedicle transfer for face and neck defects. A free submental flap has been reported for reconstruction of a contralateral facial defect. However, further anatomic investigations and wider clinical applications are needed.

The skin in the submandibular and submental regions is usually very delicate. It may be hairy in adult males, and its thickness varies with the individual. The resultant linear scar under the mandible may be inconspicuous and is reported to be acceptable. Direct skin closure may result in tightness at the front of the neck; if neck extension is thereby limited, a secondary release would be required.

There may be the risk of injury to the marginal mandibular branch of the facial nerve during flap dissection, although this can be avoided with care.

Harvesting Technique

(Fig. 12-20) The patient is positioned with the neck extended and the face turned toward the contralateral side. The flap is located in the submandibular and submental regions. Its superior margin follows the inferior border of the mandible; its anterior margin can go beyond the midline by 2 or 3 cm; and the posterior margin is located perpendicular to the anterior edge of the masseter where the facial artery can be palpated. The inferior margin depends on the width of the proposed flap. Usually, the skin defect can be directly closed after removal of a flap with a width of about 6 cm. The common size of the submental flap is approximately 6 cm × 11 cm.

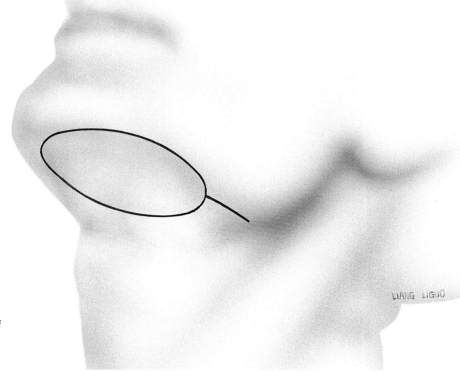

1. Submental a. and v.
2. Facial a. and v.
3. Digastric m.
4. Mylohyoid m.
5. Submandibular gland
6. Marginal mandibular branch of facial n.
7. Mandible
8. Platysma m.

(Fig. 12-21) The inferior margin of the flap is incised through the platysma [8], and the facial vein [2] can be visualized at the posterior portion of the inferior margin under the platysma. Keeping the facial vein and platysma together with the flap, the lower flap portion is elevated from the mylohyoid [4] and the anterior belly of the digastric [3], as well as from the surface of the submandibular gland [5], until the upper edge of the gland and the submental vessels [1] are identified.

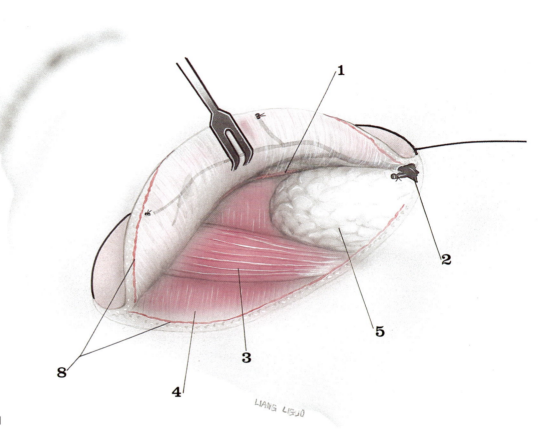

1. Submental a. and v.
2. Facial a. and v.
3. Digastric m.
4. Mylohyoid m.
5. Submandibular gland
8. Platysma m.

(Fig. 12-22) The superior margin of the flap is incised. Special attention should be paid, when dividing the platysma, to avoid injury to the marginal mandibular branch of the facial nerve [6]. After emerging from the parotid gland, this branch of the facial nerve usually runs along the lower border of the mandible under the platysma [8] and crosses the facial vessels [2] to supply the risorius and the muscles of the lower lip and chin. Sometimes, it appears above the lower border of the mandible or lies upon the submandibular gland [5].

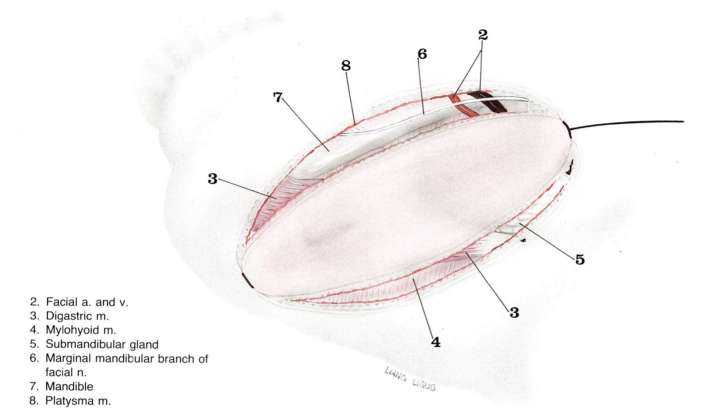

2. Facial a. and v.
3. Digastric m.
4. Mylohyoid m.
5. Submandibular gland
6. Marginal mandibular branch of facial n.
7. Mandible
8. Platysma m.

(Fig. 12-23) Under direct visualization, the marginal mandibular branch of the facial nerve [6] is preserved at the donor site, and the submental vessels [1] are included in the flap. The flap is elevated anteriorly to posteriorly, and the submental vessels are then traced to their origin from the facial vessels [2].

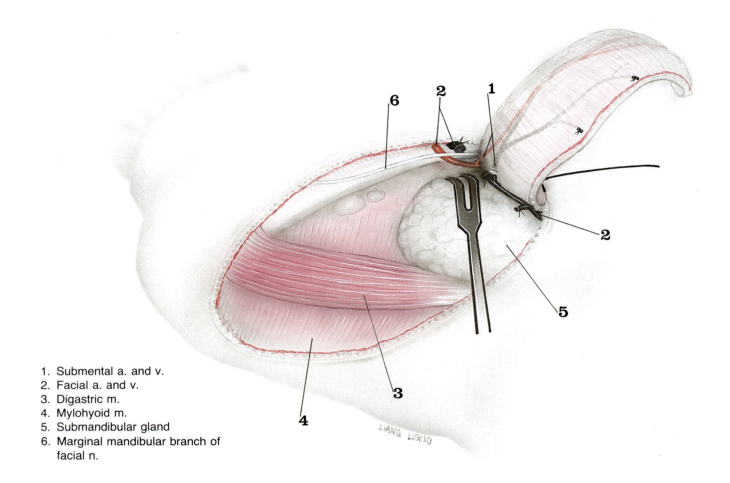

1. Submental a. and v.
2. Facial a. and v.
3. Digastric m.
4. Mylohyoid m.
5. Submandibular gland
6. Marginal mandibular branch of facial n.

(Fig. 12-24) Through a 3-cm extension incision, the submandibular gland [5] is separated from the mandible [7], and the facial artery [2] is dissected out by ligating its trunk over the mandible going toward the face and its branches to the gland.

Since the facial vein [2] lies superficially, the venous pedicle can be of sufficient length, although the length of the arterial pedicle can attain about 6 cm by further dissection.

For donor-site closure, the inferior flap edge should be undermined, pulled up toward the superior edge, with the superior edge kept intact. Tension should be avoided, to prevent distortion of the lower lip.

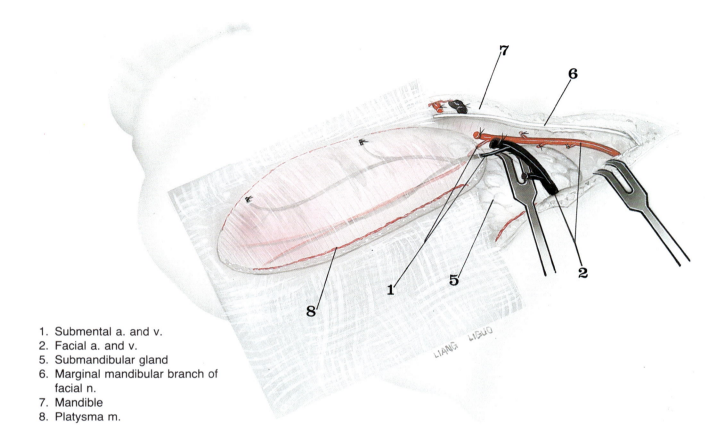

1. Submental a. and v.
2. Facial a. and v.
5. Submandibular gland
6. Marginal mandibular branch of facial n.
7. Mandible
8. Platysma m.

RECIPIENT SITE EXPOSURES

The External Carotid Artery and Its Branches

(Fig. 12-25) The patient is placed in a supine position, with the neck extended and the head turned to the contralateral side. An incision is made transversely at the upper third of the neck, on the middle portion of a curved line from the thyroid cartilage to the mastoid process.

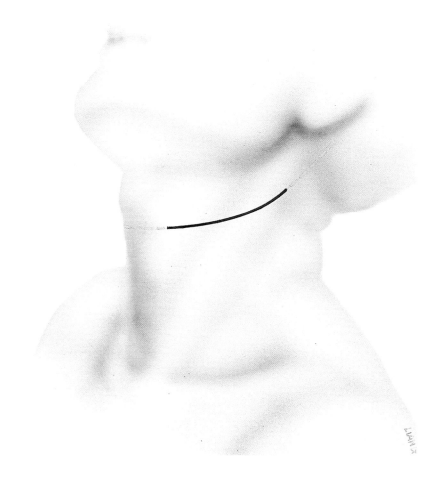

1. Parotid gland
2. Sternocleidomastoid m.
3. Facial v.
4. External jugular v.
5. Mandibular branch of facial n.
6. Platysma m.
7. Stylohyoid m.
8. Digastric m.
9. Carotid sheath
10. External carotid a.
11. Internal carotid a.
12. Internal jugular v.
13. Superior thyroid a.
14. Superior laryngeal a.
15. Lingual a.
16. Facial a.
17. Hypoglossal n.

(**Fig. 12-26**) The platysma [6] and deep cervical fascia are incised, the upper and lower skin flaps are developed and retracted, and the anterior border of the sternocleidomastoid muscle [2] is then identified. Attention should be paid not to injure the marginal mandibular branch of the facial nerve [5], which lies below the parotid [1] and mandible and under the platysma [6], and extends to supply the risorius and the muscle of the lower lip and chin.

The facial vein [3] incorporating the communication between the deep and superficial systems is ideally suited as a recipient vein.

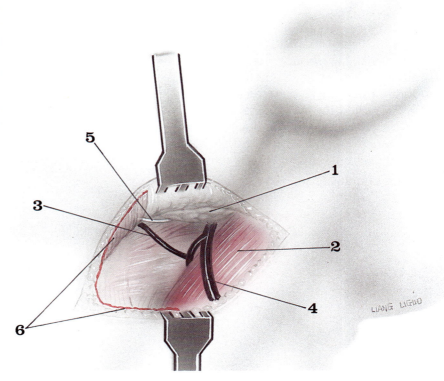

1. Parotid gland
2. Sternocleidomastoid m.
3. Facial v.
4. External jugular v.
5. Mandibular branch of facial n.
6. Platysma m.

(**Fig. 12-27**) The facial vein [3] is traced distally, ligated or microclipped. The sternocleidomastoid muscle [2] is mobilized and retracted posteriorly. The carotid sheath [9] is exposed.

2. Sternocleidomastoid m.
3. Facial v.
4. External jugular v.
7. Stylohyoid m.
8. Digastric m.
9. Carotid sheath

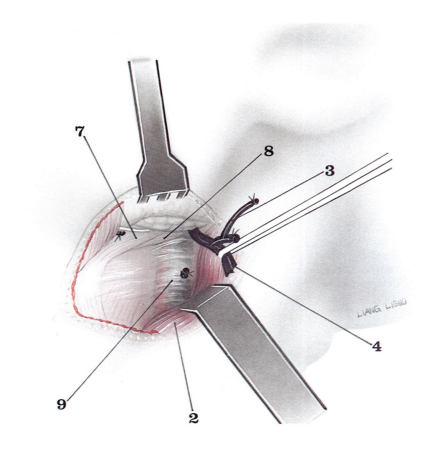

(Fig. 12-28) After the sheath is open, the internal jugular vein [12], which is usually superficial to the artery, is dissected and gently retracted with vessel loops. The external carotid artery [10], which arises from the common carotid artery at about the level of the upper border of the thyroid cartilage, is easily revealed. However, the hypoglossal nerve [17] (the 12th cranial nerve, which crosses the external and internal carotid arteries [10,11] at a level a little above the hyoid bone), should be identified and protected, before isolating the following three branches of the external carotid artery.

The superior thyroid artery [13] arises from the vessel a little above the upper margin of the thyroid cartilage and goes anteroinferiorly. The lingual artery [15] leaves the vessel at the level of the greater horn of the hyoid bone and runs deep to the hyoglossus muscle. The facial artery [16] arises a little above the lingual artery and runs upward.

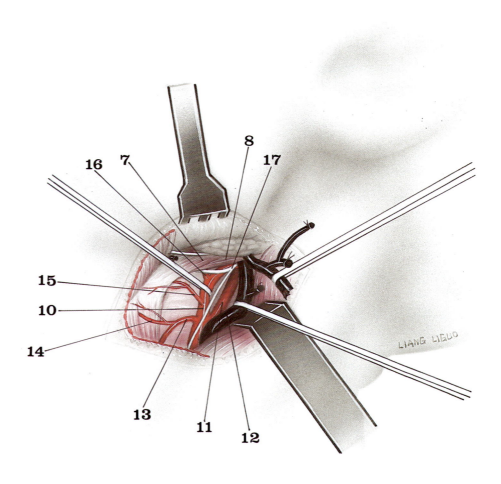

7. Stylohyoid m.
8. Digastric m.
10. External carotid a.
11. Internal carotid a.
12. Internal jugular v.
13. Superior thyroid a.
14. Superior laryngeal a.
15. Lingual a.
16. Facial a.
17. Hypoglossal n.

BIBLIOGRAPHY

Temporoparietal Flaps

Abul-Hassan HS, van Drasek-Ascher G, Acland RD: Surgical anatomy and blood supply of the fascial layers of the temporal region. Plast Reconstr Surg 77:17, 1986.

Brent B, Byrd HS: Secondary ear reconstruction with cartilage grafts covered by axial, random, and free flaps of temporoparietal fascia. Plast Reconstr Surg 72:141, 1983.

Brent B, Upton J, Acland RD, et al: Experience with the temporoparietal fascial free flap. Plast Reconstr Surg 76:177, 1985.

Carstens MH, Greco RJ, Hurwitz DJ, Tolhurst DE: Clinical applications of the subgaleal fascia. Plast Reconstr Surg 87:615, 1991.

Chiarelli A, Baldelli A, DiVincenzo A, Martini G: Utilization of the superficial temporoparietal fascia in reconstructive plastic surgery: A clinical case. Ophthal Plast Reconstr Surg 5:274, 1989.

Chowdary RP: Use of temporoparietal fascia free flap in digital reconstruction. Ann Plast Surg 23:543, 1989.

Delaere PR, Guelinckx PJ, Ostyn F: Vascularized temporoparietal fascial flap for closure of a nasal septal perforation: Report of a case. Acta Otorhinolaryngol Belg 44:47, 1990.

East CA, Brough MD, Grant HR: Mastoid obliteration with the temporoparietal fascia flap. J Laryngol Otol 105:417, 1991.

Hallock GG: The extended temporoparietal fascia "non-free" flap. Ann Plast Surg 22:65, 1989.

Hing DN, Buncke HJ, Alpert BS: Use of the temporoparietal free fascial flap in the upper extremity. Plast Reconstr Surg 81:534, 1988.

Hirase Y, Kojima T, Bang HH: Secondary reconstruction by temporoparietal free fascial flap for ring avulsion injury. Ann Plast Surg 25:312, 1990.

Hirase Y, Kojima T, Hirakawa M: Secondary ear reconstruction using deep temporal fascia after temporoparietal fascial reconstruction in microtia. Ann Plast Surg 25:53, 1990.

Jenkins AM, Finucan T: Primary nonmicrosurgical reconstruction following ear avulsion using the temporoparietal fascial island flap. Plast Reconstr Surg 83:148, 1989.

Marks MW, Friedman RJ, Thornton JW, Argenta LC: The temporal island scalp flap for management of facial burn scars. Plast Reconstr Surg 82:257, 1988.

Matsuba HM, Hakki AR, Romm S, et al: Variations on the temporoparietal fascial flap. Laryngoscope 100:1236, 1990.

Rose EH: Small flap coverage of hand and digit defects. Clin Plast Surg 16:427, 1989.

Rose EH, Norris MS: The versatile temporoparietal fascial flap: Adaptability to a variety of composite defects. Plast Reconstr Surg 85:224, 1990.

Turpin IM, Altman DI, Cruz HG, Achauer BM: Salvage of the severely injured ear. Ann Plast Surg 21:170, 1988.

Upton J, Rogers C, Durham-Smith G, Swartz WM: Clinical applications of free temporoparietal flaps in hand reconstruction. J Hand Surg 11A:475, 1986.

Superficial Cervical Flap

Dassler EH, Anson HJ: Surgical anatomy of the subclavian artery and its branches. Surg Gynec Obstet 108:149, 1959.

Freeland AP, Rogers JH: The vascular supply of the cervical skin with reference to incision planning. Laryngoscope 85:714, 1975.

Futrell JW, Rabson JA: Discussion of Coleman JJ, Jurkiewicz MJ, Nahai F, Mathes SJ: The platysma musculocutaneous flap: Experience with 24 cases. Plast Reconstr Surg 72:322, 1983.

Huelke DF: Study of the transverse cervical and dorsal scapular arteries. Anat Reconstr 132:233, 1958.

Hurwitz CJ, Rabson JA, Futrell JW: The anatomic basis for the platysma skin flap. Plast Reconstr Surg 72:302, 1983.

Kenyeres MP: A new cervical island flap: A preliminary report. Acta Chir Plast 24:90, 1982.

Lamberty BGH: The supraclavicular axial patterned flap. Br J Plast Surg 32:207, 1979.

Lamberty BGH: The cutaneous arterial supply of cervical skin in relation to axial skin flaps. Anat Clin 3:317, 1982.

Mathes SJ, Vasconez LO: The cervico humeral flap. Plast Reconstr Surg 61:7, 1978.

Morris RL, Dillman D, McCabe JS, et al: The transverse cervical neurovascular free flap. Ann Plast Surg 10:90, 1983.

Submental Flap

Baudet J, Martin D, Pascal JF, Peres JM, et al: The submental area: A new donor site. Presented at the 10th Symposium of the International Society of Reconstructive Microsurgery, Munich, Germany, September 19, 1991.

Martin D, Baudet J, Mondie JM, Peri G: A propos du lambeau cutane sous-mental en îlot: Protocole operatoire. Perspectives d'utilisation. Ann Chir Plast Esthet 35:480, 1990.

General References

Anderson JE (ed): *Grant's Atlas of Anatomy*, 8th ed. Baltimore: Williams & Wilkins, 1983.

Banks SW, Laufman H: *An Atlas of Surgical Exposures of the Extremities*, 2nd ed. Philadelphia: WB Saunders, 1987.

Chen Z-W, Yang D-Y, Chang D-S: *Microsurgery*. NY: Springer-Verlag, Shanghai Scientific and Technical Publishers, 1982.

Clemente CD: *Anatomy: A Regional Atlas of the Human Body*, 3rd ed. Baltimore: Urban & Schwarzenberg, 1987.

Cormack GC, Lamberty GH: *The Arterial Anatomy of Skin Flaps*. Edinburgh: Churchill Livingstone, 1986.

Daniller AI, Strauch B: *Symposium on Microsurgery*, vol 14. St. Louis: CV Mosby, 1976:

Gordon L: *Microsurgical Reconstruction of the Extremities*. New York: Springer-Verlag, 1988.

Harii K: *Microvascular Tissue Transfer: Fundamental Techniques and Clinical Applications*. Tokyo: Igaku-Shoin, 1983.

Henry AK: *Extensile Exposure*, 2nd ed. Edinburgh: Churchill Livingstone, 1973.

Loré JM Jr: *An Atlas of Head and Neck Surgery*, 2nd ed, vol II. Philadelphia: WB Saunders, 1973.

McVay CB: *Surgical Anatomy*, 6th ed, vol I. Philadelphia: WB Saunders, 1984.

Pho RWH: *Microsurgical Technique in Orthopaedics*. London: Butterworths, 1988.

Serafin D, Buncke HJ Jr (eds): *Microsurgical Composite Tissue Transplantation*. St. Louis: CV Mosby, 1979.

Smet HT: *Tissue Transfers in Reconstructive Surgery*. New York: Raven Press, 1988.

Strauch B, Vasconez LO, Hall-Findlay E (eds): *Grabb's Encyclopedia of Flaps*, 3 vols. Boston: Little, Brown, 1990.

Urbaniak JR (ed): *Microsurgery for Major Limb Reconstruction*. St. Louis: CV Mosby, 1987.

Urbaniak JR (ed): *Symposium on Microvascular Surgery, Hand Clinics*, vol 1, no 2. Philadelphia: WB Saunders, 1985.

Warwick R, Williams PL (eds): *Gray's Anatomy*, 35th British ed. Philadelphia: WB Saunders, 1973.

Webster MHC, Soutar DS: *Practical Guide to Free Tissue Transfer*. London: Butterworths, 1986.

Zhong S-Z: *Microsurgical Anatomy* (in Chinese). Shanghai: People's Medical Publishers, 1982.

INDEX

Abdominal flap, lower, 136–138
Abdominal wall and cavity, 448–479
　free jejunum transfer, 472–479
　greater omentum transfer, 462–471
　rectus abdominis flap, 448–461
Accessory lateral thoracic artery, 440
Anastomoses, 2
Anatomic snuff box, 88–89
Ankle and foot, 314–385
　dorsalis pedis flap, 314–319
　　osteocutaneous with second metatarsal, 326–335
　　skin, 320–325
　　tendinocutaneous with extensor tendons, 332–335
　extensor digitorum brevis flap, 336–340
　free toe and toe tissue transfer, 347–385
　medial plantar flap, 341–346
Anterior costal osteocutaneous flap, 438–439
Anterior intercostal artery, 426, 435–437
Anterior tibial artery, 298–304
Anterior tibial flap, 257–263
　anatomy, 257
　harvesting technique, 258–261
　reverse island, 262–263
Anterolateral thigh flap, 194–196
　anatomy, 194
　harvesting technique, 195–196
　innervation, 194
Anteromedial thigh flap, 197–200
　anatomy, 197
　harvesting technique, 198–200
　innervation, 197
Arcuate artery, 314
Arm *see* Forearm flaps; Shoulder, arm, and axilla
Auriculotemporal nerve, 526
Axilla *see* Shoulder, arm, and axilla
Axillary artery
　branches from, 26
　exposure of first and second parts, 28–31
　exposure of second and third parts, 31–33
　and forearm flaps, 44
　recipient exposure of, 26–27
　variations in branches from, 27
Axillary flap *see* Lateral thoracic flap

Back
　latissimus dorsi flap, 482–503
　scapular and parascapular flaps, 404–522
Bilobed temporal fascia flap, 532–533
Brachial artery
　exposure of middle part, 37–39
　and forearm flaps, 44, 45
　medial approach to proximal portion, 34–36
　posterior approach to proximal portion, 40–42
　recipient exposure of, 34
　see also Deep brachial artery

Carotid artery, external, 550–552
Circumflex scapular artery, 504
Costal bone graft *see* Revascularized costal bone graft and intercostal flap

Deep brachial artery
　and lateral arm flap, 17
　medial approach to proximal portion, 34–36
　posterior approach to, 40–42
Deep circumflex iliac artery (DCIA)
　anatomy of, 142–143
　iliac osteocutaneous flap based on, 154–158
　vascularized iliac bone graft based on, 145–153
Deep palmar arch system, 84–85, 87
Deep plantar artery, 347
Deep temporal fascia, 532
Deltoid flap, 8–11
　anatomy, 8
　harvesting technique, 10–11
　innervation, 9
　variations, 9
Descending genicular artery, 252
Digital artery, 99–100
Digital nerve, 99–100
Distal perforating artery, 347–348
Donor sites, 3
　see also specific flaps and procedures
Dorsal approach, to exposure of princeps pollicis artery, 96–97
Dorsal arterial system, 347

Dorsal cutaneous nerve, 316
Dorsalis pedis artery, 314, 379–381
Dorsalis pedis flap, 314–319
　arterial anatomy, 314
　innervation, 315
　osteocutaneous with second metatarsal, 326–335
　skin, 320–325
　tendinocutaeous with extensor tendons, 332–335
　variations, 317
　venous drainage, 315
Dorsal metatarsal artery, 314, 318

Extensor digitorum brevis flap, 336–340
　anatomy, 336
　blood supply, 336
　innervation, 336
　muscle, 337–340
External carotid artery, 550–552

Facial artery, 544
Femoral artery
　anterior approach to common and superficial, 201–202
　anterior approach to deep, 210–212
　anterior approach to superficial in Hunter's canal, 203–205
　posterior approach to deep, 213–216
　posterior approach to superficial, 206–209
Fibula
　anatomy, 220
　exposure of arched segment of anterior tibial artery by resection of, 298–300
　vascularized bone graft, 221–227
Fibular osteocutaneous flap, 233–237
Fibular osteomuscular transfer, 238–243
First dorsal metatarsal artery, 314, 318
Flap design, 4
Foot *see* Ankle and foot
Forearm flaps, 44–82
　innervation, 47
　radial, 49–56
　　osteocutaneous, 63–66
　　for penile reconstruction, 57–61
　　recipient exposure of artery, 77–79
　　reversed island, 61–62

Forearm flaps (cont.)
  tendinocutaneous, 67–68
  recipient exposure of bifurcation of radial and ulnar arteries, 74–76
  recipient exposure of ulnar artery, 80–82
  retrograde deep venous system, 47
  ulnar, 69–76
  venous drainage, 46–47
Fourth lumbar artery, 120, 139–141
Free jejunum transfer, 472–479
  anatomy, 472
  blood supply, 472
  exposure of inferior epigastric artery, 477–479
  harvesting technique, 474–476
Free scalp skin flap, 536–537
Free toe and toe tissue transfer, 347–385
  arterial anatomy, 347
  exposure of dorsalis pedis artery, 379–381
  exposure of medial plantar artery and its bifurcation with lateral plantar artery, 384–385
  exposure of posterior tibial artery behind medial malleolus, 382–383
  first web space skin flap, 361–363
  free big toe transfer, 350–355
  free pulp flap, 372
  free second toe transfer, 356–361
  second and third toe transfer en bloc, 378–379
  vascularized joint transfer, 373–377
  wrap–around flap, 364–366
    modified, 367–371

Gastrocnemius flap, 244–251
  anatomy, 244
  blood supply, 244
  innervation, 244
  lateral muscle, 250–251
  medial muscle, 245–249
Gastroepiploic arterial arch, 462
Gluteal artery, superior see Superior gluteal artery
Gluteal region, 102–118
Gluteal thigh flap, 107–110
Gluteus maximus flap, 102–103
Gracilis flap, 166–173
  anatomy, 166
  blood supply, 166
  innervation, 166
  muscle, 168–171
  myocutaneous, 171–173
Greater omentum transfer, 462–471
  anatomy, 462
  blood supply, 462
  composite flap of stomach and omentum, 468–471
  extending greater omentum, 467
  harvesting free omentum, 464–466
Groin flaps, 120–135
  composite with "tendon" transfer, 132–135
  iliac flap and inferior epigastric flap, 120, 129–130
  iliofemoral, 123–126
  lateral-to-medial procedure, 124–126, 131
  medial-to-lateral procedure, 127–128
  osteocutaneous, 130–131
  venous drainage, 120

Hand and wrist, 84–100
  deep palmar arch system, 84–85, 87
  exposure of digital artery and nerve, 99–100
  exposure of radial artery in anatomic snuff box, 88–89
  exposure of ulnar artery at wrist, 90–92
  princeps pollicis artery, 85, 93–97
  superficial palmar arch, 85–86, 97–98
Harvesting techniques, 4
  see also specific flaps and procedures
Head and neck, 526–552
  bilobed temporal fascia flap, 532–533
  free scalp skin flap, 536–537
  recipient exposure of external carotid artery and its branches, 550–552
  submental flap, 544–549
  superficial cervical flap, 538–543
  temporocalvarial osteofacial flap, 534–535
  temporoparietal flap, 526–527
    fascia, 528–531
Hunter's canal, 203–205

Iliac bone graft, vascularized see Vascularized iliac bone graft
Iliac flap, 120, 129–130
  anatomy, 139
  based on fourth lumbar artery, 139–141
  harvesting technique, 140–141
  osteocutaneous based on deep circumflex iliac artery, 154–158
Iliofemoral flap, 123–126
Inferior epigastric artery, 477–479
Inferior epigastric flap, 120
Inferior epigastric vessels, 451–455
Inferior gluteal artery, 102
Inferior gluteal nerve, 102
Inferior gluteal vessels, 107
Inferior lateral peroneal artery, 257
Intercostal flap see Revascularized costal bone graft and intercostal flap
Internal oblique flap, 159–164
  anatomy, 159
  blood supply, 159
  muscle, 160–163
  osteomuscular, 164

Jejunum see Free jejunum transfer

Knee see Lower leg and knee

Lateral arm flap, 17–21
  anatomy, 17
  harvesting technique, 18–21
  innervation, 17
Lateral intercostal skin flap, 430–432
Lateral leg skin flap see Peroneal flap
Lateral plantar artery, 341, 384–385
Lateral plantar nerve, 341
Lateral popliteal cutaneous artery, 270
Lateral tarsal artery, 314
Lateral thigh flap, 190–193
  anatomy, 190
  harvesting technique, 191–193
  innervation, 190
Lateral thoracic artery, 390, 414
Lateral thoracic flap, 440–445
  arterial anatomy, 440
  harvesting technique, 441–445
  innervation, 440
  venous drainage, 440
Lateral-to-medial procedure, 124–126, 131
Latissimus dorsi flap, 482–503
  bilobed split, 496–497
  blood supply, 482
  innervation, 482
  lateral split, 498–500
  muscle, 487–492
  myocutaneous, 493–495
  rib osteomyocutaneous, 501–503
  and scapular flap, 519–522
  variations in branching of thoracodorsal neurovascular bundle, 484
  variations of subscapular artery and vein, 485
Leg see Lower leg and knee
Lower abdominal flap, 136–138
Lower leg and knee, 218–312
  anterior tibial flap, 257–263
  exposure of popliteal artery, 275–288
  exposure of tibioperoneal trunk, 289–312
  fibula and adjacent tissue transfer, 218–228
  gastrocnemius flap, 244–251
  medial leg flap, 264–269
  peroneal flap, 228–243
  posterior leg flap, 270–274
  saphenous flap, 252–256

Medial arm flap, 12–16
  anatomy, 12
  harvesting technique, 13–16
  innervation, 12
Medial femoral cutaneous nerve, 252
Medial leg flap, 264–269
  anatomy of posterior tibial artery, 264
  harvesting technique, 265–269
Medial malleolus, 382–383
Medial pectoral nerve, 391
Medial plantar artery, 341, 384–385

Medial plantar flap, 341–346
   anatomy, 341
   harvesting technique, 342–346
   innervation, 341
Medial plantar nerve, 341
Medial tarsal artery, 314
Medial thigh flap, 187–189
   anatomy, 187
   harvesting technique, 188–189
   innervation, 187
Medial-to-lateral procedure, 127–128
Metatarsophalangeal joint, 373, 376–377
Microscope, 1–2
Microsurgery, 4–5
   anatomy and its variations, 3
   definition, 1
   donor sites, 3
   flap design, 4
   harvesting techniques, 4
   mastering instruments, 1
   training in basic techniques, 1–2
   see also specific flaps and procedures
Microvascular surgery, 1
Middle temporal artery, 526

Neck see Head and neck

Omentum see Greater omentum transfer
Osteocutaneous flap
   anterior costal, 438–439
   dorsalis pedis with second metatarsal, 326–335
   groin, 130–131, 141
   iliac, 154–158
   posterior costal, 433–434
   radial forearm, 48, 63–66
   scapular, 514–516
Osteofacial flap, 534–535

Palmar digital arteries, 85
Palmar metacarpal arteries, 85
Parascapular flap see Scapular and parascapular flaps
Paraumbilical perforators, 450
Pectoralis major flap, 390–407
   anatomy, 390
   blood supply, 390
   innervation, 390–391
   muscle, 393–397
      clavicular segment, 402–407
      myocutaneous, 398–399
      osteomyocutaneous, 400–401
Pectoralis minor muscle flap, 408–413
   anatomy, 408
   blood supply, 408
   harvesting technique, 410–413
   innervation, 408
Penile reconstruction, 57–61
Peroneal artery
   anatomy, 218
   exposure of, 308
   inferior lateral, 257
   superior lateral, 257
   variations of, 219
Peroneal flap, 228–243
   fibular osteocutaneous flap, 233–237
   fibular osteomuscular transfer, 238–243
Peroneal nerve, 316
Plantar arterial system, 347
Popliteal artery
   exposure of, 275–288
   lateral approach to proximal portion, 286–288
   lateral cutaneous, 270
   medial approach to distal portion, 281–282
   medial approach to middle portion, 278–280
   medial approach to proximal portion, 275–277
   posterior approach to, 282–285
Posterior arm flap, 22–25
   anatomy, 22
   harvesting technique, 23–25
   innervation, 22
Posterior cervical triangle, 538
Posterior circumflex humeral artery, 9
Posterior costal osteocutaneous flap, 433–434
Posterior femoral cutaneous nerve, 102
Posterior intercostal artery, 426, 427–429
Posterior leg flap, 270–274
   anatomy, 270
   harvesting technique, 272–274
   innervation, 270
Posterior tibial artery, 264, 305–307, 341, 382–383
Princeps pollicis artery, 85, 93–97
Proximal interphalangeal joint, 373

Radial artery
   anatomy of, 44, 48, 84–85
   exposure in anatomic snuff box, 88–89
   recipient exposure of bifurcation, 74–76
   recipient exposure in forearm, 77–79
   retrograde deep venous system, 47
Radial collateral artery, and lateral arm flap, 17, 18
Radial forearm flap, 49–56
   design, 50
   osteocutaneous, 63–66
   for penile reconstruction, 57–61
   reversed island, 61–62
   tendinocutaneous flap, 67–68
Radialis indicis artery, 85
Recipient vessels, 2–3
Rectus abdominis flap, 448–461
   anatomy, 448
   blood supply, 448
   innervation, 450
   muscle, 451–453
   myocutaneous, 454–455
      lower transverse, 455–457
      modified lower, 458
   paraumbilical perforators, 450
   thoracoumbilical, 459–461
Rectus femoris flap, 180–186
   anatomy, 180
   blood supply, 180
   innervation, 180
   muscle, 182–184
   myocutaneous, 185–186
Revascularized costal bone graft and intercostal flap, 426–439
   anterior costal osteocutaneous flap, 438–439
   arterial anatomy, 426
   lateral intercostal skin flap, 430–432
   posterior costal osteocutaneous flap, 433–434
   vascularized rib graft, 427–429, 435–437
Rib graft, vascularized, 427–429, 435–437

Saphenous artery, 252
Saphenous flap, 252–256
   anatomy, 252
   harvesting technique, 253–256
   innervation, 252
   variations, 252
Saphenous vein, 252, 316
Scapular and parascapular flaps, 504–522
   anatomy, 504
   combined, 517–518
   parascapular, 512–513
   scapular, 506–511
      lateral exposure of vascular emergence, 507
      and latissimus combined flap, 519–522
      measurement of scapula, 514–516
      medial exposure of vascular emergence, 508–511
      osteocutaneous, 514–516
Serratus anterior flap, 414–425
   anatomy, 414
   blood supply, 414
   costo-osteomuscular, 424–425
   innervation, 414
   muscle, 415–419
      composite serratus-latissimus, 422–423
      myocutaneous, 420–421
Shoulder, arm, and axilla, 8–42
   deltoid flap, 8–11
   exposure of first and second portions of axillary artery, 28–31
   exposure of middle part of brachial artery, 37–39
   exposure of second and third portions of axillary artery, 31–33
   lateral arm flap, 17–21
   medial approach to proximal portion of brachial artery and deep brachial artery, 34–36
   medial arm flap, 12–16
   posterior approach to deep brachial

Shoulder, arm, and axilla (*cont.*)
    artery and proximal portion of brachial artery, 40–42
    posterior arm flap, 22–25
    recipient exposure of axillary artery, 26–27
    recipient exposure of brachial artery, 34
Soleus muscle, 238–243
Stomach *see* Abdominal wall and cavity
Submental artery, 544
Submental flap, 544–549
    anatomy, 544
    harvesting technique, 545–549
    innervation, 544
    venous drainage, 544
Subscapular artery, 440, 485
Subscapular vein, 485
Superficial cervical artery, 538, 539
Superficial cervical flap, 538–543
    arterial anatomy, 538
    harvesting technique, 540–543
    innervation of posterior cervical triangle, 538
    variations in superficial cervical artery, 539
Superficial circumflex iliac artery (SCIA), 120–125, 128–132, 135, 137
Superficial circumflex iliac vein (SCIV), 120–121, 127, 137
Superficial epigastric artery (SEA), 120–122, 125, 128, 137
Superficial epigastric vein (SEV), 120–121, 127, 137
Superficial inferior epigastric flap, 136–136
Superficial palmar arch, 85–86, 97–98
Superficial temporal fascia, 528
Superficial temporal vein, 526
Superior gluteal artery, 102
    anatomy of deep branch, 111
    recipient site exposure, 116–118

Superior gluteal vessels, 111
Superior gluteus myocutaneous flap, 104–106
Superior lateral peroneal artery, 257
Superior ulnar collateral artery, 12, 13
Supraclavicular nerves, 538
Suture selection, 2

Temporocalvarial osteofacial flap, 534–535
Temporoparietal fascia flap, 528–531
Temporoparietal flap, 526–527
Tendinocutaneous flap, 67–68
"Tendon" transfer, 132–135
Tensor fascia lata flap, 174–179
    anatomy, 174
    blood supply, 174
    innervation, 174
    myocutaneous, 176–178
    osteomyocutaneous, 179
Thigh region
    anterolateral thigh flap, 194–196
    anteromedial thigh flap, 197–200
    gracilis flap, 166–173
    lateral thigh flap, 190–193
    medial thigh flap, 187–189
    recipient site exposure, 201–216
    rectus femoris flap, 180–186
    tensor fascia lata flap, 174–179
Thoracoacromial artery, 390
Thoracodorsal artery, 414, 440
Thoracodorsal neurovascular bundle, 484
Thoracoumbilical flap, 459–461
Thorax, 390–445
    lateral thoracic flap, 440–445
    pectoralis major flap, 390–407
    pectoralis minor muscle flap, 408–413
    revascularized costal bone graft and intercostal flap, 426–439
    serratus anterior flap, 414–425
Tibioperoneal trunk
    exposure of, 289–312

    anterior tibial artery, 301–304
    arched segment of anterior tibial artery by resection of fibula, 298–300
    peroneal artery, 308–312
    posterior tibial artery, 305–307
    lateral approach, 295–297
    medial approach, 289–291
    posterior approach, 292–294
Toe *see* Free toe and toe tissue transfer
Transverse facial arteries, 526

Ulnar artery, 44, 48
    anatomy of, 85
    exposure at wrist, 90–92
    recipient exposure of bifurcation, 74–76
    recipient exposure in forearm, 80–82
    retrograde deep venous system, 47
Ulnar forearm flap, 69–73

Vascularized iliac bone graft, 111–115, 142–145
    anatomy of deep branch of superior gluteal artery, 111
    anatomy of deep circumflex iliac artery, 142
    anatomy of iliac bone, 144
    based on deep circumflex iliac artery, 145–153
    donor closure, 152–153
    harvesting techniques, 112–115
    variations in ascending branch of deep circumflex iliac artery, 143
    venous drainage, 142
Volar approach, to exposure of princeps pollicis artery, 93–95

Wrist *see* Hand and wrist